# MEDICAL TERMINOLOGY
## EXERCISES IN ETYMOLOGY

### EDITION II

# MEDICAL TERMINOLOGY
## EXERCISES IN ETYMOLOGY

## EDITION
## II

## CHARLES W. DUNMORE
**ASSOCIATE PROFESSOR OF CLASSICS**
**NEW YORK UNIVERSITY**

## RITA M. FLEISCHER
**LATIN/GREEK INSTITUTE**
**CITY UNIVERSITY OF NEW YORK**

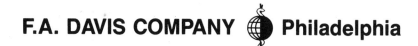

F.A. DAVIS COMPANY · Philadelphia

Last digit indicates print number   10   9   8   7   6

**Library of Congress Cataloging in Publication Data**

Dunmore, Charles William.
    Medical terminology.

    Bibliography: p.
    Includes indexes.
    1. Medicine—Terminology—Problems, exercises, etc.
2. Greek language—Medical Greek—Problems, exercises,
etc.  3. Latin language—Medical Latin—Problems,
exercises, etc.  I. Fleischer, Rita M.  II. Title.
[DNLM: 1. Nomenclature.  W 15  D992m]
R123.D86  1985    610'.14    85-4350
ISBN 0-8036-2946-X

# PREFACE

In this second edition, the main body of the text remains little changed. Major changes are in the exercises, where many words that were thought awkward to deal with have been removed and, in many instances, replaced. Some vocabulary words have been removed, and a few have been added, along with derivatives of these new words in the exercises.

A substantial amount of new material has been added to the book and incorporated as Supplementary Lessons I–V. The former Lesson 13 on hematology has been revised and is now Supplementary Lesson I, The Hematopoietic and Lymphatic Systems. In Supplementary Lesson II, The Musculoskeletal System, Latin word order, as well as the form of Latin adjectives, is explained. This information is useful not only for the understanding of Supplementary Lesson III, Biological Nomenclature, but for the Latin names of nerves given in Supplementary Lesson IV, The Nervous System, as well. Supplementary Lesson V, The Endocrine System, has been relegated to last place because the material in it does not lend itself to etymological exercises.

We should like to thank the F.A. Davis Company for permission to use illustrations from their publications. All the words in the exercises of this edition can be found in *Taber's Cyclopedic Medical Dictionary* (ed 14), F.A. Davis Company, Philadelphia, 1981.

New York 1985                                                                                    C.W.D.

R.M.F.

# PREFACE TO THE FIRST EDITION

Medical terminology is based largely upon a vocabulary drawn from ancient Greek, with a smaller number of words derived from Latin. As new advances were made in the field of medicine during and following the Renaissance (and continuing up to the present day), words had to be found to express these new discoveries. The medical scientists turned to the early Greek and Roman physicians, especially Hippocrates, Galen, and Celsus, and borrowed words outright from their medical treatises. (See the Appendix for a discussion of these physicians.) These ancient scientists had an extensive medical vocabulary which they used to describe their observations and theories. Hippocrates, for example, used the words *apoplexy, hypochondria, dysentery, ophthalmia, epilepsy, asthma, diarrhea,* etc. to describe certain physical conditions that he observed. Where the modern medical scientist could not find an appropriate word—for a disease, for example, that was unknown to the early physicians—he turned to the everyday vocabulary of the ancient languages and coined a term. Words were fashioned in this manner in America, England, and in most of the countries of Europe; thus, the language of medicine is truly an international language, recognized and used by medical men of diverse nationalities. To cite some examples: the words for hematology, embolism, and nephritis are *hématologie, embolisme,* and *néphrite* in French; *ematología, embolísmo,* and *nephritica* in Italian; *hematología, embolia,* and *nefritis* in Spanish.

Words from Greek and Latin that have been most productive of medical terminology are presented in the vocabularies of this book, along with the prefixes and suffixes in common use. Examples of medical terms derived from these words are found in the accompanying exercises.

To the memory of
Richard Mansfield Haywood

# TABLE OF CONTENTS

# INTRODUCTION

Learning the language of medical terminology is like learning any other language: The vocabulary must be systematically memorized. In this way students build up a vocabulary which, combined with a knowledge of the meaning of prefixes and suffixes, will enable them to recognize at a glance the meaning of most of the words in common use in today's medical terminology.

The Etymological Notes in the lessons are put there for the student's interest, and it is not expected that any part of these notes will be memorized. Words of importance in medical terminology that are found in these notes are repeated in the exercises at the end of each lesson. In the same way, the essays on the body systems that are found in Lessons 10 through 15 are put there for the students whose knowledge of human physiology might be hazy; this is not a textbook of physiology, and students should use these essays as a means of understanding the significance of the terminology found here.

The reason for the inclusion of quotations from the ancient physicians is mainly that of antiquarian interest: to show the acuity of their observations and the extent of their medical knowledge and, conversely, to show how, in many respects, they were bound by what we would call superstition and "old wives' tales." References to the texts of these ancient writers are from the Loeb Classical Library, William Heinemann Ltd., London. Translations are wholly our own.

The pronunciation of medical terms follows the same rules that govern the pronunciation of all English words. The consonants c and g are "soft" before the vowels e, i, and y—that is, they are pronounced like the c and g of the words *cement* and *ginger*; before a, o, and u, they are "hard" and are pronounced like the c and g of *cardiac* and *gas*. k is always "hard," as in *leuko-cyte*. The long vowels *eta* and *omega* of Greek words are marked with macrons: $\bar{e}$, $\bar{o}$; this indicates that they are pronounced like the e and o of *hematoma*. Long i is pronounced "eye," as in the *-itis* of *appendicitis*. The accent falls upon the penult, the syllable before the last, if that syllable contains a diphthong, a long vowel, or even a short vowel if it is followed by two consonants. If the penult is short, the accent falls upon the antepenult, the second syllable from the end of the word.

Students should have access to or, preferably, own a standard medical dictionary. *Taber's Cyclopedic Medical Dictionary*, F.A. Davis Company, Philadelphia, is recommended.

# BIBLIOGRAPHY

Definitions in this manual have been taken from the following sources:

**Latin words:** Lewis, CT and Short, C (eds): *Harper's Latin Dictionary*. The American Book Company, New York, 1907.

**Greek words:** Liddell, HG and Scott, R: *A Greek–English Lexicon*. Oxford University Press, London, 1953.

**Medical terms:** Thomas, Clayton L (ed): *Taber's Cyclopedic Medical Dictionary*, ed 14. FA Davis, Philadelphia, 1981.

Some of the statements included in the exercises have been taken from the following works:

Bauer, J: *Differential Diagnosis of Internal Disease*. Grune & Stratton, New York, 1967.

Benson, RC: *Handbook of Obstetrics and Gynecology*. Lange Medical Publications, Los Altos, California, 1980.

Boggs, DR and Winkelstein, A: *White Cell Manual*. FA Davis, Philadelphia, 1975.

Geschickter, CF: *The Lung in Health and Disease*. JB Lippincott, Philadelphia, 1973.

Harker, LA: *Hemostasis Manual*. FA Davis, Philadelphia, 1974.

Harvey, AM and Cluff, LE et al: *The Principles and Practice of Medicine*, ed 17. Appleton-Century-Crofts, New York, 1968.

Hillman, RS and Finch, CA: *Red Cell Manual*. FA Davis, Philadelphia, 1974.

Holvey, DN (ed): *The Merck Manual of Diagnosis and Therapy*, ed 12. Sharp & Dohme Research Laboratories, Rahway, New Jersey, 1972.

Houston, JC, Joiner, CL, and Trounce, JR: *A Short Textbook of Medicine*. The English Universities Press Ltd., London, 1972.

*Journal of the American Medical Association*. Chicago, 1974, 1975, 1976.

Keefer, CS and Wilkins, RW: *Medicine, Essentials of Clinical Practice*. Little, Brown & Co, Boston, 1970.

Lewis, AE: *The Principles of Hematology*. Appleton-Century-Crofts, New York, 1970.

*Nomenclature and Criteria for Diagnosis of Diseases of the Heart and Great Vessels*, ed 7. The Criteria Committee of the New York Heart Association. Little, Brown & Co, Boston, 1973.

Vaughan, D, Asbury, T, and Cook, R: *General Ophthalmology*. Lange Medical Publications, Los Altos, California, 1971.

# THE GREEK ALPHABET

| UPPER CASE | LOWER CASE | NAME OF LETTER | ENGLISH EQUIVALENT |
|:---:|:---:|:---:|:---:|
| A | $\alpha$ | alpha | a |
| B | $\beta$ | beta | b |
| Γ | $\gamma$ | gamma | g |
| Δ | $\delta$ | delta | d |
| E | $\epsilon$ | epsilon | e |
| Z | $\zeta$ | zeta | z |
| H | $\eta$ | eta | $\bar{e}$ |
| Θ | $\theta$ | theta | th |
| I | $\iota$ | iota | i |
| K | $\kappa$ | kappa | k |
| Λ | $\lambda$ | lambda | l |
| M | $\mu$ | mu | m |
| N | $\nu$ | nu | n |
| Ξ | $\xi$ | xi | x |
| O | $o$ | omicron | o |
| Π | $\pi$ | pi | p |
| P | $\rho$ | rho | r |
| Σ | $\sigma, \varsigma$ | sigma | s |
| T | $\tau$ | tau | t |
| Υ | $\upsilon$ | upsilon | y |
| Φ | $\phi$ | phi | ph |
| X | $\chi$ | chi | ch |
| Ψ | $\psi$ | psi | ps |
| Ω | $\omega$ | omega | $\bar{o}$ |

# GREEK NOUNS AND ADJECTIVES

*A man who is wise should consider health the most valuable of all things to mankind and learn how, by his own intelligence, to help himself in sickness.* [Hippocrates, *Regimen in Health* 9]

In the mid-eighth century B.C., the Greeks borrowed the art of writing from the Phoenicians, a Semitic-speaking people of the Levant inhabiting the region in the area of modern Lebanon. The Phoenician system of writing had to be adapted to the Greek language, as there were characters representing sounds in that Semitic language that did not exist in Greek, and sounds in Greek for which there were no characters in the Semitic system. In their adaptation of these Phoenician characters, the Greeks began to make a distinction between long and short vowels, representing long and short *e* by *eta* [H] and *epsilon* [E] respectively, and long and short *o* by *omega* [Ω] and *omicron* [O]. But the distinction was carried no further, and no differentiation in writing was made between the long and short vowels *a*, *i*, and *u*. In transliterating Greek words, a macron will be used to mark the long vowels *ē* and *ō* in this text:

| | |
|---|---|
| *xēros* | dry |
| *splēn* | spleen |
| *phōnē* | voice |
| *thōrax* | chest cavity |

During and following the first century B.C., many Greek words were borrowed by the Romans and, in the process of the borrowing, they assumed the spelling of Latin words. It has been the practice since then, in the coining of English words from Greek, to use the form and spelling of Latin, even if the word never actually appeared in the Latin language.

The letter *k* was little used in Latin,[1] and Greek *kappa* was transliterated in that language as *c*, which always had the hard sound of *k*. Most English words derived from Greek words containing a *kappa* are spelled with *c*:

| | | |
|---|---|---|
| *kyanos* | blue | **cyanotic** |
| *mikros* | small | **microscope** |
| *kolon* | colon | **colitis** |
| *skleros* | hard | **arteriosclerosis** |

---

[1]*k* is found only in the word *Kalendae*, the Calends, the first day of the month, and its derivative words *Kalendalis*, *Kalendaris*, *Kalendarium*, and *Kalendarius*, in the word *Karthago*, Carthage, the Phoenician city in North Africa, and in two archaic words, *kalo*, call, and *koppa*, the name of the Greek symbol for 90.

But there are exceptions, and the *kappa* is retained as *k* in some words:

| | | |
|---|---|---|
| *leukos* | white | **leukemia** |
| *kinēsis* | motion | **dyskinesia** |
| *karyon* | kernel | **karyogenesis** |
| *kēlē* | swelling | **keloid** |

Some words are spelled with either *k* or *c*: **keratocele, ceratocele** (*kerat-*, horn); **synkinesis, syncinesis** (*kin-*, move).[1]

Greek words beginning with *rho [r]* were always accompanied by a strong expulsion of breath called the *rough breathing*. In transliterating Greek words and in the spelling of English derivatives this rough breathing is indicated by an *h* following the *r:*

| | | |
|---|---|---|
| *rhombos* | rhombus | **rhombencephalon** |
| *rhodon* | rose | **rhodopsin** |
| *rhiza* | root | **rhizoid** |
| *rhythmos* | rhythm | **rhythmic** |

But there are exceptions: **rhachialgia, rachialgia; rhachischisis, rachischisis** (*rhachis*, spine).

Words beginning with *rho [r]* usually double the *r* when following a prefix or another word element, and the rough breathing *[h]* follows the second *r:*

| | | |
|---|---|---|
| *rhe-*[2] | flow | **diarrhea** |
| *rhag-* | burst forth | **hemorrhage** |
| *rhaph-* | sew | **cystorrhaphy** |

When Greek words containing diphthongs were borrowed into Latin, the diphthongs *ai, ei, oi,* and *ou* were changed to the Latin spelling of these sounds, but these Latin diphthongs usually undergo a further change in English:

| GREEK | LATIN | ENGLISH | EXAMPLES | | |
|---|---|---|---|---|---|
| *ai* | *ae* | e | *haima* | blood | **hematology**[3] |
| | | | *aitia* | cause | **etiology** |
| *ei* | *ei* | ei or i | *cheir* | hand | **cheirospasm, dyschiria** |
| | | | *leios* | smooth | **leiomyofibroma** |
| | | | *meiŏn* | less | **miocardia** |
| *oi* | *oe* | e | *oidēma* | swelling | **edema**[3] |
| | | | *oistros* | desire | **estrogen** |
| *ou* | *u* | u | *gloutos* | buttock | **gluteal** |
| | | | *boulē* | will | **hypobulia**[4] |

In the Greek language, words beginning with the sound of the rough breathing *[h]* often lost their aspiration when another word-element preceded the aspirated word (except after the prefixes *anti-, apo-, epi-, hypo-, kata-,* and *meta-*). But the spelling of English derivatives of such words varies, and the aspiration is often retained:

| | | |
|---|---|---|
| *haima* | blood | **an-emia, an-hemolytic** |
| *hidros* | sweat | **chrom-idrosis, an-hidrotic** |

---

[1]Cf. cinema, kinematics (*kinēma*, motion).

[2]These forms are from Greek verbs.

[3]British spelling usually retains the Latin diphthongs *ae* and *oe*: haematology, aetiology, oedema, oestrogen, and so forth.

[4]But note that the diphthong is retained in some words: aboulia (also spelled abulia).

| | | |
|---|---|---|
| *helkos* | ulcer | enter-**elcosis**, gastro-**helcosis** |
| *haphē* | touch | hyper-**aphia**, an-**haphia** |

Greek is an inflected language. This means that words have different endings to indicate their grammatical function in a sentence. The inflection of nouns, pronouns, and adjectives is called declension. Greek nouns are declined in five grammatical cases in both singular and plural: nominative, genitive, dative, accusative, and vocative. There are three declensions of Greek nouns, each having its own set of endings for the cases. Nouns are cited in dictionaries and vocabularies in the form of the nominative singular, often called the dictionary form.

Nouns of the first declension, mostly feminine, end in -*ē* or -*ā*, sometimes in short -*a*. Second-declension nouns, mostly masculine or neuter, end in -*os* if masculine, and in -*on* if neuter. The base of nouns of the first and second declensions is found by dropping the ending of the nominative case, and it is to the base, called in this text the *combining form*, that suffixes and other combining forms are added to form words.

| | | |
|---|---|---|
| *nephros* | kidney | **nephr**-itis |
| *neuron* | nerve | **neur**-otic |
| *psōra* | sore | **psor**-iasis |
| *psychē* | mind | **psych**-osis |

Rarely, the entire word is used as the combining form: **colonalgia** (*kolon*, colon), **enteronitis** (*enteron*, intestine).

If a suffix or a combining form that commences with a consonant is affixed to a combining form that ends in a consonant, a vowel, called the *combining vowel*, usually *o*, sometimes *i* (especially with words derived from Latin), is inserted between the two forms:[1]

> **leuk-o-cyte**
> **neur-o-blast**
> **psych-o-neurosis**
> **col-i-plication**[2]

Exceptions occur when suffixes beginning with *s* or *t* follow an element ending with *p* or *c*:

> **eclamp-sia**
> **epilep-tic**
> **apoplec-tic**
> **emphraxis** (for **emphrac-sis**)

Adjectives agree in gender, number, and case with the noun that they modify. They are cited in dictionaries and vocabularies in the form of the nominative singular masculine. The dictionary form of most Greek adjectives ends in -*os*, and the combining form is found by dropping this ending. There are some adjectives that end in -*ys*, and the combining form of these is found by dropping the -*s*, rarely the -*ys*:

| | | |
|---|---|---|
| *leukos* | white | **leuk**-emia |
| *kyanos* | blue | **cyan**-osis |
| *tachys* | swift | **tachy**-pnea |
| *glykys* | sweet | **glyc**-emia |

---

[1]Medical dictionaries and dictionaries of English usually give the combining vowel as part of the combining form, as in *leuko-*, *neuro-*, *psycho-*, and so forth.

[2]Latin *plica*, fold

3

When Greek nouns are borrowed into English, they usually appear in one of four ways:

in the original vocabulary form:

| | |
|---|---|
| *kolon* | colon |
| *mania* | mania |
| *omphalos* | omphalos |
| *psychē* | psyche |

with the ending changed to the form of Latin:

| | |
|---|---|
| *aortē* | aorta |
| *bronchos* | bronchus |
| *kranion* | cranium |
| *tetanos* | tetanus |

with the ending changed to silent -*e*:

| | |
|---|---|
| *gangraina* | gangrene |
| *kyklos* | cycle |
| *tonos* | tone |
| *zōnē* | zone |

with the ending dropped:

| | |
|---|---|
| *organon* | organ |
| *orgasmos* | orgasm |
| *spasmos* | spasm |
| *stomachos* | stomach |

# PREFIXES 1[1]

Prefixes modify or qualify in some way the meaning of the word to which they are affixed. It is often difficult to assign a single specific meaning to each prefix, and often it is necessary to adapt a meaning that will fit the particular use of a word.

**a-** (**an-** before a vowel or *h*): not, without, lacking, deficient:

| | |
|---|---|
| **a**-biogenesis | **an**-algesia |
| **a**-sthenia | **an**-hemolytic |
| cardi-**a**-sthenia | **an**-hidrosis |

**anti-** (**ant-** often before a vowel or *h*; hyphenated before *i*): against, opposed to, preventing, relieving:

| | |
|---|---|
| **anti**-biotic | **anti**-icteric |
| **anti**-histamine | **ant**-algesic |
| **anti**-toxin | **ant**-hemorrhagic |

---

[1]A complete list of prefixes will be found in the Index of Prefixes and Suffixes.

4

dys-: difficult, painful, defective, abnormal:

| | |
|---|---|
| **dys**-menorrhea | **dys**-pepsia |
| **dys**-ostosis | **dys**-trophy |

ec- (ex- before a vowel):[1] out of, away from:

| | |
|---|---|
| **ec**-tasis | **ex**-angia |
| **ec**-topic | **ex**-odontia |

ecto- (ect- often before a vowel): outside of:

| | |
|---|---|
| **ecto**-derm | **ecto**-plasm |
| **ecto**-enzyme | **ect**-ostosis |

en- (em- before *b*, *m*, and *p*): in, into, within:

| | |
|---|---|
| **en**-cephalitis | **em**-metropia |
| **em**-bolism | **em**-physema |

endo-, ento- (end-, ent- before a vowel): within:

| | |
|---|---|
| **endo**-genous | **ento**-zoon |
| **endo**-metritis | **end**-odontics |
| **ento**-cele | **ent**-optic |

epi- (ep- before a vowel or *h*): upon, over, above:

| | |
|---|---|
| **epi**-cardium | **ep**-arterial |
| **epi**-dermis | **ep**-hidrosis |

exo-: outside, from the outside, toward the outside:

| | |
|---|---|
| **exo**-cardia | **exo**-metritis |
| **exo**-hysteropexy | **exo**-toxin |

hemi-: half, partial; (often) one side of the body:

| | |
|---|---|
| **hemi**-cardia | **hemi**-paralysis |
| **hemi**-gastrectomy | **hemi**-plegia |

hyper-: over, above, excessive, beyond normal:

| | |
|---|---|
| **hyper**-galactia | **hyper**-lipemia |
| **hyper**-glycemia | **hyper**-parathyroidism |

hypo- (hyp- before a vowel or *h*): under, deficient, below normal:

| | |
|---|---|
| **hypo**-chondria | **hyp**-algia |
| **hypo**-dermic | **hyp**-hidrosis |

---

[1]The prefix *ex-* in most words is derived from Latin: excrete, exhale, extensor, exudate, and so forth.

**peri-**: around, surrounding:

| | |
|---|---|
| **peri**-angiitis | **peri**-laryngitis |
| **peri**-cecitis | **peri**-odontology |

**syn-** (sym- before *b*, *p*, and *m*; the *n* assimilates or is dropped before *l* and *s*): together, with, joined:

| | |
|---|---|
| syn-apse | sym-pathy |
| syn-dactylism | sym-melia |
| syn-thetic | syl-lepsis |
| sym-biosis | sy-stolic |

Note that words can have more than one prefix and that a prefix can follow a combining form:

| | |
|---|---|
| **anti-dys**-uric | cardi-**ec**-tomy |
| cardi-**a**-sthenia | **dys-anti**-graphia |

# SUFFIXES 1[1]

Suffixes are elements that are added to combining forms. They form nouns, adjectives, or verbs. Most of these nouns are abstract, that is, they indicate a state, quality, condition, procedure, or process. In the terminology of medicine most of the conditions indicated by these suffixes are pathological or abnormal: *psoriasis*, *hepatitis*, *pneumonia*, *myopia*, *astigmatism*, and so forth. Some nouns indicating procedures or processes are *abdominocentesis*, *appendectomy*, *gastroscopy*, and *hysteropexy*.

**-a**: forms abstract nouns: *state, condition:*

| | |
|---|---|
| dyspne-**a** | hyposarc-**a** |
| erythroderm-**a** | rhinorrhe-**a** |

**-ac** (rare): forms adjectives: *pertaining to, located in:*

| | |
|---|---|
| cardi-**ac** | ile-**ac** |
| celi-**ac** | ischi-**ac** |

**-ia**: forms abstract nouns; often the suffix **-ia** appears as **-y**: state, condition:

| | |
|---|---|
| anem-**ia** | hypertroph-**y** |
| pneumon-**ia** | melanchol-**y** |

**-iac** (rare): forms nouns: *person afflicted with:*

| | |
|---|---|
| hemophil-**iac** | insomn-**iac** |
| hypochondr-**iac** | man-**iac** |

**-iasis**: forms abstract nouns: *disease, abnormal condition;* often used with the name of a parasitic organism to indicate infestation of the body by that organism. When used with **lith-**

---

[1]A complete list of suffixes will be found in the Index of Prefixes and Suffixes.

(Greek *lithos*, stone): formation and/or presence of calculi in the body:

| | |
|---|---|
| elephant-**iasis** | ancylostom-**iasis** |
| nephrolith-**iasis** | schistosom-**iasis** |

-**ic**: forms adjectives:[1] *pertaining to, located in:*

| | |
|---|---|
| analges-**ic** | hypoderm-**ic** |
| gastr-**ic** | tox-**ic** |

-**in**, -**ine**: form names of substances:

| | |
|---|---|
| adrenal-**in** | chlor-**ine** |
| antitox-**in** | epinephr-**ine** |

-**ist**: forms nouns: *a person interested in:*

| | |
|---|---|
| cardiolog-**ist** | hematolog-**ist** |
| dermatolog-**ist** | orthodont-**ist** |

-**itic**: forms adjectives:[1] *pertaining to; pertaining to inflammation:*

| | |
|---|---|
| antineur-**itic** | arthr-**itic** |
| antiprur-**itic** | nephr-**itic** |

-**itis**: forms nouns indicating an inflamed condition: *inflammation:*

| | |
|---|---|
| gastr-**itis** | laryng-**itis** |
| hepat-**itis** | periton-**itis** |

-**ium** (rarely -**eum**): forms nouns: *membrane, connective tissue:*[2]

| | |
|---|---|
| endometr-**ium** | pericard-**ium** |
| epicran-**ium** | periton-**eum** |

-**ma**: forms nouns: (often) *abnormal* or *diseased condition.* The combining form for nouns ending in -**ma** is -**mat**-. Sometimes the final -**a** drops off the noun.

| | |
|---|---|
| ede-**ma** | ede-**mat**-ous |
| trau-**ma** | trau-**mat**-ic |
| phleg-**m** | phleg-**mat**-ic |
| sper-**m** | sper-**mat**-ic |

-**osis**: forms abstract nouns: *abnormal* or *diseased condition:*[3]

| | |
|---|---|
| nephr-**osis** | scler-**osis** |
| neur-**osis** | sten-**osis** |

---

[1]It should be noted that many words in -*ic*, -*itic*, and -*tic* that structurally are adjectives often can be used as both adjectives and nouns: analgesic, antineuritic, antiseptic, plastic, and so forth.

[2]In a few words -*ium* names a region of the body: *epigastrium, hypogastrium, hypochondrium.*

[3]See the Etymological Notes to this lesson for other uses of -*osis*.

...ectives from nouns in -osis: *pertaining to:*

| | |
|---|---|
| nephr-**otic** | scler-**otic** |
| neur-**otic** | sten-**otic** |

-**sia**: forms abstract nouns: *state, condition:*

| | |
|---|---|
| amne-**sia** | dyspha-**sia** |
| ecta-**sia** | hypacu-**sia** |

-**sis**: forms abstract nouns: *state, condition:*

| | |
|---|---|
| antisep-**sis** | paraly-**sis** |
| eme-**sis** | prophylaxis (prophylac-**sis**) |

-**tic**: forms adjectives from nouns in -sis:[1] *pertaining to:*

| | |
|---|---|
| antisep-**tic** | paraly-**tic** |
| eme-**tic** | prophylac-**tic** |

-**y**: forms abstract nouns. See -**ia**.

Words can have more than one suffix. Sometimes the suffix -**iac** or -**ic** is affixed to the noun-forming suffix -**sia** or -**sis**. When this occurs, the only vestige left of the noun-forming suffix is the -s:

| | |
|---|---|
| amne-**sia** | amne-s-**ic**, amne-s-**iac** |

A suffix can appear in the middle of a word affixed to a combining form:

hemat-**in**-uria
hepat-**ic**-o-enterostomy

# VOCABULARY

| GREEK WORD | COMBINING FORM | MEANING |
|---|---|---|
| *algos* | ALG- | pain |
| *algēsis* | ALGES- | sensitivity to pain |
| *angeion* | ANGI- | (blood) vessel, duct |
| *arteria* | ARTERI- | [air passage] artery[3] |
| *arthron* | ARTHR- | joint |
| *bios* | BI- | life |
| *bradys* | BRADY- | slow |
| *kardia* | CARDI- | heart |
| *kephalē*[2] | CEPHAL- | head |
| *kranion* | CRANI- | skull |
| *kytos* | CYT- | [hollow container] cell |

---

[1] See page 7, footnote 1.

[2] The mark over the *e* of this word is called a macron and indicates that this was an *eta*, a long *e*, rather than an *epsilon*, a short *e*. See the Greek alphabet facing page 1.

[3] Sometimes the original meaning of a Greek word differs from its meaning in modern medical terminology. When this is the case, the original meaning of the word will be put in brackets.

| | | |
|---|---|---|
| *enkephalon*[1] | ENCEPHAL- | brain |
| *erythros* | ERYTHR- | red, red blood cell |
| *leukos* | LEUK- | white, white blood cell |
| *lithos* | LITH- | stone, calculus |
| *logos* | LOG- | word, study |
| *malakos* | MALAC- | soft |
| *nephros* | NEPHR- | kidney |
| *neuron* | NEUR- | [tendon] nerve, nervous system |
| *osteon* | OSTE- | bone |
| *skleros* | SCLER- | hard |
| *stenos* | STEN- | narrow |
| *tachys* | TACHY- | rapid |
| *toxon* | TOX(I)- | [bow, archery] poison |

*(handwritten: (steos?)    ?    STE    calcium)*

## SUFFIX FORMS

Many combining forms are used in combination with certain suffixes so commonly that this combination can be called a *suffix form*. Some suffix forms in common use are listed below:

| COMBINING FORM | SUFFIX FORM | MEANING |
|---|---|---|
| LOG- | -logy | study, science: **cardiology** |
| | -logist | one who specializes in a certain study *or* science: **neurologist** |
| MALAC- | -malacia | softening (of tissues): **nephromalacia** |
| SCLER- | -sclerosis | hardening (of tissues): **arteriosclerosis** |
| STEN- | -stenosis | narrowing (of a part of the body): **angiostenosis** |
| TOX- | -toxic | poisonous (to an organ): **nephrotoxic** |

*(handwritten: -steosis    calcification (of tissues): angiosteosis)*

## ETYMOLOGICAL NOTES

Throughout its history, the English language has become enriched by borrowings from other languages, particularly Latin, Greek, and French. Borrowing from French began as early as the period of the Norman conquest of England and reached its high point during and immediately after the Renaissance.[2] As the French language itself is a modified form of Latin, many of these borrowed words ultimately come from Greek, since many words from this language had passed into Latin. One such word is **migraine**, a severe form of headache, usually unilateral. The French word *migraine* is derived from Latin *hemicrania*, which was borrowed from Greek *hemikrania*, pain on one side of the head, from the prefix *hēmi-*, half, and *kranion*, skull.[3]

The ancient Greeks used to smear poison on their arrowheads for use in hunting, and this

---

[1] This word is a combination of the prefix *en-*, in, within, and the noun *kephalē*, head.
[2] See the Appendix for a brief history of the English language.
[3] Cf. British *megrim* and Italian *emicrânia*.

poison was called *toxicon pharmakon* (*toxon*, bow, archery; *pharmakon*, drug); thus, the meaning of the modern word **toxic**. A **toxicologist** is one skilled in the study of poisons, while a **toxophilite** is a lover (*philos*) of archery.

The suffix -osis indicates an abnormal condition: **neurosis, psychosis** (*psychē*, mind). When affixed to a combining form indicating an organ or part of the body, it usually indicates a non-inflammatory diseased condition: **nephrosis, gastrosis** (*gastēr*, stomach). Following the combining form CYT-, cell, it means an abnormal increase in number of the type of cell indicated: **leukocytosis, erythrocytosis.** Following the combining form for an adjective, it indicates the abnormality characterized by the meaning of the adjective: **stenosis**: narrowing of a passage; **sclerosis**: hardening of tissues; **cyanosis** (*kyanos*, blue): bluish discoloration of a part.

There are a few words ending in -osis that have specialized meanings: **anastomosis**: a surgical or pathological connection between two passages; **exostosis**: a bony growth arising from the surface of a bone; **aponeurosis**: a sheet of tissue connecting muscles to bones; **symbiosis**: the living together in close association of two organisms of different species; **antibiosis**: the association between two organisms in which one is harmful to the other. The adjectival form for words in -osis is -otic: **neurosis, neurotic; psychosis, psychotic; nephrosis, nephrotic; symbiosis, symbiotic.**

The word **etiology** is from the Greek noun *aitia*, cause, origin, with the suffix form **-logy.** The etiology of a disease or abnormal condition is its cause or origin. In medical dictionaries it is usually abbreviated ETIOL.

# EXERCISE 1

A. Analyze and define each of the following words. In this, and in succeeding exercises, analysis should consist of separating the words into prefixes (if any), combining forms, and suffixes (if any), giving the meaning or force of each. Define the word. Care should be taken to differentiate between nouns and adjectives in your definitions. Consult the medical dictionary for the current meanings of these words.

1. abiosis   *lack of life.*

2. analgia   *condition of lack of pain.*

3. analgesia   *condition of lack of sens. to pain.*

4. analgesic[1]   *agent used to decrease sensitivity to pain.*

5. angiostenosis   *ab. cond. of stretching out of the blood vessels. (narrowing)*

6. angiosteosis   *ab. cond. of calcification of a vessel*

7. antitoxin   *substance that works against a poison.*

8. arteriomalacia   *ab. cond. - softening of the arteries,*

9. arthrosclerosis   *ab. cond - hardening of the arteries.*

---
[1] Adjectives ending in *-ic* or *-tic* often are used as nouns with the meaning of an agent or drug used for some particular purpose. Sometimes such words are used to refer to a person suffering from a certain disability: neurotic, paraplegic.

10

10. biotoxin _Substance poisonous to life._

11. cephalalgia _pain in the head. (Headache)_

12. dysarthrosis _____

13. encephalalgia _____

14. encephalosis _____

15. endosteum _____

16. epicranium _____

17. erythrocytosis _Abnormal condition of red blood cells._

18. exocardia _____

19. hemialgia _pain in ½ of the body._

20. hyperalgesia _ab. high sens to pain._

21. hypalgesia _(ab. low sens. to pain._)

22. leukocyte _white blood cell_

23. lithiasis[1] _____

24. nephrolithiasis _____

25. neuritis _____

26. osteoarthritis _____

27. perineuritis _____

28. periosteum _____

29. toxicosis _____

B. Give the word derived from Greek elements meaning each of the following. It is not necessary to give combining forms for words in parentheses. Verify your answer in the medical dictionary.[2]

---

[1]Pronounced lith-eye'-a-sis
[2]See the Selective Glossary of English-Greek/Latin.

1. Inflammation around a blood vessel _____

2. (Abnormal) softening (of the tissues) of the kidney _____

3. Hardening of the arteries _____

4. Pertaining to the heart _____

5. The state of living together _____

6. The membrane around the heart _____

7. Poisonous _____

8. (Abnormal) narrowing (of a passage) _____

9. (Abnormal) rapidity of heart (action) _____

10. Pain of a nerve _____

C. Give a clear, concise definition of each of the following italicized words.

1. *Bradycardia* may be an innocuous constitutional trait running in the family.

2. The clinical picture presented by *encephalitis* depends upon the area of the central nervous system involved, rather than the type or kind of virus which causes the damage.

3. Malignant *nephrosclerosis* is differentiated from glomerulonephritis by the rapidity of onset of severe hypertension, quickly followed by renal involvement.

4. The disturbance of calcium and phosphorus metabolism caused by vitamin D deficiency causes beriberi in infants and children and *osteomalacia* in adults.

5. In such varied and unique situations as a quarter-mile run, parturition, an epileptic seizure, an episode of pain, or an emotional disturbance, a transient *leukocytosis* of 20,000 to 30,000 cells per cubic millimeter may be found.[1]

6. The earliest known diseases to which prehistoric man was exposed were necrosis, exostoses, and other bony lesions, the *arthritides*,[2] including rheumatoid arthritis and spondylitis deformans, and diseases of the teeth.

D. Answer each of the following questions.

1. What is the meaning of *antibiosis*? What is an *antibiotic*?

2. What is the *endocardium*? the *epicardium*?

3. What is the *endoneurium*? the *epineurium*?

4. What is meant by an *endotoxin*? an *exotoxin*?

5. What is *epinephrine*? Why was it so named? What is another name for it?

---

[1] Normally, 1 cu. mm. of blood contains 5,000 to 10,000 leukocytes.

[2] *-itides* is the plural form for words ending in *-itis*.

6. What is the meaning of *craniostosis*? What is an *exostosis*?

7. What is meant by the *etiology* of a disease?

8. What is the name given to a person who is an expert in each of the following fields?

The heart _____ The nervous system _____

Poisons _____

9. What is the name of the study of each of the following?

The structure and function of bones _____

The structure and function of cells _____

10. What is an *antiantitoxin*? _____

## DRILL AND REVIEW

E. The meaning of each of the following words can be determined from its etymology. Determine the meaning of each. Verify your answer in the medical dictionary if necessary.

| | |
|---|---|
| 1. acardia | 16. endangiitis[1] |
| 2. atoxic | 17. angiocarditis |
| 3. antalgesic | 18. cardioangiology |
| 4. antiarthritic | 19. cytobiology |
| 5. dysostosis | 20. craniology |
| 6. hemianalgesia | 21. craniomalacia |
| 7. hyperalgia | 22. arteriolith |
| 8. hyperleukocytosis | 23. angiolith |
| 9. hypalgia | 24. nephrolith |
| 10. endocranium | 25. antilithic |
| 11. arteritis | 26. malacosis |
| 12. endarteritis | 27. malacotic |
| 13. periarteritis | 28. sclerotic |
| 14. periarthritis | 29. osteosclerosis |
| 15. angiitis | 30. encephalosclerosis |

---

[1]Also spelled endangeitis, where the -e- is from the Greek diphthong -ei- of *angeion*

31. stenocephaly
32. stenotic
33. nephralgia
34. ostalgia
35. arthroneuralgia
36. toxin
37. erythrotoxin
38. neurotoxin
39. neurotoxic
40. encephalic
41. sclerencephalia
42. encephalolith
43. periarthric
44. pericranium
45. perinephrium
46. pericarditis
47. periencephalitis
48. perinephritis
49. periosteitis
50. cytotoxin
51. anticytotoxin
52. toxicology
53. endangium
54. angiosclerosis
55. angiosis
56. angiosteosis

# LESSON 2
# NOUNS OF THE THIRD DECLENSION

*The learning of medicine can be compared to the growth of plants in the earth. Our inherent ability is the soil. The precepts of our teachers are the seeds. Learning from childhood is like the seeds falling into the plowed land at the proper season. The place of learning is like the nourishment that arises from the surrounding air to the seeds that are planted. Love of work is the labor. Time strengthens all of these things so that their nurture is completed.* [Hippocrates, *Law* 3]

Nouns of the third declension are somewhat different from those of the first and second declensions in that this class of nouns usually has two combining forms, one formed from the nominative singular, the dictionary form, and the other from some case other than the nominative. For this reason, dictionaries and vocabularies of Greek cite the genitive singular, which usually ends in *-os*, along with the nominative case of these nouns. The combining form is found by dropping the ending *-os*. Sometimes the base of the genitive case is the same as the nominative case: *cheir, cheiros*, hand, and there will be but one combining form. But usually they differ:

| | |
|---|---|
| *derma, dermatos*, skin: | **derm**-algia |
| | hypo-**derm**-ic |
| | **dermat**-o-logy |
| | **dermat**-itis |
| *gastēr, gastros*, stomach: | **gastr**-ic |
| | **gastr**-itis |
| | arch-i-**gaster** |

Sometimes the nominative singular, the dictionary form, of a noun is itself a word, without prefix or suffix:

| | |
|---|---|
| **derma:** | the skin |
| **hepar:** | the liver |
| **meninx:** | one of the coverings of the brain and spinal cord |
| **soma:** | the body |

## PREFIXES 2

eso-: within, inner, inward:

eso-gastritis                    eso-phylaxis
eso-phoria                       eso-tropia

**eu-**: good, normal, healthy:

eu-cholia                        eu-phoria
eu-pepsia                        eu-tocia

**meta-** (**met-** before a vowel or *h*): change, after:

**meta**-bolism                  met-encephalon
**meta**-morphosis               met-hemoglobin

**para-** (often **par-** before a vowel): alongside, around, abnormal:

**para**-hepatitis               **par**-acusia
**para**-metrium                 **par**-onychia

**pro-**: before:

**pro**-dromal                   **pro**-gnosis
**pro**-gnathous                 **pro**-phylaxis

There are a few other prefixes that are so little used as not to merit inclusion in this list. When a word using one of these prefixes is found in the exercises, a footnote will indicate its meaning.

**amphi-**, **ampho-**: on both sides, around, both: **amphi**-bious, **ampho**-tonia
**ana-**: up, back, again: **ana**-tomy
**apo-** (**ap-** before a vowel): away from: **apo**-cope, **ap**-enteric
**cata-** (**cat-** before a vowel or *h*): downward, disordered: **cata**-bolism, **cat**-hode
**di-** (rarely **dis-**): twice, double: **di**-phonia, **dis**-diaclast
**dia-** (**di-** before a vowel): through, across, apart: **dia**-gnosis, **di**-optometer
**pros-**, **prosth-**: in place of: **pros**-thesis, **prosth**-odontics

# SUFFIXES 2

-**al**: a Latin-derived adjectival suffix: *pertaining to, located in:*
bronchi-**al**                   parenter-**al**
hypogloss-**al**                 psychologic-**al**

-**ase**: forms names of enzymes:
amyl-**ase**                     lip-**ase**
lact-**ase**                     malt-**ase**

-**asia**, -**asis** (rare): form abstract nouns: *state, condition:*
hyperchrom-**asia**              xer-**asia**
phlegm-**asia**                  blepharochal-**asis**

-ema: forms abstract nouns: *state, condition*. The combining form of nouns in -ema is -emat-:

| | |
|---|---|
| emphys-**ema** | emphys-**emat**-ous |
| eryth-**ema** | eryth-**emat**-ous |

-esis, -esia: form abstract nouns: *state, condition, procedure*:

| | |
|---|---|
| amniocent-**esis** | diur-**esis** |
| diaphor-**esis** | ano-**esia** |

-etic: forms adjectives, often from nouns in -esis: *pertaining to*:

| | |
|---|---|
| diaphor-**etic** | gen-**etic** |
| diur-**etic** | sympath-**etic** |

-ics, -tics: form nouns indicating a particular science or study: *science* or *study of*:

| | |
|---|---|
| geriatr-**ics** | ortho-**tics** |
| pediatr-**ics** | therapeu-**tics** |

-ism: forms abstract nouns: *state, condition, quality*:

| | |
|---|---|
| astigmat-**ism** | phototrop-**ism** |
| melan-**ism** | synerg-**ism** |

-ismus: forms abstract nouns: *state, condition; muscular spasm*:

| | |
|---|---|
| chir-**ismus** | strab-**ismus** |
| laryng-**ismus** | pachycolp-**ismus** |

-oid, (rarely) -ode, -id: form words (both nouns and adjectives) indicating a particular shape, form, or resemblance: *resembling*:

| | |
|---|---|
| aden-**oid** | nemat-**ode** |
| arachn-**oid** | lip-**id** |

-oma: forms abstract nouns: usually *tumor*; occasionally *disease*. The combining form for words in -oma is -omat-; the plural often is -omata.

| | |
|---|---|
| carcin-**oma** | carcin-**omat**-ous |
| xanth-**oma** | xanth-**omata** |

-ose: a Latin-derived adjectival suffix; also used to form names of chemical sustances: *full of, resembling*:

| | |
|---|---|
| hemat-**ose** | fruct-**ose** |
| varic-**ose** | gluc-**ose** |

-ous: a Latin-derived adjectival suffix: *pertaining to, characterized by*:

| | |
|---|---|
| adipogen-**ous** | atrich-**ous** |
| amorph-**ous** | pyogen-**ous** |

-tics: See -ics.

-us: a Latin noun-forming ending: *condition, person* (sometimes a malformed fetus):

| | |
|---|---|
| abrachi-**us** | microphthalm-**us** |
| hydrocephal-**us** | tetan-**us** |

There are many suffixes used to form names of chemical substances. Some of these are:

-**ate** (chlor-**ate**)
-**ide** (brom-**ide**)
-**ite** (nitr-**ite**)
-**one** (testoster-**one**)

# VOCABULARY

| GREEK WORD | COMBINING FORM(S) | MEANING |
|---|---|---|
| | ACR- | [highest point] extremities (particularly the hands and feet) |
| *karkinos*[1] | CARCIN- | carcinoma, cancer |
| *kēlē* | -CEL-[2] | hernia, tumor |
| *cheir* | CHEIR-, CHIR- | hand |
| *cholē* | CHOL(E)- | bile, gall |
| *kolon* | COL(I)-,[3] COLON- | colon |
| *kyanos* | CYAN- | blue |
| *kystis* | CYST(I)-, -CYSTIS | bladder, cyst[4] |
| *enteron* | ENTER- | (small) intestine |
| *ergon* | ERG- | action, work |
| *gastēr, gastros* | GASTR-[5] | stomach |
| *haima, haimatos* | HEM-, HEMAT-, -EM-[6] | blood |
| *hēpar, hēpatos* | HEPAT- | liver |
| *lipos* | LIP- | fat |
| *makros* | MACR- | (abnormally) large *or* long |
| *megas, megalou*[7] | MEGA-, MEGAL- | (abnormally) large *or* long |
| *melas, melanos* | MELAN- | dark, black |
| *mikros* | MICR- | (abnormally) small |
| *odynē* | ODYN- | pain |
| *onkos* | ONC- | tumor |
| *pachys* | PACHY- | thick |
| *pyon* | PY- | pus |
| *sarx, sarcos* | SARC- | flesh, soft tissue |
| *spasmos* | SPASM- | spasm, involuntary muscular contraction |
| *splēn* | SPLEN- | spleen |
| *stoma, stomatos* | STOM-, STOMAT- | mouth, opening |

---

[1]The Greek word *karkinos*, as well as the Latin word *cancer*, meant crab. The Greek and Roman medical writers used these words to name any spreading, ulcerous growth on the body. The Greek physician Hippocrates used also the word *karkinōma* (carcinoma) to refer to a growth of this sort.

[2]Words indicating the presence of a hernia end in -cele: gastrocele, nephrocele. Some words in -cele indicate tumors, or swellings, caused by accumulations of fluids: galactocele (*gala, galaktos*, milk).

[3]Words in coli- refer to the colon bacillus, *Escherichia coli*, named after the German physician Theodor Escherich (1857–1911). Colinephritis is inflammation of the kidney caused by the presence of the *Escherichia coli* (usually abbreviated *E. coli*).

[4]Words in cyst(i)- usually refer to the urinary bladder. Forms in cholecyst- refer to the gallbladder. In the terminology of ophthalmology, the dacryocyst is the lacrimal sac, and the phacocyst is the capsule of the crystalline lens of the eye. Some words in cyst- refer to the growth called a cyst: cystoid. See the Etymological Notes to this lesson.

[5]Some words in -gaster refer to embryonic structures: archigaster, epigaster.

[6]Combining forms preceded by a hyphen are found only following a prefix or another combining form: anemia, leukemia, and so forth.

[7]The forms of this adjective are irregular.

# ETYMOLOGICAL NOTES

The word **surgeon** has come into English indirectly from two Greek words, *cheir*, hand, and *ergon*, action, work. The Greek verb *cheirourgoun* meant to work with the hands, and the noun *cheirourgos*, one who works with his hands, was applied to the surgeon. The word was borrowed into Latin as *chīrurgus*. Celsus, the Roman writer of the first century A.D., had this to say about the surgeon:

*A surgeon (chirurgus) should be a young man, or certainly one not long out of youth. He should have a strong and steady hand, one which never trembles, and he should be able to use both the right and left hand equally well. He must have a sharp and keen eye and be of a firm spirit, feeling a sense of pity deep enough that he wishes to cure his patient, but not so sensitive as to be so influenced by his cries of pain that he acts in haste or cuts less than necessary; on the contrary, he should go about everything just as if he were not at all affected by the moans that he hears.* [*De Medicina*, Preface 4]

The Latin word *chirurgus* came into Old French as *cirurgien* and was borrowed into English as early as the thirteenth century in the form *sorgien*. Among the subsequent forms of the word in English were *surgeyn, surgyen, surgien*, and ultimately *surgeon*. But a collateral form of the word also developed, giving rise to the spelling *chirurgeon*. In 1760, Samuel Johnson wrote to Boswell concerning a friend, "*I am glad that the chirurgeon at Coventry gives him so much hope.*" The modern French word for surgeon is *chirurgien*, and the Italian is *chirúrgo*.

The Greek noun *ergon* has given us the word **synergism**. *Taber's Cyclopedic Medical Dictionary*[1] defines synergism as: *The harmonious action of two agents, such as drugs or organs, producing an effect that neither could produce alone or an effect that is greater than the total effects of each agent operating by itself.* From the same root are the words **synergia, synergic, synergetic**, and **synergist**.

The Greek word *stoma*, mouth, opening, has a specialized use in the terminology of medicine. In surgical procedures, an **anastomosis** (*ana-*, up, back) is the formation of a passage between any two normally distinct spaces or organs. An **arteriovenous anastomosis** is a communication opened between an artery and a vein. Words ending in -stomy indicate such surgical procedures. An **enteroenterostomy** is the creation of a communication between two noncontinuous segments of the intestine. A **colostomy** is the formation of a more or less permanent passage between the colon and the surface of the abdomen. This opening is known as a **stoma**. The plural of **stoma** is **stomata** or, less preferably, **stomas**.

The suffix **-oma** often indicates an abnormal or diseased condition, such as **trachoma**, a chronic contagious form of conjunctivitis, or **glaucoma**, a destructive disease of the eye caused by increased intraocular pressure. But it usually denotes an abnormal growth of tissue (neoplasm), or a tumor (Latin *tumor*, swelling). *Taber's Cyclopedic Medical Dictionary* defines a tumor as: *A spontaneous new growth of tissue forming an abnormal mass which performs no physiologic function. It is with few exceptions of unknown cause, noninflammatory, and develops independent of, and unrestrained by normal laws of growth and morphogenesis.* Tumors are generally benign, but there are exceptions. **Sarcoma** is a malignant tumor originating in connective tissue such as muscle (**myosarcoma**; Greek *mys*, muscle) or bone (**osteosarcoma**). If the tumor arises in the muscular tissue of a blood vessel it is called **angiosarcoma** or **hemangiosarcoma**. A sarcoma containing nerve cells is called **neurosarcoma**.

The word-element to which the suffix **-oma** is affixed indicates either the location of the growth or its nature: **hepatoma**, tumor of the liver; **nephroma**, tumor of a kidney; **cholangioma**, a tumor of bile ducts; **hemangioma**, a tumor of blood vessels—that is, the swelling consists of dilated blood vessels; **hematoma**, a swelling that contains blood; this occurs when ruptured blood vessels flood the nearby tissues. **Melanoma** is a malignant tumor composed of cells of

---

[1]FA Davis Company, Philadelphia, 15th edition, 1985.

melanin, the substance that gives pigmentation to the hair, skin, and other tissues. **Melanomatosis** is the formation of numerous melanomas on or beneath the skin.

The Greek noun *onkos* meant bulk, mass. This word has given us the combining form indicating a swelling or tumor: **arthroncus**, tumor of a joint; **mastoncus**, tumor of the breast (*mastos*, breast); **nephroncus**, tumor of a kidney (another word for **nephroma**). **Oncology** is the branch of medicine dealing with tumors.

Another combining form indicating an abnormal swelling comes from the noun *kēlē*. The form *-cele*, which is generally used as a suffixed element of a word, usually means hernia, the protrusion of an organ or part of an organ through the wall of the cavity which normally contains it: **gastrocele**, hernia of the stomach; **cystocele**, hernia of the bladder; **splenocele**, hernia of the spleen. Sometimes a word in *-cele* indicates a swelling caused by an abnormal accumulation of fluid, as in **urocele**, an accumulation of urine in the scrotal sac; **hydrocele**, an accumulation of serous fluid; or **galactocele**, a milk-filled tumor caused by obstruction of a milk duct. **Celology** is the study of hernias, and a **keloid** is a scarlike growth of tissue on the skin. (*kel-* is an alternate form of *cel-*, from Greek *kēlē*.)

The term **cyst** refers either to a cyst or to the bladder. *Taber's Cyclopedic Medical Dictionary* defines a cyst as: *A closed sac or pouch with a definite wall which contains fluid, semifluid, or solid material. It is usually an abnormal structure resulting from developmental anomalies, obstruction of ducts, or from parasitic infection.* Cysts are of many types and include the following: **dermoid cyst**, a cyst containing elements of hair, teeth, or skin; **ovarian cyst**, a sac that develops in the ovary; **sebaceous cyst**, a cyst of the sebaceous, or oil-secreting, glands of the skin. **Cystalgia** is pain in the bladder, and **cholecystitis** is inflammation of the gallbladder.

## EXERCISE 2

A. Analyze and define each of the following words.

1. acromegaly _____

2. anastomosis[1] _____

3. anemic _____

4. anergic _____

5. anodyne _____

6. arthroncus _____

7. arthropyosis _____

8. carcinomatous _____

9. cheirospasm _____

10. chirismus _____

_____
[1]Greek *ana-*, up, back

22

11. colostomy _____

12. coloenteritis _____

13. colicystitis _____

14. colitoxemia _____

15. cyanosis _____

16. cystolithiasis _____

17. dysarthrosis _____

18. dysentery _____

19. endogastritis _____

20. enterocholecystostomy _____

21. enterodynia _____

22. erythrism _____

23. gastrolithiasis _____

24. hematoma _____

25. hepatolithiasis _____

26. hepatosplenitis _____

27. lipemia _____

28. macrocephalous _____

29. melanoma _____

30. microcephalia _____

31. microbe[1] _____

---

[1]Note that the *b* of microbe is the only surviving part of the Greek noun *bios*. The final -*e* is an English noun-forming suffix.

32. nephrocystanastomosis _____

33. nephropyosis _____

34. neurergic _____

35. neurospasm _____

36. ostemia _____

37. pachismus _____

38. pachyacria _____

39. stomatitis _____

40. synergy _____

41. asynergy _____

B. Give the word derived from Greek elements meaning each of the following. It is not necessary to give combining forms for words in parentheses. Verify your answer in the medical dictionary.

1. Hernia of the bladder _____

2. (Unnaturally) dark (color of the) blood _____

3. Abnormal enlargement of the liver _____

4. Resembling pus _____

5. Abnormal smallness of the spleen _____

6. Hernia of the stomach _____

7. Inflammation around the gallbladder _____

8. Surgical opening of a passage between the stomach, intestine, and colon _____

9. A fat cell _____

C. Give a clear, concise definition of each of the following italicized words.

1. Pain is the outstanding clinical feature of cholecystitis and is usually present in the *epigastrium*.

2. The etiology of *acrocyanosis* is unknown, but a local sensitivity of the arterioles to cold is thought to be the cause.

3. Any *hepatotoxin* can initiate this type of disease.

4. In cases of erythremia, *hyperemia* is observed in all organs and may account for the hepatomegaly.

5. It has been estimated that 15 million people in the USA are afflicted with *cholelithiasis*.

6. Differentiation of *splenomegaly* from a very large left lobe of the liver or from an enlarged kidney is often difficult.

7. It is obvious that in cases of *pyonephrosis* the danger of propagation of microorganisms is involved.

8. *Sarcoid* skin lesions occur in various forms which may resemble leprosy.

9. Researchers suggest that the Pill presents not just one more risk to its users but is *synergetic* in its effect.

D. Answer each of the following questions.

1. What is *eubiotics?*

2. For what purpose is *heparin* used? How do you explain the form of the word?

3. What is a *synarthrosis?*

4. What is a *sarcobiont?*[1]

5. What are *microbiota? macrobiota?*[2]

6. What is the meaning of the term *parenteral?*

7. What is a *lipoma?*

8. What is the meaning of *synergism?*

9. What is *sarcostosis?*

---

[1] *biont-* is the present participial stem of the Greek verb *bioun,* live; thus, the participle means "[a] living [creature]."

[2] The Greek word *biota* is the neuter plural form meaning "living things."

10. What is the function of *lipase* in the body?

11. What is a *microcyte*? a *macrocyte*?

## DRILL AND REVIEW

E. The meaning of each of the following words can be determined from its etymology. Determine the meaning of each. Verify your answer in the medical dictionary if necessary.

1. acromicria
2. acroarthritis
3. paracolitis
4. paracystium
5. parahepatitis
6. cystospasm
7. hemoid
8. splenoid
9. leukocytoid
10. cardiomegaly
11. enteromegaly
12. gastromalacia
13. stomatomalacia
14. hepatomalacia
15. antidysenteric
16. antianemic
17. macrocephalia
18. macrostomia
19. pyocele
20. lipocele
21. splenocele
22. arthrodynia
23. cephalodynia
24. hepatodynia
25. stomatodynia
26. cystolith
27. enterolithiasis
28. microlithiasis
29. gastrology
30. hematology
31. spasmology
32. hemocytology
33. megacardia
34. megacephalic
35. megalgia

36. cholangioma
37. hemangioma
38. endostoma
39. periosteoma
40. dyscholia
41. eucholia
42. melanomatosis
43. carcinomatosis
44. eparterial
45. microchiria
46. macrocheiria
47. chiromegaly
48. periangiocholitis
49. cholecystenterostomy
50. colinephritis
51. colitis
52. colonalgia
53. colonic
54. colonitis
55. pericolonitis
56. cystoid
57. megalocystis
58. epicystitis
59. endocystitis
60. enterocystocele
61. enteroenterostomy
62. enteroneuritis
63. enterostenosis
64. gastrogastrostomy
65. dysemia
66. epinephrinemia
67. hemangiomatosis
68. hemarthrosis
69. hemonephrosis
70. toxemia

71. pachyemia
72. pyemic
73. pyotoxinemia
74. cholemia
75. hypererythrocythemia
76. melanin
77. melanism
78. hepatomelanosis
79. oncology
80. oncosis
81. osteoncus
82. nephroncus
83. acropachy

84. pachyostosis
85. ostempyesis
86. pyocephalus
87. pyarthrosis
88. apyous
89. stenostomia
90. microstomia
91. lipocardiac
92. liposis
93. hyperliposis
94. hypoliposis
95. anergia
96. hemisynergia

# GREEK VOCABULARY

*For those who have a fever, if jaundice occurs on the seventh, the ninth, the eleventh, or the fourteenth day, it is a good sign, provided the right hypochondrium does not become rigid. Otherwise it is a bad sign.* [Hippocrates, *Aphorisms* 4.64]

## VOCABULARY

| GREEK WORD | COMBINING FORM(S) | MEANING |
|---|---|---|
| *arachnē* | ARACHN- | spider, web; arachnoid membrane |
| *chlōros* | CHLOR- | green |
| *chondros* | CHONDR- | cartilage |
| *daktylos* | DACTYL- | finger, toe |
| *derma, dermatos* | DERM(AT)-, -DERMA | skin |
| *helkos* | (H)ELC- | ulcer |
| *hidrōs, hidrōtos* | HIDR(OT)-,-IDR- | sweat |
| *histos* | HIST(I)-[1] | [web] tissue |
| *hydōr, hydatos* | HYDR-[2] | water, fluid |
| *hypnos* | HYPN- | sleep |
| *ikteros* | ICTER- | jaundice |
| *isos* | IS- | equal |
| *mēninx, mēningos* (plural, *mēninges*) | MENING-, -MENINX | meningeal membrane, meninges |
| *mys, myos* | MY(S)- | [mouse] muscle |
| *mykēs, mykētos* | MYC(ET)- | [mushroom] fungus |
| *myelos* | MYEL- | bone marrow, spinal cord |
| *narkē* | NARC- | stupor, numbness |
| *nekros* | NECR- | corpse; dead |
| *oligos* | OLIG- | few, deficient |
| *onyx, onychos* | ONYCH- | fingernail, toenail |
| *pous, podos* | POD- | foot |

---

[1]The combining form HISTI- is from the diminutive noun *histion*.

[2]This combining form is slightly irregular.

| polios | POLI- | [gray] gray matter of the brain and spinal cord |
| polys | POLY- | many, excessive |
| psychē | PSYCH- | [soul] mind |
| sōma, sōmatos | SOM(AT)-, -SOMA | body |
| sthenos | STHEN- | strength |
| xanthos | XANTH- | yellow |

## ETYMOLOGICAL NOTES

Arachne, in Greek mythology, was a young girl of Maeonia, a land of Asia Minor, who became so skilled in the art of weaving that she challenged Athena, a goddess unequaled at the loom, to a contest. Ovid, the first-century B.C. Roman poet, tells us the story in the *Metamorphoses*, a long poem that deals with mythological metamorphoses.

Athena took up the challenge, and the two, goddess and low-born girl, began to weave their tapestries. The goddess began by depicting the Acropolis in Athens with the twelve Olympian gods seated on their lofty thrones in serene majesty, with Jove in their midst. Then, so that Arachne might know what reward she could expect for her mad presumption, she wove in the four corners scenes showing punishments meted out to mortals who had dared challenge the gods.

Arachne, in her tapestry, wove pictures of the gods in various disguises seducing mortal women. Athena could find no flaw in Arachne's work, but, indignant at her success, tore the web showing the celestial crimes, and with her shuttle struck Arachne again and again. The wretched girl could bear the punishment no longer and bound a noose around her neck and hanged herself. Ovid tells us that as Arachne hung there, Athena felt pity and lifted her, saying,

*Live, wicked girl, but hang forever; and so that you may never feel secure in time to come, let this same punishment fall upon all your generations, even to remote posterity.*

*And as the goddess turned to leave, she sprinkled Arachne with the juices from Hecate's herb, and the girl's hair, touched by the poison, fell off, and her nose and ears fell off, and her head became shrunken, and her whole body was tiny. There was nothing left but belly and slender fingers clinging to her side as legs. And as a spider she still spins and practices her ancient art.*
[Ovid, *Metamorphoses* 6.136–145]

The arachnoid membrane, or **arachnoidea**, is a thin, delicate membrane, the intermediate of the three that enclose the brain and spinal cord. The outer, tough, fibrous membrane is the dura mater (Latin, hard mother), sometimes called the **pachymeninx**, or simply the dura. The innermost of the three meninges is the pia mater (devout mother). The arachnoidea is separated from the dura by the subdural (Latin *sub*, under) space, and from the pia by the subarachnoid space. **Subdural hematoma** is caused by venous blood oozing into the subdural space of the brain. It is usually the result of trauma, and even a comparatively trivial injury can result in severe and steady headache and sometimes coma. Symptoms of subdural hematoma may not be apparent for a period of several days or even several weeks following the initial injury.

**Meningitis** is the inflammation of the meninges of the brain or spinal cord and is of several types, the most common being acute bacterial meningitis. This may be caused by one of several bacteria, but, regardless of the causative organism, the resulting disorders are similar. Classic symptoms are headache, fever, stiff neck, and lethargy. Unfortunately, typical manifestations of the disease are not seen in infants aged 3 months to 2 years, and, although antibiotics have reduced the fatality rate to less than 10 percent for cases recognized early, undiagnosed meningitis remains a lethal disease, with the prognosis for life progressively more bleak the younger the patient.

The combining form MYEL- *(myelos)* refers to either bone marrow or the spinal cord. A **myeloma** is a tumor originating in the bone marrow. **Myelomeningitis** is inflammation of the spinal cord and the meninges. **Poliomyelitis**, inflammation of the gray matter of the spinal cord, is known also as infantile paralysis, or simply polio. Until recently this was a dread paralytic infection of childhood, but in recent years it has become rare due first to the development of the Salk vaccine by Dr. Jonas E. Salk (1914–      ), and later the Sabin vaccine, an oral vaccine taken on sugar cubes, developed by Dr. Albert B. Sabin, an American physician born in Russia in 1906.

    **Jaundice** is a condition that manifests itself externally by a yellow staining of the skin caused by deposition of bile pigments. The word jaundice is from the French *jaunisse*, which is from Latin *galbinus*, yellowish-green in color. Another term for jaundice is **icterus**, from the Greek *ikteros*, jaundice. Pliny the Elder, the Roman writer of the first century A.D., whose *Natural History* in thirty-seven books provides us with an encyclopedia of geography, botany, zoology, and so forth, writes on jaundice, which was called the royal disease (*rēgius morbus*):

*There are certain remedies for jaundice: a dram of dirt from the ears and teats of sheep mixed with a pinch of myrrh and two cups of wine; the ashes of the head of a dog mixed with honey wine; a millipede in a half-cup of wine; earthworms in vinegar mixed with myrrh; wine in which a hen's feet have been rinsed—but the feet must be yellow and be washed in water first; a partridge's or an eagle's brain in three cups of wine; the ashes of a pigeon in honey wine; the intestines of a pigeon in wine; the ashes of sparrows in honey wine and water.*

*There is a bird that is called* icterus *because of its color. People say that if one with jaundice looks at this bird the disease leaves him. But the bird dies. I think that this bird is the one that in Latin is called* galgulus *(the golden oriole).* [Pliny, *Natural History* 30.28]

    The **hypochondrium** is the soft part of the abdomen beneath the cartilage of the lower ribs and located on either side of the **epigastrium**, the upper central region of the abdomen over the pit of the stomach. This area, in which are situated the gallbladder, liver, and spleen, was thought of as being the seat of melancholy. The form **hypochondria**, properly the plural of hypochondrium, entered the English language in the seventeenth century as an abstract noun meaning a melancholy state for which there is no apparent cause.

# EXERCISE 3

A. Analyze and define each of the following words.

1. achlorhydria _____

2. anisocytosis _____

3. asthenia _____

4. angiosclerotic myasthenia _____

5. anhypnia _____

6. antihypnotic _____

7. arachnoidea encephali[1] _____

---

[1]The ending *-ea* forms nouns. *encephali* is the Latin form of the genitive singular case. *arachnoidea encephali* means the arachnoidea of the encephalon.

8. arteriomyomatosis _____

9. chondroporosis[1] _____

10. dermatocyst _____

11. dermatomycosis _____

12. enterelcosis _____

13. ephidrosis _____

14. epidermomycosis _____

15. gastrohelcosis _____

16. helcoid _____

17. histiocyte _____

18. histiocytosis _____

19. hyperchlorhydria _____

20. hypnalgia _____

21. hypnoidal _____

22. macrodactylia _____

23. melanoleukoderma _____

24. meningitis _____

25. mycethemia _____

26. myoendocarditis _____

27. narcosis _____

28. narcotism[2] _____

---

[1]Greek *poros*, passage
[2]A shortened form of "narcoticism"

29. necrocytotoxin _____

30. necrologist _____

31. necrosis _____

32. neuromyositis[1] _____

33. oligoerythrocythemia _____

34. onychomycosis _____

35. pachydermia _____

36. pachyonychia _____

37. perionychia _____

38. poliomyelitis _____

39. polioencephalomeningomyelitis _____

40. psychosis _____

41. somatopsychosis _____

42. sympodia _____

43. toxicoderma _____

44. xanthoma _____

45. xanthosis _____

B. Give the word derived from Greek elements that means each of the following. Verify your answer in the medical dictionary.

1. Preventing perspiration _____

2. Condition of (having) fingers or toes of equal (length) _____

3. Cartilaginous and fatty tumor _____

---

[1]The -s- between myo- and -itis has been inserted to avoid hiatus, an awkward gap between two vowels. This is known as an epenthetic consonant: fibromyositis, fibrositis, neurofibrositis, and so forth.

4. Abnormally large (size of) fingers and toes _____

5. Disease of the stomach due to fungus _____

6. A tissue tumor _____

7. (Accumulation of) fluid around the kidney _____

8. Hernia of the meninges _____

8. Deficient (volume of) blood _____

10. (Abnormal) redness of the skin _____

11. The study of the (human) body _____

12. Yellowness of the skin _____

13. (Containing) no water _____

14. Ulceration of (the mucosa of) the kidney _____

15. The study of ulcers _____

16. The study of sleep _narcology_____

17. Membrane around a cartilage _____

18. An enzyme (which digests) tissue _____

19. Diminished (secretion of) sweat _hypohidrosis_____

20. Inhibiting (the growth of) fungi _antimycosis_____

21. State of having supernumerary fingers _____

22. Hardening of the skin _dermatosclerosis./scleroderma/scleriasis_

23. Inflammation of cartilage _____

24. Softness of cartilage _____

C. Give a clear, concise definition of each of the following italicized words.

1. For generalized *hyperhidrosis*, treatment of the underlying systemic disease or psychotherapy is necessary.

2. Several syndromes associated with arteritis have been separated from *polyarteritis* on the basis of *histological* and/or clinical differences.

3. In heavy blood stream invasions there may be a true pyemia with multiple abscesses throughout the body, the *osteomyelitis* being only a part of the general infection.

4. There is no special treatment of typical *psychosomatic* diseases as opposed to other diseases; in the treatment of all illnesses certain therapeutic procedures are appropriate for psychological as well as for *somatic* components.

5. Early [thiamine] deficiency produces *neurasthenia* with fatigability, irritability, poor memory, sleep disturbances, precordial pain, anorexia, abdominal discomfort, and constipation.

6. Lagging or regenerative activity behind the physiologic wear and tear of tissues characterizes senescence. Senile *osteoporosis*[1] is in fact the most common variety of osteoporosis.

7. Arthrosis of the knee joint may in rare instances be simulated by osteoma or *osteochondroma* of the joint.

8. *Polymyositis*[2] is more common in females than in males and may occur at any age.

---

[1] Greek *poros*, passage
[2] See page 33, footnote 1.

9. It is now recognized that in a small proportion of patients with *polycythemia* (about 9 percent) there is an underlying renal lesion, neoplastic cyst, or *hydronephrosis*.

10. In the skin the *xanthomata* of primary hypercholesteremic *xanthomatosis* consist of large and small aggregates of xanthoma, or foam cells.

*Xan<u>thomata</u>     omata = plural of oma*

*(usually) yellow nodules (on the eyelid)*

11. *Leukonychia* is often present in cases of cirrhosis of the liver and in myelomatosis.

D. Answer each of the following questions.

1. What is the difference between a *myoma* and a *myeloma*?

2. What is the meaning of each of the following?

   perimysium _____

   epimysium _____

   endomysium _____

3. For what purpose is an *icteric index* used?

   *to quantify the severity of jaundice by measuring the bilirubin in the blood.*

4. What is the meaning of each of the following?

   arachnidism _____

   arachnoiditis _____

   arachnodactyly _____

5. What is the difference between *psychic* and *psychotic?*

36

6. What is *leukomyelitis?*

7. What is a *polyp?*[1]

8. What is the meaning of the word *mycetes?*

9. What is the meaning of *mycetism* (also spelled *mycetismus*)?

10. What is meant by the condition called *acrocephalosyndactylia* (also known as Apert's syndrome)?[2]

## DRILL AND REVIEW

E. The meaning of each of the following words can be determined from its etymology. Determine the meaning of each. Verify your answer in the medical dictionary.

| | |
|---|---|
| 1. mycoid | 20. myelasthenia |
| 2. myeloid | 21. myasthenia gastrica[3] |
| 3. icteroid | 22. anonychia |
| 4. chondrodynia | 23. hyperonychia |
| 5. dermatodynia | 24. melanonychia |
| 6. myodynia | 25. scleronychia |
| 7. pododynia | 26. perionychium |
| 8. histocyte | 27. megalonychosis |
| 9. chondrocyte | 28. chondralgia |
| 10. xanthocyte | 29. dermalgia |
| 11. lipochondroma | 30. podalgia |
| 12. chondroangioma | 31. somatalgia |
| 13. dermatomyoma | 32. anhidrosis |
| 14. polyarthritis | 33. dyshidrosis |
| 15. polyneuritis | 34. polyhidrosis |
| 16. polyemia | 35. cyanhidrosis |
| 17. enteromycosis | 36. acrohyperhidrosis |
| 18. paronychomycosis | 37. hematidrosis |
| 19. somasthenia | 38. megalodactylous |

---

[1]The final *-p* of this word is from Greek *pous*, foot.
[2]named for Eugène Apert, French physician (1868–1940)
[3]*gastrica* is the feminine form of this adjective, agreeing with the feminine noun *myasthenia.*

39. toxicodermatitis
40. epidermis[1]
41. epidermal
42. neurohistology
43. anhydremia
44. anhydromyelia
45. anti-icteric
46. icterohepatitis
47. icteroanemia
48. splenicterus
49. meningoarteritis
50. meningomyelocele
51. meningoencephalitis
52. meningoencephalomyelitis
53. meningomalacia
54. amyosthenia
55. myolipoma
56. myoneural
57. myosclerosis
58. endomyocarditis
59. hematomyelia
60. neuromyelitis
61. podology
62. podarthritis
63. antasthenic
64. hypnotic
65. myonarcosis
66. antinarcotic
67. oligocholia
68. oligodactylia
69. oligoleukocythemia
70. xanthous
71. xanthemia
72. xanthoderma
73. microsoma
74. macrosomia
75. hypermegasoma
76. syndactylism

---

[1]-*is* is a Latin ending for nouns of the third declension.

# GREEK VERBS

*In the winter eat as much as possible and drink as little as possible. The drink should be undiluted wine, and the food should be bread and roasted meat. Eat as few vegetables as possible during this season. In this way the body will be most dry and hot.* [Hippocrates, *Regimen in Health* 1]

Greek verbs are conjugated. This means that there are different endings for person and number, and sometimes for the tenses, moods, and voices. A Greek verb normally has six different forms, called principal parts, and it is on these parts that the various tenses are built. Many verbs are lacking one or more of the principal parts, and often verbs are irregular, and knowing the dictionary form of a verb does not always allow one to predict the other forms.

Greek dictionaries and grammars cite verbs in the first person singular, but dictionaries of the English language and medical dictionaries usually cite verbs in the form of the present infinitive, and it is in this form that they will be given in this text. The present infinitive of most verbs ends in *-ein*, but there are other infinitival endings in *-ai*, *-an*, *-oun*, and *-sthai*. Not all of the principal parts of a verb are used in forming English derivatives, and in this text only the combining forms of principal parts that have been productive of English derivatives will be given.

Often the entry form of a verb has not yielded any English derivatives. The principal parts of the verb *gignesthai*, come into being are:

*gignomai, genēsomai, egenomēn, gegenēmai, gegona, egenēthēn*

The third principal part, which supplies one of the past tenses (the aorist), furnishes the combining form GEN-, as in the words pathogenic, genesis, carcinogen, and so forth. Greek grammars often cite the verb *lyein*, loosen, destroy, as an example of a model verb:

*lyō, lysō, elysa, lelyka, lelymai, elythēn*

The combining form of *lyein* is LY(S)-, as in analysis or hemolysin.

# VOCABULARY

| GREEK WORD | COMBINING FORM(S) | MEANING |
|---|---|---|
| *autos* | AUT- | self |
| *aisthēsis* | ESTHE(S)- | sensation, sensitivity, sense |
| *gignesthai* | GEN(E)-, -GEN | come into being; produce |
| *graphein* | GRAPH- | write, record |
| | GRAM- | [something written] a record |
| | IATR- | healer, physician; treatment |
| ~~*autos*~~ | IDI- | ~~of one's~~ self |
| *kinein* | KINE- | move |
| *kinēsis* | KINES(I)- | movement, motion |
| *lyein* | LY(S)- | destroy, break down |
| *myxa* | MYX- | mucus |
| *orthos* | ORTH- | straight, erect; normal |
| *ous, ōtos* | OT- | ear |
| *pathos* | PATH- | [suffering] disease |
| *piptein* | PT- | fall, sag |
| *pyr, pyros* | PYR- | [fire] fever, burning |
| *pyretos* | PYRET- | fever |
| *pyressein* | PYREX- | be feverish |
| *rhein* | RHE- | [run] flow, secrete |
| *rhēgnynai* | RHAG- | [burst forth] flow profusely, hemorrhage |
| *rhēxis* | RHEX- | rupture |
| *rhis, rhīnos* | RHIN- | nose |
| *skopein* | SCOP- | look at, examine |
| *sēpein* | SEP- | [be putrid] be infected |
| *tasis* | TA- | stretching |
| *telos* | TEL- | end, completion |
| *tenōn, tenontos* | TEN-, TENON(T)- | tendon |
| *therapeuein* | THERAP(EU)- | treat medically, heal |
| *tomē* | TOM- | a cutting, slice |
| *tonos* | TON- | [a stretching] (muscular) tone, tension |

*[handwritten: ptosis]* *[handwritten: prolapse]*

## COMPOUND SUFFIX-FORMS

Some combining forms of verbs, usually with the addition of a suffix and/or prefix, have become so commonly used in a certain form and meaning as to remain fixed as **compound suffix-forms:**

-ectasia, -ectasis: dilation, enlargement: **cardiectasia, nephrectasis**

-gen:[1] substance that produces (something): **antitoxinogen, carcinogen**

-genesis: formation, origin: **lipogenesis, pathogenesis**

-genic, -genous: causing, producing, caused by, produced by *or* in: **pathogenic, neurogenic, hepatogenous**[2]

---

[1]Strictly speaking, *-gen, -gram,* and *-graph* are not suffix-forms, as there is no suffix on the combining form. It seemed desirable, however, that *-gen, -genesis, -genic,* and *-genous,* as well as *-gram, -graph,* and *-graphy,* should be listed together so as to show the relationship between words using these forms.

[2]Since these suffix-forms can mean either producing *or* produced by, the meaning of some few words is ambiguous: *pyretogenous* means either producing fever *or* produced by fever.

-**gram**:[1] a record of the activity of an organ (often an x-ray): **cardiogram, angiogram**

-**graph**:[1] an instrument for recording the activity of an organ: **polygraph, cardiograph**

-**graphy**: 1. the recording of the activity of an organ (usually by x-ray examination): **cholangiography, cystography**; 2. a descriptive treatise (on a subject): **neurography, osteography**

-**lysis**: dissolution, reduction, decomposition: **hemolysis, pyretolysis**

-**lytic**: pertaining to dissolution or decomposition (forms adjectives from words in *-lysis*): **hemolytic, bacteriolytic**

-**pathy**: disease: **neuropathy, hemopathy**

-**ptosis**: dropping, sagging (of an organ or part): **gastroptosis, coloptosis**

-**rrhagia**:[2] profuse discharge, hemorrhage: **pyorrhagia, cystorrhagia**

-**rrhea**: profuse discharge, excessive secretion: **otopyorrhea, gastromyxorrhea**

-**rrhexis**: bursting (of tissues), rupture: **angiorrhexis, enterorrhexis**

-**scope**: an instrument for examining: **rhinoscope, otoscope**

-**scopy**: examination: **endoscopy, cystoscopy**

-**tome**: a surgical instrument for cutting: **histotome, gastrotome**

-**tomy**: surgical incision: **cholecystotomy, enterotomy**

-**ectomy**: surgical excision; removal of all (total excision) or part (partial excision) of an organ: **gastrectomy, nephrectomy**

## ETYMOLOGICAL NOTES

*There is no disease more grievous or severe than that which, by a certain stiffness of the nerves, now draws the head back toward the shoulder blades, now draws the chin down toward the chest, and now holds the neck stretched out immobile. The Greeks call the first* opisthotonos, *the second* emprosthotonos, *and the third* tetanos. [Celsus, *De Medicina* 4.6]

The name of the disease **tetanus** (Greek *tetanos*) is related linguistically to the nouns *tasis*, stretching, and *tonos*, tension; this acute disease was known to the ancient physicians. Hippocrates writes, *Spasm or tetanus following severe burns is a bad sign.* [*Aphorisms* 7.13] Signs of tetanus are stiffness of the muscles of the jaw, esophagus, and neck, and, for this reason, the disease is often called lockjaw. In the advanced stage these and other muscles become fixed in a rigid position. If the body is stretched backward in a tetanic spasm, the position is called **opisthotonos** (Greek *opisthen*, in back); if stretched forward, it is called **emprosthotonos** (*emprosthen*, in front); if stretched to the side, **pleurothotonos** (*pleurothen*, on the side), and if the body is held rigidly stretched in a straight line, the condition is called **orthotonos** (*orthos*, straight, upright).

The causative agent of tetanus is the bacillus *Clostridium tetani*, which takes its name from *klōstēr*, spindle, from the rodlike shape of these bacilli. The suffix *-id* indicates a member of a genus, and *-ium* is a Latin diminutive ending, from the Greek *-ion*. The word *klōstēr* is derived from the verb *klōthein*, spin. Clotho, the Spinner, is the one of the three sisters, the Fates (in Greek *Moirai*, in Latin *Parcae*), who spins the thread of life for each of us; her sister Lachesis, the Apportioner, determines the length of the thread, and the third sister, Atropos, Irreversible, cuts it.

The adjective *idios* meant of one's self, pertaining to one's own interest. Galen, the Roman physician of the second century A.D., used the term *idiopatheia*, **idiopathy**, to refer to an ailment having a local origin—that is, originating within the body. We can speak of an **idiopathic**

---

[1]Strictly speaking, *-gen*, *-gram*, and *-graph* are not suffix-forms, as there is no suffix on the combining form. It seemed desirable, however, that *-gen*, *-genesis*, *-genic*, and *-genous*, as well as *-gram*, *-graph*, and *-graphy*, should be listed together so as to show the relationship between words using these forms.

[2]Words beginning with the letter *r*- [Greek *rho*] usually double this letter following another element. There are exceptions: perirhinal, craniorhachischisis (sometimes spelled craniorrhachischisis).

disease—one without a recognizable cause. There was a noun *idiōma*, meaning a peculiarity or particular feature of something. Our word idiom is ultimately derived from this noun. An *idiōtēs* was a person in private life, as opposed to one holding public office. It came to mean one who was unlearned or unskilled. The word idiot entered the English language early in the fourteenth century in the sense of a person who was so unskilled in mental ability as to be incapable of acting in a rational way: an idiot. In the sixteenth century the term an idiot mistakenly came to be a nidiot, and then through the influence of the pronunciation of the term the spelling was changed to nidget or nigit. Thomas Heywood, the seventeenth-century English dramatist, wrote in *The Wise Woman of Hogsdon* (1638), "I think he saith we are a company of fooles and nigits."

The **parotid** gland, which runs alongside the ear, is one of the glands that supply saliva to the mouth. Inflammation of this gland, **parotitis,** is the acute, contagious disease commonly known as mumps. The Roman physician Celsus knew of mumps, although there was no Latin name for it.

*Parotid swellings* (parotides) *are likely to occur below the ears, sometimes in periods of health when inflammation occurs here, and sometimes after long fevers when the force of the disease has turned in that direction.* [De Medicina 6.16]

He recommends as a remedy for these swellings a mixture of pumice, liquid pine resin, frankincense, soda scum, iris, wax, and oil. Pliny, the Roman encyclopedist, recommends as beneficial a mixture of foxes' testicles and bull's blood, dried and pounded together and mixed with the urine of a she-goat, all of this to be poured drop-by-drop into the ear and followed by an external application of she-goat's dung mixed with axle grease. [*Natural History* 28.49]

**Rheum,** a watery discharge, is from *rheuma, rheumatos,* a word related to the verb *rhein* and meaning "that which flows." The ancient Greek writers used the word to refer to the current of a river, the eruption of lava from a volcano, or to anything that flowed. Hippocrates used it in the sense of a discharge of liquid from the body: *Those of us with a cold in the head and a discharge* (rheuma) *from the nostrils generally find that this discharge is more acrid than that which formerly accumulated there and daily passed from the nostrils.* [Ancient Medicine 18] **Rheumatism** *(rheumatismos)* was thought to be caused by a flowing of the humors in the body and was thus named.

The word **ptomaine,** the generic name for certain alkaloid bodies found in decaying animal and vegetable matter, some of which are exceedingly toxic, was coined in 1876 by the Italian scientist Franz Salmi from the Greek *ptōma, ptōmatos,* fallen body, corpse, from the verb *piptein,* fall. Not only was the word incorrectly formed, as it should have been *ptomatine (ptomat- + ine),* but popular usage has given it an incorrect pronunciation, rhyming it with *domain;* it should be pronounced in three syllables, pto-ma-ine.

The ancient Greeks were unaware of the existence of capillaries in the human body simply because they did not have the optical devices with which to see these microscopic vessels. It was not until the seventeenth century that their existence was demonstrated by the Italian anatomist Marcello Malpighi as a result of his discovery of capillary anastomosis in the lungs. The word **capillary** is from Latin *capillāris,* pertaining to hair *(capillus).* But many terms for abnormal conditions of the capillaries have been formed from the Greek elements *tel-,* end, and *angi-,* vessel, as both the arterial and the venous systems terminate in capillaries. **Telangiosis** is any disease of capillaries, and **telangioma** is a tumor made up of dilated capillaries.


# EXERCISE 4

*For those who have a fever* (pyretos), *if deafness occurs, if blood flows from the nose, or if the bowels become disordered, the disease will be cured.* [Hippocrates, *Aphorisms* 4.40]

A. Analyze and define each of the following words.

1. acroosteolysis _____

2. amyxia _____

3. angiogram _____

4. anticytolysin _____

5. arachnolysin _____

6. atelocardia _____

7. autocytolysin _____

8. autohemolysis _a destruction of the red blood cells by its plasma_

9. cardiotomy _____

10. dysgraphia _____

11. dyskinesia _____

12. endoscope _____

13. gastromyxorrhea _____

14. gastrorrhagia _____

15. gastroscope _____

16. gastroscopy _____

17. gastrotome _____

18. genetics _____

19. hemidysesthesia _____

20. hepatogenous _____

21. hepatorrhexis _____

22. hypertonus _____

43

23. idiogenesis _____

*obsolete*
24. idioneurosis _____

*profuse*
25. leukorrhagia *flow of whitish discharge* _____

26. leukorrhea _____

27. myatonia _____

28. myectomy _____

29. myelatelia _____

30. myotatic _____

31. myotenositis[1] _____

32. myxoma _____

33. necrogenous _____

34. nephrectomy _____

35. neurotmesis[2] _____

36. onychorrhexis _____

37. orthosis _____

38. otomycosis _____

39. pachyrhinic _____

40. pathogenic _____

41. ptosis _____

42. pyrexia _____

43. pyrexin *substance from inflammatory exudate which causes fever.*

---

[1]The -s- between *myo-* and *-itis* has been inserted to avoid hiatus, an awkward gap between two vowels. This is known as an epenthetic consonant.

[2]The -tm- in this word is from Greek *temnein*, cut.

44. pyrogen _Substance that produces fever._

45. rhinomycosis _____

46. septicemia _____

47. spasmolytic _____

48. splenectasia _____

49. syntasis _____

50. telangioma _____

51. telangiosis _____

52. tenodynia _____

53. tenonitis _____

54. tenontomyotomy _incision into a tendon + muscle w/ removal of part or all of the muscle._

55. tenostosis _____

56. therapeutics _____

57. toxicotherapy _use of treatment by means of poison._

58. toxolysin _____

B. Give the word derived from Greek elements that means each of the following. Verify your answer in the medical dictionary.

1. Causing cancer _____

2. Originating outside (of an organ or part) _____

3. X-ray examination of the bile ducts _cholangiography_

4. Slowness of movement _____

5. Hemorrhage from the urinary bladder _____

6. A flowing through _diarrhea._

45

7. Discharge of pus (from) the ear ___Otopyorrhea___

8. Falling of the intestine ___enteroptosis___

9. The study of the ear and nose _____

10. Surgical removal of a kidney _____

11. Incomplete development of the foot _____

12. Instrument for examining the nose _____

13. Causing fever _____

14. Thickness of the ear _____

15. Hemorrhage from the nose _____

16. (Any substance capable of) producing disease _____

17. Disintegration of tissue ___histolysis___

18. Fat producing ___lyposeus / lypogenic___

19. Resembling mucus _____

20. Lack of feeling (in the) extremities _____

21. Arterial dilation ___arterioectasis___

22. Ulceration of the ear ___othelcosis___

23. Treatment (of disease) by water ___hydrotherapy___

24. Rupture of a (blood) vessel _____

C. Give a clear, concise definition of each of the following italicized words as it is used in the sentence below.

1. *Hyperpyrexia* is a serious threat to life, and heroic measures must be instituted immediately.

2. Subtotal *gastrectomy* may result in achlorhydria and may be associated with iron deficiency anemia and occasionally with ascorbic or folic acid deficiencies.

3. Onset of *rhinoscleroma* is insidious and the patient may have only cosmetic complaints.

4. A common complaint in acute gastritis is *pyrosis* along the course of the esophagus.

5. People with peripheral *neuropathies* may develop symptoms that include *paresthesia, dysesthesia, hyperesthesia,* and *hypesthesia.*

6. Myelopathic anemias constitute a heterogeneous group of conditions of diverse cause and uncertain *pathogenesis.*

7. Congenital *amyotonia* is a hereditary disease of infancy.

8. It should never happen as it does that an innocuous [heart] murmur casually found in a perfectly healthy young person becomes the origin of *iatrogenic* invalidism and mental crippling.

    *pertaining to being produced by treatment.*

9. To diagnose *psychogenic* backache and institute the only correct treatment, that is, adequate *psychotherapy,* is often of decisive importance.

    ↳ *treatment bmo mental means*
    
    *b mental means*

10. *Hyperkinesis* is a common feature in minimal brain dysfunction.

11. Acute *myelogenous* leukemia developed in a 19-year-old Marshallese man who had been exposed to radioactive fallout at 1 year of age.

12. The possible cure was a marrow transplant from a healthy donor, but a rare combination of *antigens* in the patient's blood made the odds of finding a perfect match a million to one.

13. Certain foods, including wheat germ, vitamin E, and brewer's yeast, are erroneously thought to be *ergogenic*.

14. In patients with hereditary familial *telangiectasia* involving the nasal mucosa, it may be necessary to remove the involved mucous membrane and replace it with a skin graft. Submucosal injection of a mild sclerosing agent just beneath the telangiectasis is often of value and is the treatment of choice.

D. Answer each of the following:

1. What is the difference in meaning between *antipyretic* and *antipyrotic*?

2. What is the common name for the disease *parotitis*? Why is parotitis so named?

3. What exactly is an *idiopathic* condition?

4. What is the difference in etymology and meaning between the words *dermatoma* and *dermatome*?

5. What is muscular *tone*?

6. What is *antisepsis*?

7. What is the difference in meaning between the following pairs of words: *cholangiotomy* and *cholangiostomy*; *cholecystocolotomy* and *cholecystocolostomy*?

8. What is meant by *osteography*?

9. What is the *peritoneum* and why is it so named?

membrane stretched around the viscera. enclosing

10. What is the difference between a substance that is *pyogenic* and one that is *pyrogenic*?

pus-producing    fever-producing

11. What is *entomology*, and why was this study so named?

12. What is an *autogenous* vaccine?

13. What is *autism*?

14. What is *orthotics*?

15. What is meant by *endogenous* disease? *exogenous* disease? Give an example of each.

16. What is *eugenics*?

17. What is a *polygraph* and why is it so named?

18. What is the etymology of the word *symptom*? What is the meaning of *asymptomatic*?

19. What is meant by the term *orthocephalic? brachycephalic?*[1] *dolichocephalic?*[2]

20. What is meant by *orthobiosis*?

## DRILL AND REVIEW

E. The meaning of each of the following words can be determined from its etymology. Determine the meaning of each. Verify your answer in the medical dictionary if necessary.

1. euesthesia
2. ectogenous

3. mycetogenetic
4. hypnogenetic

---

[1] Greek *brachys*, short
[2] Greek *dolichos*, long

5. anhepatogenic
6. otogenic
7. osteogen
8. pyretogen
9. antipyogenic
10. antitoxinogen
11. oncogenesis
12. otoncus
13. iatric
14. iatrology
15. podiatrist
16. psychiatry
17. angiocardiography
18. encephalography
19. akinesia
20. eukinesia
21. autokinesis
22. oncolysis
23. osteolysis
24. sarcolysis
25. hypomyxia
26. myxangitis
27. myxomyoma
28. myxolipoma
29. myxochondroma
30. entotic
31. parotic
32. epiotic
33. macrotia
34. microtia
35. polyotia
36. endopathy
37. exopathic
38. myopathy
39. toxicopathy
40. poliomyelopathy
41. polioencephalopathy
42. osteoarthropathy
43. encephalomyelopathy
44. coloptosis
45. splenoptosis
46. othemorrhea
47. hidrorrhea
48. otorrhagia
49. encephalorrhagia
50. meningorrhagia
51. myorrhexis
52. arteriorrhexis

53. erythrocytorrhexis
54. rhinalgia
55. rhinogenous
56. rhinolithiasis
57. rhinorrhea
58. rhinostenosis
59. rhinotomy
60. endorhinitis
61. endotoscope
62. cystoscope
63. pyreticosis
64. pyretotherapy - treatment benegns of fever
65. apyretic
66. apyrexia
67. apyrogenic
68. gastrectasia
69. enterectasia
70. hemangiectasis
71. telangiitis
72. atelostomia
73. atelocheiria
74. atelencephalia
75. tenalgia
76. tenonectomy
77. chondrectomy
78. nephrolithotomy
79. onychotomy
80. tenotomy
81. histotome
82. toxipathy
83. kinesiotherapy
84. kinesialgia
85. kinesiatrics
86. hepatolysin
87. anhemolytic
88. lipolytic
89. mycosis
90. otopyosis
91. neuropathogenesis
92. histopathology
93. antihemorrhagic
94. autoantitoxin
95. septicopyemia
96. aseptic peritonitis
97. autosepticemia
98. myotasis
99. gastric atony
100. hypotonia

# LESSON 5
# GREEK VOCABULARY

γνῶθι σαυτόν. *Know thyself.* [Thales, sixth-century B.C. philosopher, as quoted by Diogenes Laertius (third century A.D.) in *Lives of the Philosophers.*]

γνῶθι σαυτόν

## VOCABULARY

| GREEK WORD | COMBINING FORM(S) | MEANING | |
|---|---|---|---|
| *akouein* | ACOU(S)-, ACU(S)- | hear | |
| *amnion* | AMNI- | fetal membrane, amniotic sac | |
| *kentein* | CENTE- | pierce | *centesis : surgical puncture* |
| *chrōma, chrōmatos* | CHROM-, CHROMA-, CHROMAT- | color, pigment | |
| *oidēma, oidēmatos* | EDEMA, EDEMAT- | swelling | |
| *dipsa* | DIPS- | thirst | |
| *emein* | EME- | vomit | |
| *gignōskein* | GNO(S)- | know | *diagnosis* |
| *lalein* | LAL- | talk | |
| *lapara* | LAPAR- | abdomen, abdominal wall | |
| *legein* | LEX- | read | |
| *mimnēskein* | MNE- | remember | |
| *neos* | NE- | new | |
| *nous* | NO- | mind, mental activity, comprehension | |
| *oregein* | OREC-, OREX- | have an appetite | |
| *oxys* | OX(Y)-[1] | acute, pointed; rapid; oxygen | *acid* |
| *phēnai* | PHA- | speak, communicate | |
| *phagein* | PHAG- | swallow, eat | |

---

[1]The combining form OX- indicates the presence of oxygen: anoxia, hypoxia, hypoxemia, and so forth. In a few words OXY- means rapid: oxylalia, oxytocia. Oxycephalous denotes a head that is pointed and dome-like. In some words OXY- has the meaning of acid: oxygen. These words do not appear in the exercises of this text. In a few words OXY- has the meaning of sharp: oxyphonia means an abnormally sharp sound to the voice.

| | | |
|---|---|---|
| *pharmakon* | PHARMAC(EU)-[1] | medicine, drug |
| *phēmē* | PHEM- | speech |
| *phobos* | PHOB- | (abnormal) fear |
| *phonē* | PHON- | voice, sound |
| *phrassein* | PHRAC-[2], PHRAG- | enclose, obstruct |
| *phrazein* | PHRAS- | speak |
| *phrēn* | PHREN- | mind; diaphragm[3] |
| *phylattein* | PHYLAC-[4] | protect (against disease) |
| *phyma, phymatos* | PHYM-, PHYMA, PHYMAT- | growth, swelling |
| *physis* | PHYS(I)- | nature, appearance |
| *phyton* | PHYT- | plant (organism), growth |
| *poiein* | POIE- | produce, make |
| *sapros* | SAPR- | rotten, putrid, decaying |
| *stear, steatos* | STEAR-, STEAT- | fat, sebum,[5] sebaceous glands |

## ETYMOLOGICAL NOTES

On August 1, 1774, Joseph Priestley, a British clergyman and experimental chemist, focused the rays of the sun through a magnifying glass onto red oxide of mercury and produced a vapor which he named dephlogisticated air. It was a commonly held belief among the scientists of that time that all matter contained a substance called phlogiston (from the Greek *phlogistos*, inflammable), which was released during burning. Priestley, after discovering that his lungs felt particularly light and easy for some time after breathing the vapor, asked, "Who can tell but that, in time, this pure air may become a fashionable article in luxury? Hitherto, only two mice and myself have had the privilege of breathing it."[6] Priestley journeyed to Paris in the fall of 1774 and described his experiment to the French scientist Antoine Lavoisier, who renamed the newly discovered vapor *oxygen*, meaning acid-producing.

Oedipus, the tragic hero of Sophocles' *Oedipus the King*, owes his name to the verb *oidein*, become swollen. An oracle had told Laius, king of Thebes, that if his wife bore him a son, this child would eventually kill him. When a son was born to the queen, Laius pierced the infant's feet and tied them together and gave him to a shepherd to expose on the mountainside. But instead, the child was given to the king of Corinth, who, childless, brought him up as his own son, naming him *Oidipous*, swollen foot. As is well known, Oedipus (to give his name the Latin spelling) did eventually kill his father and, furthermore, marry Jocasta, his own mother; hence the Freudian term Oedipus Complex.

The Greek noun *oidēma*, swelling, from the verb *oidein*, become swollen, has given us the word **edema**, a swelling caused by an accumulation of tissue fluid. If the condition is generalized—that is, existing over large areas of the body—it is sometimes called **hydrops** (from Greek *hydrōps*, from *hydōr*, water) or **dropsy**.

The Greek noun *askos* meant skin or hide, but more usually a bag or sack made of skin, especially a wineskin. Homer tells us that when Odysseus and his men departed from the island of Aeolia, where Aeolus, the Keeper of the Winds had entertained them for a full month, Aeolus

---

[1]The combining form PHARMACEU- is from the Greek adjective *pharmakeutikos*, concerning drugs.

[2]Words in -emphraxis are from PHRAC- and -*sis*.

[3]See the Etymological Notes to this lesson.

[4]Words in -phylaxis are from PHYLAC- and -*sis*.

[5]Sebum, from Latin *sebum*, grease, fat, is the fatty secretion of the sebaceous glands of the skin.

[6]Copyright 1974 by The New York Times Company. Reprinted by permission.

gave Odysseus a bag (*askos*) made of the hide of an ox nine years old in which he bound the blustering winds, allowing the breath of only the West Wind to blow, thus affording Odysseus and his men a sure passage across the sea. [*Odyssey* 10.19 ff] The ancient Greeks knew of the condition that we call **ascites**, and named it *ascitēs*, the baggy disease, from the baggy aspect of the human body resulting from the accumulation of serous fluid in the peritoneal cavity.

In Greek mythology, Mnemosyne, Memory, was a Titaness, one of the children of Sky and Earth. The eighth-century B.C. poet, Hesiod, tells us of the union of Mnemosyne and Zeus:

*For nine nights did all-wise Zeus lie with her, entering her holy bed far away from the immortals. And when a year had passed and the seasons turned as the months waned, and many days were fulfilled, she bore nine daughters, all of like mind, whose hearts are turned to song and whose spirits are free from care, a little way from the highest peak of snow-clad Olympus.* [*Theogony* 56 ff]

These were the nine Muses: Clio, Euterpe, Thalia, Melpomene, Erato, Terpsichore, Polyhymnia, Urania, and Calliope, patron goddesses of the Arts.

There was a Greek verb *mimnēskein*, remember, related to the name of this goddess of memory, Mnemosyne, and from it we get such words as **amnesia, amnesty, mnemonic**, and so forth. The Latin nouns *memoria* and *mēns, mentis*, mind, are related to this Greek verb and have given us our words **memory** and **mental**.

The Greek word *amnos*, lamb, had a diminutive form, *amnion*, meaning the innermost of the membranes surrounding the human fetus, and this is the modern meaning of the word. The **amnion** is a thin, transparent sac which holds the fetus suspended in it surrounded by the amniotic fluid, or *liquor amnii*, which protects the fetus from injury. The Greek diminutive form, *amnion*, little lamb, was probably so named because this membrane resembles the extremely thin and delicate skin of the newborn lamb. **Amniocentesis** is the puncturing of the abdomen with a long, thin, hollow needle and the removal of a small amount of the amniotic fluid surrounding the fetus. This fluid contains some fetal cells which are grown in the laboratory. Some weeks later these cells are examined microscopically, and it can be determined if there is any abnormality in the chromosome number. Each human somatic cell contains 23 pairs of chromosomes, the genetic and hereditary determinants of human beings, and abnormalities in the number of chromosomes in the cells can indicate genetic defects in the unborn fetus.

The fear of water implicit in the word **hydrophobia** is caused by the excruciatingly painful spasms of the muscles of the throat that are precipitated by any attempt on the part of the unfortunate victim of this fatal disease to drink—even though he is at the point of death from dehydration. The incubation period of this dread disease varies from ten days to three months. If it is treated promptly, and the carrier of the virus, often dog, squirrel, or bat, is identified so that treatment may begin immediately, recovery is normal. But once the period of incubation has commenced there is virtually no alternative to death. The Latin word *rabiēs*, which is commonly used for this disease, meant simply madness. Celsus has written about hydrophobia and its cure:

*Certain physicians, after the bite of a rabid dog, send the victims directly to the bath, and there allow them to sweat as long as their strength permits, with the wound kept exposed so that the poison may readily drip from it. Then much undiluted wine is drunk, as this is an antidote to all poisons. After three days of this treatment the patient is thought to be out of danger. But if the wound is not sufficiently treated there arises a fear of water which the Greeks call hydrophobia, an exceedingly distressing disease in which the sufferer is tormented simultaneously by thirst and dread of water. There is little hope for those who are in this state. However, there remains one last remedy: throw the patient unexpectedly into a pool of water when he is not looking. If he cannot swim, allow him to sink and drink the water and then raise him up; but if he can swim, keep pushing him under so that he becomes filled with water, although unwillingly. In this way both his thirst and his fear of water are removed at the same time.* [*De Medicina* 5.27.2]

The ancients believed that the midriff was the seat of the emotions, and thus the word *phrēn* was applied to this area as a physical part of the body and also as the center of the emotions, the heart or the mind. Homer tells us in the *Odyssey* that Odysseus, after the Cyclops had made a meal of two of his companions, pondered how to deal with this monster:

*And I formed a plan to steal near to him and, drawing my sharp sword from beside my thigh, to strike him in the breast, at the point where the midriff* (phrēn) *holds the liver* (hēpar). [*Odyssey* 9.299–301]

Later in the poem Odysseus becomes enraged when one of his companions speaks slightingly of him.

*So he spoke, and I pondered in my mind* (phrēn) *whether or not to draw my long sword from beside my thigh and strike off his head and bring it to the ground, even though he was a kinsman of mine by marriage.* [*Odyssey* 10.438–441]

Thus, derivative words of *phrēn* in medical terminology refer to either the diaphragm or the mind or the mental processes. The **phrenic nerve** serves the diaphragm, while **tachyphrenia** means abnormally rapid mental activity.

The Greek verb *gignōskein* meant to know, understand; a secondary meaning was to examine, form an opinion, determine. From this verb were derived the nouns *gnōsis*, knowledge, *diagnōsis*, means of discerning, opinion, diagnosis, and *gnōmōn*, one who knows, judge. The verb *phyein* meant to grow according to the laws of nature. From this verb was derived a noun, *physis*, natural growth, outward form or appearance of anything. The word *physiognōmia* meant the study of one's appearance, a judgment of one's character from his appearance. Our word is **physiognomy**, the human countenance. From *gnōsis* and *diagnōsis* we get **physiognosis**, diagnosis from one's facial appearance, and **leukodiagnosis**, diagnosis from an examination of leukocytes. Other derivatives of the noun *physis* include **physic**, **physics**, **physical**, and **physician**. The Greek nouns *phyton*, plant, growth, and *phyma*, a growth upon the body, tumor, have given us **phytogenesis**, the origin and development of plants; **phytotoxin**, a poison derived from plants; **dermatophyte**, a fungal (that is, plant) organism growing in or on the skin; **osteophyma**, a growth of bone; and **ecphyma**, an outgrowth on the skin.

Horace, the Roman poet of the first century B.C., mentions in two of his poems a girl whom he calls Lalage. She is otherwise unknown, and Horace may have made up the name from the Greek verb *lalein*, talk, as his Lalage seems to be fond of chattering.

> *pone me pigris ubi nulla campis*
> *arbor aestiva recreatur aura,*
> *quod latus mundi nebulae malusque*
>   *Iuppiter urget;*
>
> *pone sub curru nimium propinqui*
> *solis in terra domibus negata:*
> *dulce ridentem Lalagen amabo,*
>   *dulce loquentem.*
>
> [*Odes* 1.22.17–24]

> Place me on a barren plain
> where no tree grows in the summer breeze,
> a land overhung by mists and gloomy skies;
>
> place me in a land too close to the chariot
> of the sun, a land barren of homes.
> I will love my sweetly laughing,
> sweetly chattering Lalage.

# EXERCISE 5

*In cases where there are swellings (phymata) and pains in the joints following fevers, those afflicted are eating too much food.* [Hippocrates, *Aphorisms* 7.45]

A. Analyze and define each of the following words.

1. achromacyte _discolored red blood cell._
    *matocye*

2. achromatosis _____

3. acouesthesia _sensation of hearing_____

4. agnosia _____

5. amniotitis[1] _____

6. anacusia _____

7. anoxia _lack of oxygen._____

8. arthrophyte _____

9. cephalocentesis _____

10. cholemesis _____

11. chromoscope _____

12. chromoscopy _____

13. dermatophyte _____

14. diagnosis _____

15. diaphragm _____

16. diaphragmatocele _____

17. dipsogen _____

18. dysacusia _____

---

[1]The *-ot-* of this word is from the suffix *-otic*.

19. dyschromia _____

20. dyslexia _____

21. dysmnesia _____

22. dysphasia _difficulty in producing the right words- caused by brain lesion._

23. dysphemia _"_ "_ caused by psychoneurological prob._

24. dysphonia _difficulty with voice._

25. ecphyma _____

26. edema _____

27. emetic _____

28. emphraxis _____

29. entophyte _____

30. esophylaxis _____

31. hematopoiesis _____

32. hematopoietic _____

33. histodiagnosis _____

34. hydrophobophobia _____

35. hyperchromatism _____

36. hypophrenia _____

37. lalorrhea _____

38. laparocholecystotomy _____

39. laparogastrostomy _____

40. leukodiagnosis _____

41. leukopoiesis _____

42. logagnosia _____

43. micracusia _____

44. mnemasthenia _____

45. myelopoiesis _____

46. neogenesis _____

47. neopathy _____

48. neostomy _____

49. nephremphraxis _____

50. odynophagia _____

51. oligochromemia _____

52. oligodipsia _____

53. osteophyma _____

54. oxyacusis _____

55. oxycephalia _____

56. oxyrhine _(ADJ) having a pointed/sharp nose_

57. oxyesthesia _____

58. paracentesis _____

59. paranoia _condition of having persistant persecutory delusions._

60. paranoiac _____

61. paranoid _____

62. parorexia _____

63. periphrenitis _____

64. phage _____

65. phagocyte _____

66. phagocytosis _____

67. pharmaceutics _____

68. pharmacodiagnosis _____

69. pharmacography _____

70. phobophobia _Abnormal fear of acquiring a fear_____

71. phoniatrics _____

72. phrenicotomy _Cutting of the phrenic nerve._____

73. phyma _____

74. phymatoid _____

75. phymatosis _____

76. physiognomy[1] _____

77. physiognosis _____

78. physiology _____

79. physical _____

80. phytotoxin _____

81. polyphrasia _____

82. polydipsia _____

83. psychochromesthesia _sensation of seeing color caused by something other than visual apparatus._

---

[1]Greek *gnōmōn*, judge

84. pyemesis _____

85. rhinolalia _____

86. sapremia *condition of rotten blood.*
*septicemia – infected blood.*_____

87. saprogenic _____

88. saprophyte _____

89. stearodermia _____

90. steatoma _____

91. steatonecrosis _____

92. steatolysis _____

93. steatopygia[1] _____

94. tachyphasia _____

95. toxophylaxin _____

B. Give the word derived from Greek elements that means each of the following. Verify your answer in the medical dictionary.

1. Deafness in one ear _____

2. Excessive vomiting _____

3. Incision of the spleen through the abdominal wall _____

4. Abnormally excessive memory _____

5. Difficulty in swallowing _____

6. Absence of color _____

7. Fear of new (things) _____

8. Having no appetite _____

---

[1]Greek *pygē*, buttock

9. Fear of spiders _____

10. Fear of corpses _____

11. Lack of strength of the voice _____

12. Inability to swallow _____

C. Define each of the following italicized words.

1. The most common type of *anorexia* is found in acute indigestion and acute gastritis.

2. *Angioedema* can be due to drug allergy, insect stings or bites, desensitization injections, or ingestion of certain foods (particularly eggs, shellfish, nuts, and fruits).

3. Effects depend on the type and degree of *hypoxia*, the rapidity of its development, its duration, and the relative physiological competency of the involved cells at the onset.

4. In cases of cirrhosis, if the major complications of *hematemesis*, hepatic coma, ascites, and jaundice have appeared, *prognosis* is poor, with one-year survival rates of only 30 percent.

5. *Anaphylaxis*[1] occurs within minutes after introduction of the offending agent and is manifested by collapse, profound hypotension, wheezing, and cyanosis.

6. Since exploratory *laparotomy* is of value in determining the cause of illness in some instances, it is important to consider when such a procedure is indicated.

---

[1]Greek *ana-*, up, back

7. *Hyperorexia* is often found in convalescence from acute diseases.

8. *Ascites*[1] is a spectacular abnormality, often bringing patients to clinical attention.

D. Answer each of the following questions.

1. What is meant by *laparoscopy*?

2. What is a *phylactic* agent?

3. What is *prophylaxis*? How is it applied in dentistry?

4. What is *anaphylactic* shock?

5. What is an *emphractic* agent?

6. What is an *agnogenic* disease?

7. What is an *orexigenic* agent?

---

[1]Greek *askitēs*, dropsy, from *askos*, bag

8. What is *mnemonics*?[1]

9. What is *aphasia*? Using the medical dictionary, determine the meaning of *amnesic aphasia*, *auditory aphasia*, and *optic aphasia*.

10. What is a *paroxysm*?

11. What is *oxyhydrocephalus*?

12. What is the United States *Pharmacopeia*?

13. What is *erythropoietin*?[2]

14. What is a *scopophobiac*?

15. What is *physiatrics*?

16. What is *orthophrenia*?

---

[1]Greek *mnēmōn*, remembering
[2]The -*t*- in this word is from *erythropoietic*.

# DRILL AND REVIEW

E. The meaning of each of the following words can be determined from its etymology. Determine the meaning of each, and verify your answer in the medical dictionary.

1. hypacousia
2. paracusia
3. odynacusis
4. amniorrhea
5. amniorrhexis
6. amniotome
7. amniotomy
8. amnioscope
9. amniography
10. alalia
11. dyslalia
12. oxylalia
13. bradylalia
14. tachylalia
15. tachyphagia
16. bradyphagia
17. polyphagia
18. pyophagia
19. onychophagy
20. erythrophage
21. microbiophobia
22. graphophobia
23. hypnophobia
24. algophobia
25. polyphobia
26. dipsesis
27. dipsotherapy
28. adipsia
29. splenemphraxis
30. angiemphraxis
31. paraphonia
32. oxyphonia
33. bradyphrasia
34. tachyphrasia
35. tachyphrenia
36. hyperphrenia
37. aphrenia
38. gastrophrenic
39. paraphrenitis
40. laparomyitis
41. laparohepatotomy
42. laparogastrotomy
43. laparoenterotomy
44. laparoenterostomy
45. edematous
46. acroedema
47. hypernoia
48. eunoia
49. anoesia
50. anoetic
51. anhematopoiesis
52. hematopoietic
53. cholepoiesis
54. dyshematopoiesia
55. erythropoiesis
56. leukopoietic
57. pyopoiesis
58. pyopoietic
59. isochromatic
60. anisochromatic
61. chromatogenous
62. chromotherapy
63. chromogenesis
64. chromogenic
65. chromidrosis
66. antemetic
67. lalophobia
68. lalopathy
69. bradylexia
70. alexia
71. mnemic[1]
72. hypomnesia
73. dysorexia
74. aphemia
75. hypoxemia
76. hematophagous
77. necrophagous
78. sarcophagy
79. phagocytolysis
80. pharmaceutical
81. pharmacophobia
82. pharmacotherapy
83. pharmacology
84. diaphragmodynia
85. phonopathy
86. prophylactic
87. phytogenesis
88. hematophyte
89. arthrocentesis
90. cardiocentesis
91. pericardiocentesis
92. steatolysis
93. steatopathy
94. steatorrhea

---

[1]Greek *mnēma*, memory

# GREEK VOCABULARY

NIΨONANOMHMAMHMONANOΨIN: Νίψον ἀνόμημα μὴ μόναν ὄψιν. *Wash your sins, not only your face.* [A palindromic inscription on the sacred font in the courtyard of Hagia Sophia in Istanbul.]

## VOCABULARY

| GREEK WORD | COMBINING FORM(S) | MEANING |
|---|---|---|
| *alexein* | ALEX(I)- | ward off (disease) |
| *anēr, andros* | ANDR- | man, male |
| *ankylos* | ANKYL-, ANCYL- | fused, stiffened; hooked |
| *Aphrodisios* | APHRODIS(I)- | [of *or* pertaining to Aphrodite, Greek goddess of love] sexual desire |
| *dēmos* | DEM- | people, population |
| *dromos* | DROM- | a running |
| *Erōs, Erōtos* | ER-, EROT- | [Eros, son of Aphrodite, Greek goddess of love] sexual desire |
| *gynē, gynaikos* | GYN(EC)- | woman, female |
| *helmins, helminthos* | HELMINT(H)- | (intestinal) worm |
| *nēma, nēmatos* | NEMAT- | thread (worm) |
| *nosos* | NOS- | disease, illness |
| *odous, odontos* | ODONT- | tooth |
| *palin* | PALI(N)- | back, again |
| *pas, pantos* | PAN(T)- | all, entire, every |
| *phoros* | PHOR- | bearing, carrying[1] |
| *phōs, phōtos* | PHOS-, PHOT- | light, daylight |
| *plēssein* | PLEC-,[2] PLEG- | strike, paralyze |
| *rhachis* | R(H)ACHI- | spine |
| *schizein* | SCHIZ-, SCHIST-, -SCHISIS | split |

---

[1]The words euphoria and dysphoria are formed from the Greek compound nouns *euphoria*, a sense of well-being or comfort, and *dysphoria*, a sense of discomfort.

[2]Words in -plexy are from -PLEC- + *-sia*.

| *spondylos* | SPONDYL- | vertebra |
| *staxis* | -STAXIS, -STAXIA | dripping, oozing (of blood) |
| *thanatos* | THAN(AT)- | death |
| *tithenai* | THE- | place, put |
| *thrix, trichos* | TRICH- | hair |
| *trophē* | TROPH- | nourishment |

## ETYMOLOGICAL NOTES

Trichinosis (Greek *trichinos*, of hair) is a disease caused by the ingestion of the larvae of the parasitic worm *Trichinella spiralis* through eating raw or insufficiently cooked pork or, rarely, infested bear meat. The larvae penetrate the mucous lining of the intestinal tract and, in a few days, mature and mate, after which the males die. The females begin to discharge their young larvae after about a week, a process that continues for up to 6 weeks. These tiny larvae enter the blood stream of the host and are carried to the tissues and organs of the body to lodge eventually in muscle tissue, causing, among other symptoms, pain, nausea, diarrhea, edema, fever, chills, and general weakness. The majority of those afflicted with trichinosis recover, although involvement of the respiratory muscles can lead to death.

The name *Trichinella spiralis* is New Latin. This term is applied to words and names that have been coined in modern times in the form of and on the analogy of Latin words, or, in some instances, to the use of new meanings applied to extant Latin words. In the name *Trichinella spiralis*, *-ella* is a Latin diminutive ending added to the stem of the Greek adjective *trichinos*, and *spiralis* is a modern adjectival formation from the Latin noun *spira*, coil, spiral, borrowed from the Greek noun *speira*, anything coiled or twisted. In the binomial system of biological nomenclature, the generic name is indicated by a capitalized noun, while the species is indicated by an adjective agreeing with this noun in gender and number.[1]

The Greek word *trophē*, nourishment, has given us such words as **trophic**, concerned with nourishment, and **trophology**, the science of nutrition. Most of the words in medical terminology that use the form TROPH- have to do with the nourishment that is carried to the cells of the body by the circulating blood. Any impediment to the flow of blood to a part will result in **hypotrophy** and eventually **atrophy**. **Hypotrophy** is the gradual degeneration and loss of function of tissues—usually muscle tissue—resulting from a decrease in the flow of blood to that part. **Atrophy** is a decrease in size of a part resulting from lack of cell nourishment. **Hypertrophy** is an increase in the size of an organ or part as a consequence of an increase in the absorption of nutrition. This is usually caused by an increase in functional activity, as in **cardiac hypertrophy**, an increase in the size of the heart resulting from overgrowth of the tissues of the heart muscle due to continued stress beyond normal.[2] **Hypermyatrophy** is unusual wasting of muscle tissue, and **hemihypertrophy** is hypertrophy of the tissues of one side of the body. **Amyotrophy** is muscular atrophy. **Dystrophy** is the name given to any disorder of the body caused by defective nutrition, such as **muscular dystrophy**, a familial disease characterized by progressive atrophy of muscles. **Hemidystrophy** is dystrophy of one side of the body.

Paris, the handsome Trojan prince who carried away Helen, the wife of Menelaus, the king of Sparta, and thus precipitated the Trojan War, was a son of King Priam of Troy and his wife

---

[1]See Supplementary Lesson III, Biological Nomenclature, and the Appendix.

[2]One of the four signs of the tetralogy of Fallot (a congenital disorder caused by a defect in the heart that allows blood to pass from the left ventricle to the right) is hypertrophy of the right ventricle. This is caused by the extra stress placed upon this part of the heart muscle by the burden of pumping the additional blood that accumulates there.

Hecuba, and was surnamed Alexander (Greek *Alexandros*, Defender of Men). Apollodorus, the (probably) first-century A.D. writer of Greek mythology, has given us a brief, unadorned version of how Paris came to be called Alexander:

*The first son born to Hecuba was Hector. When a second child was about to be born, Hecuba dreamed that she had borne a firebrand and that this had spread over all the city and burned it. When Priam learned of the dream from Hecuba, he sent for his son Aesacus, who was an interpreter of dreams, having learned this art from his mother's father Merops. Aesacus declared that the child would cause the destruction of his country and advised that it be exposed. When the child was born, Priam gave it to a servant to expose on Mount Ida. This man was named Agelaus. Thus exposed, the child was nursed by a bear for five days. When Agelaus found it safe, he took it up and brought it up as his own son on his farm and named him Paris. When the child grew to be a young man, he excelled many in beauty and strength and afterwards was surnamed Alexandros because he drove away robbers and was a defender* (alexein) *of the flocks. Soon afterwards he discovered his parents.* [*Library* 3.12.5]

An **alexic** or **alexeteric** (Greek *alexētēr*, protector) agent is one that is protective against infection. An **alexipyretic** is an agent that lessens fever, and **alexin** is a defensive substance in serum which, in the presence of a specific sensitizer, exerts a lytic action on bacteria and other cells.

The Greek adjective *ankylos* meant crooked or curved, and the noun *ankylē* meant a joint that was bent and stiffened by disease; both words are derivatives of the noun *ankos*, bend or hollow. **Ankylosis** is abnormal immobility of a joint due to some pathological changes in the joint or its surrounding tissue. The combining form ANKYL- means a fusion of parts normally separate, as in **ankylochilia** (*cheilos*, lip), **ankyloproctia** (*prōktos*, anus), or **ankylocolpos** (*kolpos*, vagina).

The Greek word *Aphrodisia* meant sexual pleasures, things connected with Aphrodite, the goddess of love. There was an adjective *Aphrodisiakos*, from which we get the word **aphrodisiac**. Aphrodite did not confine her amorous attentions to Hephaestus, her husband and god of the forge, but had numerous affairs with immortals and mortals alike. One such relationship, that with Hermes, a god of many functions in Greek mythology, resulted in the birth of a son who grew to be a handsome young man resembling both his mother and his father. His name was Hermaphroditus. Ovid, the Roman poet of the first century B.C., tells us an anecdote about this young man.

As the story goes, there was once a naiad, a nymph of the water, named Salmacis, who dwelled in a pool in Caria, a land of Asia Minor. One day Hermaphroditus, who was then fifteen years old, came to the place, and Salmacis fell in love with him on sight. He, a shy young man, refused her advances. But she waited until he went bathing in the pool, and, casting off all her garments, dived in, crying, *I win, he is mine!*

*Hermaphroditus resists and denies the nymph the pleasures she has hoped for, but she clings to him, pressing her whole body to him as if they were grown together.* Struggle as hard as you wish, you wicked boy, *she says*, but you will not escape. May the gods grant me this, that no day ever come that will take him from me. *The gods heard her. Their two bodies were joined together, one face and one form for both. Just as one grafts a twig onto a branch and sees them join and grow together, so were these two bodies joined in close embrace, no longer two beings, yet no longer either man or woman, but neither, and yet both.* [*Metamorphoses* 4.368 ff]

Hesiod, the Greek poet of the mid-eighth century B.C., tells us in his *Theogony* (Origin of the Gods) that in the beginning of Creation, Chaos first came into being, then Earth, dark Tartarus in the depths of Earth, and then Eros, "fairest among the deathless gods, who unnerves the limbs and overcomes the counsels of a prudent mind of all gods and men" (*Theogony* 120–123). But in the sense in which he is usually conceived, that of the Latin Cupid, he is the creation of later Greek poets. Far from remaining the primeval deity of Hesiod, he grows younger, and from the handsome youth of the sixth–fifth centuries B.C., he becomes a wanton, lascivious boy in the Alexandrian period (third to first centuries) whose arrows kindle passion in the heart. The parentage of the second Eros is in some dispute, but the most commonly held belief makes Aphrodite his mother and either Hermes or Ares, the god of war, his father. Cicero holds to the latter view (*On the Nature of the Gods* 3.23). His Latin name, Cupid (*cupido*, desire), gives us the word **cupidity**, while his Greek name gives us **erotic, eroticism**, and so forth.

To the ancient Greeks, Thanatos was the god of death. He appears as a character on the stage in the opening scene of Euripides' tragedy *Alcestis*, where he comes to claim Alcestis, the lovely young wife of King Admetus, for whom she has offered to die. Admetus had offended the goddess Artemis, and she decreed that he must die on a certain date—unless someone would voluntarily die for him. When he could find no one to make this sacrifice, Alcestis agreed to take his place. But this was a tragedy with a happy ending, for the great hero Heracles went to the underworld and succeeded in taking Alcestis away from Thanatos, and the drama ends with Heracles' leading Alcestis back to her husband.

Homer, in the *Iliad* (16.666 ff), tells us that when Zeus' son, Sarpedon, was killed in the fighting before the walls of Troy, the god ordered Apollo to remove Sarpedon's body from the field of battle and entrust it to Sleep (Hypnos) and his twin brother Death (Thanatos), who will return it to Sarpedon's home, in Lycia. This is the subject matter of the painting on a famous ancient Greek vase, the Euphronios vase, now in the Metropolitan Museum of Art in New York City. Sleep and Death are depicted lifting the body of Sarpedon, while Apollo looks on.

## EXERCISE 6

A. Analyze and define each of the following words.

1. alexin _____

2. alexipyretic _____

3. antaphrodisiac _____

4. androgen _____

5. androgynous _____

6. ankylosis _____

7. ankylodactylia _____

8. apoplexy[1] _____

9. apothanasia _____

10. atrophy _____

11. chromatophore _____

_____
[1]Greek *apo-*, away

70

12. cystistaxia _____

13. dermonosology _____

14. diaphoresis _____

15. diplegia[1] _____

16. dysphoria _____

17. dystrophy _____

18. erogenous _____

19. euphoria _____

20. euthanasia _____

21. gastroschisis _____

22. gynandroid _____

23. gynecopathy _____

24. helminthiasis _____

25. hemidiaphoresis _____

26. hermaphrodite[2] _____

27. hypertrichosis _____

28. idiotrophic _____

29. myatrophy _____

30. nematocide[3] _____

31. nematology _____

32. nosophyte _____

[1]Greek di(s)-, twice, double
[2]Hermaphroditus, son of Hermes and Aphrodite; see the Etymological Notes to this lesson.
[3]Latin caedere, kill

33. nosotherapy _____

34. odontonecrosis _____

35. osteosynthesis _____

36. palingenesis _____

37. paliphrasia _____

38. pancarditis _____

39. pantatrophy _____

40. paraplegia _____

41. pathophoric _____

42. phosphoridrosis _____

43. photobiotic _____

44. photodysphoria _____

45. photolysis _____

46. photosynthesis _____

47. prosthesis[1] _____

48. rachicentesis _____

49. rachioplegia _____

50. schistocyte _____

51. schistocytosis _____

52. spondylolysis _____

53. thanatology _____

54. trichogen _____

_____

[1]Greek *pros-*, in place of

B. Give the word derived from Greek elements that means each of the following. Verify your answer in the medical dictionary.

1. Resembling a male _____

2. Pertaining to all the people _____

3. Excessive muscle nourishment _____

4. The study of (diseases of) women _____

5. Inflammation of every (structure of a) bone _____

6. Fear of everything _____

7. Pain in a vertebra _____

8. Inflammation of the spine _____

9. Fear of death _____

10. Hemorrhage from a tooth (socket) _____

11. The study of hair _____

12. The study of (intestinal) worms _____

13. Pain (produced by) light _____

C. Give a clear, concise definition of each of the following italicized words as it is used in the sentences below.

1. Some studies on the *epidemiology*[1] of cervical carcinoma suggest that, in some individuals, tissue exposed to chronic irritation will progress from cervicitis and epithelial dysplasia to carcinoma.

2. In *schizophrenia*, thinking or the organization of communications is disturbed, resulting in profound alterations of the individual's self-experience and his perception of the world. During the *prodromal* phase, the patient frequently experiences brief episodes when he feels that he has marked insight into the meaning of life, or brief periods of perceptual hyperclarity, in which colors and objects become vivid.

---

[1]The *-i-* following *-dem-* in this word is from the *-ic* of *epidemic*.

3. *Epistaxis* is a common emergency that usually results from a local disturbance but may be associated with a serious systemic disorder.

4. Acute promyelocytic leukemia is characterized by a bleeding *diathesis* that is more severe than the bleeding of other acute leukemias.

5. *Rachitic* tetany is caused by hypocalcemia and may accompany either infantile or adult vitamin D deficiency.

6. Common symptoms of a stroke are *hemiplegia* (affecting the arm more than the leg) and cortical sensory loss in the affected limbs.

7. When measles is at its height, the temperature may be over 104°F, with swelling of the face, conjunctivitis, *photophobia*, a hacking cough, extensive rash, and mild itching.

8. In contrast to rheumatoid arthritis, which produces unstable joints, *ankylosing spondylitis* is truly ankylosing.

9. A 44-year-old man had hematemesis a few hours before admission. For three days prior to admission he had been ingesting 12 aspirin per day. The blood pressure was 88/42 mm Hg. He was *diaphoretic* and pale. The pulse rate was 120 beats per minute.

D. Answer each of the following questions.

1. What are *antidromic* nerve impulses?

2. *Rachischisis, schistorrhachis, rachicele, myeloschisis,* and *spina bifida*[1] are all names for the same condition. What do these terms mean?

3. With what is the science of *prosthetics* concerned? What is *enthesis*?

4. What is the difference between *trichinosis* and *trichonosis*?

5. What is meant by *palindromic* rheumatism?

6. What is *Schizomycetes*? What is the significance of the etymology of this name?

7. Schistosomiasis is a disease widespread throughout Africa due to infestation by a parasitic worm of the genus *Schistosoma*. What is the etymology of this name?

8. Define the word *syndrome*.

9. What is *periodontology? exodontology? endodontics? orthodontia? prosthodontics?*[2]

10. What is the difference between an *endemic* disease and an *epidemic* disease?

---

[1]Latin *bi-*, two, FID-, split

[2]Greek *prosth-*, in place of

11. Ancylostomiasis is a disease that is common in tropical and semi-tropical areas and caused by infestation by the larvae of nematode worms of the genus *Ancylostoma* through contact with bare skin, usually the feet. What is the etymology of this name? What is a *nematode* worm?

12. What is *scoliosis*?[1]

13. What is *photic* sneezing?

14. What is the purpose of an *alexeteric*[2] agent?

15. What is a *nosocomial*[3] infection?

16. What is *amyotrophic lateral*[4] sclerosis?

## DRILL AND REVIEW

E. The meaning of each of the following words can be determined from its etymology. Determine the meaning of each and verify your answer in the medical dictionary.

1. andropathy
2. androgynoid
3. andriatrics
4. trophic
5. atrophic

6. antatrophic
7. hypertrophy
8. nephrohypertrophy
9. hypotrophy
10. chondrodystrophy

---

[1]Greek *skolios*, curved
[2]Greek *alexētēr*, protector
[3]Greek *nosokomeion*, hospital
[4]Latin *lateralis*, from *latus, lateris*, side

11. osteochondrodystrophy
12. onychatrophia
13. neurotrophy
14. neuratrophy
15. amyotrophia
16. trophology
17. nematoid
18. nematodiasis
19. nosogenesis
20. nosography
21. nosohemia
22. nosology
23. toxonosis
24. myonosus
25. arthronosos
26. aphrodisiac
27. anaphrodisiac
28. hypaphrodisia
29. gynander
30. gynecophonus
31. gynephobia
32. gyniatrics
33. panhidrosis
34. panarthritis
35. panasthenia
36. panotitis
37. panoptosis
38. pantalgia
39. pantachromatic
40. autoeroticism
41. erotogenic
42. erotophobia
43. palilalia
44. palingraphia
45. perispondylitis
46. spondylarthritis
47. spondylopathy
48. spondylopyosis
49. spondyloschisis
50. trichoschisis
51. craniorachischisis
52. schizonychia
53. rhachialgia
54. rachitome
55. rachiotomy
56. rachianesthesia
57. hydrorrhachis
58. thanatoid
59. endodontitis
60. periodontal
61. odontodynia
62. odontology
63. odontoma
64. odontopathy
65. odontogenesis
66. exodontia
67. oligodontia
68. megodontia
69. megalodontia
70. microdontism
71. polyodontia
72. antodontalgic
73. orthodontics
74. atrichia
75. hypotrichosis
76. trichopathy
77. trichophagia
78. sclerotrichia
79. melanophore
80. chromophoric
81. hemophoric
82. synthetic
83. apoplectic[1]
84. gastroplegia
85. enteroplegia
86. phrenoplegia
87. helminthoid
88. helminthemesis
89. anthelmintic
90. photesthesis
91. photokinetic
92. photogenic
93. photonosus
94. phototherapy
95. phototoxic
96. toxoalexin
97. gastrostaxis
98. metrostaxis[2]

---

[1]Greek *apo-*, away

[2]Greek *mētro-*, uterus

# GREEK VOCABULARY

*The art of medicine would never have been discovered, nor would there have been any medical research—for there would have been no need for medicine—if sick men had benefited by the same manner of living and by the same food and drink of men in health.* [Hippocrates, *Ancient Medicine* 3]

## VOCABULARY

| GREEK WORD | COMBINING FORM(S) | MEANING |
|---|---|---|
| *adēn* | ADEN- | gland |
| *aēr* | AER- | air, gas |
| *blennos* | BLENN- | mucus |
| *koilia* | CEL(I)- | abdomen |
| *cheilos* | CH(E)IL- | lip |
| *klān* | CLA(S)-, -CLAST[1] | break (up), destroy |
| *desis* | -DESIS | binding |
| *desmos* | DESM- | [binding] ligament |
| *dynamis* | DYNAM- | force, power |
| *gnathos* | GNATH- | (lower) jaw |
| *ischein* | ISCH-, -SCHE- | suppress, check |
| *leios* | LEI- | smooth |
| *lēpsis* | LEP- | attack, seizure |
| *mainesthai* | MAN- | be mad |
| *melos* | MEL- | limb |
| *metron* | METR-, -METER[2] | measure |
| *morphē* | MORPH- | form, shape |
| *nomos* | NOM- | law |
| *omphalos* | OMPHAL- | navel, umbilicus |
| *pais, paidos* | PED-[3] | child |
| *penia* | PEN- | decrease, deficiency |
| *pexis* | -PEX- | fixing, (surgical) attachment |

---

[1]Words in -clast indicate an instrument or device for breaking or crushing: lithoclast.

[2]Words in -meter indicate instruments for measuring: cephalometer.

[3]Note that British spelling retains the Latinized diphthong: paediatrics, orthopaedics, and so forth.

| | | |
|---|---|---|
| *plassein* | PLAS(T)-[1] | form, develop |
| *prostatēs* | PROSTAT- | [one who stands before] prostate gland[2] |
| *ptyein* | PTY- | spit |
| *ptyalon* | PTYAL- | saliva |
| *rhaptein* | -RRHAPH- | suture |
| *sitos* | SIT- | food |
| *histanai* | STA(T)-[3] | stand, stop |
| *taxis* | TAX- | (muscular) coordination |
| *thermē* | THERM- | heat, (body) temperature |
| *tropē* | TROP-[4] | turning |

# ETYMOLOGICAL NOTES

The verb *mainesthai*, be mad, is one of several words in both Greek and Latin that have the root MN-, all having to do with mental processes: Greek *mimnēskein*, remember (cf. *Mnemosyne*, Memory), *manteia*, prophetic power, *manthanein*, learn, *ma(n)thēmatikos*, mathematical, *mantis*, prophet, prophetic; Latin *mēns, mentis*, mind, *mentiō, mentiōnis*, mention, *mentīrī*, lie, cheat. In the beginning of the *Iliad*, when Apollo is raining his arrows upon the Greek camp because Agamemnon, the leader of the Greek army, will not return the girl whom he has taken captive to her father, a priest of Apollo, Achilles rises in the assembly and speaks:

*Come, let us consult some seer* (mantis) *or priest, or some interpreter of dreams—for dreams are sent by Zeus—who can tell us why Phoebus Apollo has conceived such anger.* [*Iliad* 1.62–64]

Tiresias, the famed blind prophet of Thebes, had a daughter, Manto, who also became famed as a seer. This is also the name of an Italian nymph who had the gift of prophecy and who founded the city of Mantua in Lombardy, the birthplace of Vergil.

Theocritus, the third-century B.C. Greek bucolic poet, called the orthopterous insect *Mantis religiosa* (praying mantis) the prophetic grasshopper (*mantis kalamaia*). Perhaps this insect was given its Latin name because of its posture, holding its forelegs in a position suggesting hands folded in prayer. [*Idylls* 10.18]

The narcotic drug morphine takes its name from Morpheus, the Graeco-Roman god of dreams (Greek *morphē*, form, shape), one of the thousand sons of Sleep, because of the dreams induced by it and especially by opium, from which it is derived. The Roman poet Ovid tells us that Morpheus is the cleverest of all of Sleep's sons in imitating the form of humans:

*No other is more skilled than he in simulating the gait, the countenance, and the speech of mortals, or in assuming their clothing and the words that each is accustomed to use.* [*Metamorphoses* 11.635–638]

The *Metamorphoses* is the greatest of the works of Ovid, written after his banishment for reasons unknown to Tomis on the Black Sea in A.D. 8 by the emperor Augustus. A long poem

---

[1]Words in -plasty refer to plastic, or restorative, surgery: rhinoplasty.

[2]The prostate gland was called *prostatēs* (pro-, in front of, *histanai*, stand) by the early Greek physicians because of its location in front of the bladder and urethra.

[3]Words in -stat indicate a device or agent for stopping the flow (of something): hemostat. (The term stat as used in hospitals is from Latin *statim*, immediately.)

[4]Words in -tropism refer to the turning of living organisms toward (positive tropism) or away from (negative tropism) an external stimulus: phototropism, thermotropism.

(11,990 lines), it tells in fifteen books stories from Greek mythology and Near Eastern legend, all involving a change in shape or form, beginning with the creation of the universe and ending with the transformation of Julius Caesar into a star after his death. The poet declares his intentions at the opening of the work:

*My purpose is to tell of bodies changed*
*to new forms. Gods—for it is you who*
*made the changes—give me inspiration*
*for this poem that runs from the beginning*
*of the world down to our own days.*

The verb *ptyein* and its derivative noun *ptyalon*, both meaning spit, are examples of onomatopoeia (*onoma, onomatos*, name, and *poiein*, make), the formation of words in imitation of sounds. One of the best-known examples of this from antiquity is found in a fragment of the *Annales* of Ennius, a second-century B.C. Roman poet, whose works are mostly lost:

*At tuba terribili sonitu taratantara dixit.*
But the trumpet, with a terrible sound, went *taratantara.*

## EXERCISE 7

A. Analyze and define each of the following words.

1. adenectomy _____

2. adenoid _____

3. adenoids _____

4. aerendocardia _____

5. aerobe[1] _____

6. aerocystoscopy _____

7. aerotropism _____

8. amyotaxy _____

9. ankylochilia _____

10. aplasia _____

11. arthroclasia _____

[1]The *b* of this word is the only surviving part of *bios*, life. The final *-e* is an English noun-forming suffix.

12. arthrodesis _____

13. arthrodysplasia _____

14. ataxophemia _____

15. athermic _____

16. blennadenitis _____

17. celiocentesis _____

18. celioenterotomy _____

19. celiomyalgia _____

20. celoschisis _____

21. celoscope _____

22. cheiloschisis _____

23. cholestasia _____

24. cystopexy _____

25. cytometer _____

26. dermatoplasty _____

27. desmitis _____

28. desmography _____

29. dysmelia _____

30. dysmorphophobia _____

31. dysstasia _____

32. enteropexy _____

33. ergometer _____

34. erythromelalgia _____

35. erythropenia _____

36. exomphalos _____

37. gastroblennorrhea _____

38. hematomphalocele _____

39. hematopexin _____

40. hemiataxia _____

41. hemostat _____

42. hidroschesis _____

43. hyperthermalgesia _____

44. hypoplasia _____

45. hypothermia _____

46. idiotropic _____

47. ischesis _____

48. leiodermia _____

49. leiomyoma _____

50. leukopenia _____

51. lipopexia _____

52. lithoclast _____

53. macrocheilia _____

54. macrognathia _____

55. metamorphosis _____

56. metaplasia _____

57. morphology _____

58. myotenontoplasty _____

59. narcolepsy _____

60. oligoptyalism _____

61. omphaloncus _____

62. oncotropic _____

63. opisthognathism[1] _____

64. orthopedics _____

65. orthostatism _____

66. osteoclast _____

67. pancytopenia _____

68. paradenitis _____

69. parasite _____

70. pedatrophy _____

71. pediatrics _____

72. pedodontist _____

73. pericardiorrhaphy _____

74. polioclastic _____

75. polyadenomatosis _____

76. prognathous _____

_____

[1]Greek *opisthen*, backward, receding

77. prostatitis _____

78. rhinoplasty _____

79. sitophobia _____

80. stasis _____

81. syndesis _____

82. syndesmopexy _____

83. thermanesthesia _____

84. thermoplegia _____

85. toxicomania _____

86. tropism _____

B. Give the word derived from Greek elements that means each of the following. Verify your answer in the medical dictionary.

1. Having many forms _____

2. Inflammation of stomach glands _____

3. Resembling mucus _____

4. Treatment by (application of) air and water _____

5. Suture of (a wound in) the abdomen _____

6. Suture of (a wound in) a muscle _____

7. Muscular force _____

8. Defective formation of the spinal cord _____

9. Plastic surgery of the nose and (upper) lip _____

10. Ulceration of the prostate (gland) _____

11. (Abnormal) smallness of the (lower) jaw _____

12. The (connective tissue) membrane surrounding a ligament _____

13. Pain in the jaw _____

14. (Abnormally) large size of the limbs _____

15. Mind-turning _____

16. Inequality between (two paired) limbs _____

17. An abdominal tumor _____

18. Umbilical hemorrhage _____

C. Give a clear, concise meaning of each of the following italicized words.

1. It was found that no good evidence existed to classify Treponema pallidum as *anaerobic*.

2. Genitourinary *neoplasms* constitute a major segment of malignant disease in children, adults, and the elderly.

3. *Adenocarcinoma* of the *prostate* accounts for the greatest number of malignancies in men over 65.

4. Chromophobic *adenomas* of the pituitary are usually manifested by headache.

5. Blood-borne *metastases* are identified by bone marrow aspiration.

6. Bladder malignancies that *metastasize*[1] to lymphatics of the bony pelvis or to sites outside the pelvis are essentially incurable.

_____

[1]*-ize* is a Greek-derived suffix which forms verbs.

7. *Cheilosis* may result from vitamin $B_6$ deficiency.

8. A significant proportion of patients who suffer a brain infarct have a history of previous brief episodes, "little strokes," of transient cerebral *ischemia*.

9. Chronic *mania* is uncommon before age 40.

10. It stands to reason that starvation, anemia, stenosis of the aortic ostium, heart block, and cerebral arteriosclerosis, but especially *autonomic* nervous imbalance, predispose to episodes of cerebral anoxia.

11. The term *idiopathic epilepsy* indicates that study of the patient has failed to disclose any etiology.

12. There is an acute conjunctivitis, known as inclusion *blennorrhea* in the newborn, and swimming pool conjunctivitis in the adult.

13. This medication minimizes the *orthostatic* effect of the drug.

14. Extreme *aerophagia* may produce abdominal distention, a sensation of smothering, palpitation, dyspnea, cardiac pain, and even a fear of impending death.

15. *Ataxia* is usually tested by observing the patient's gait, especially if he is asked to walk along a straight line, by ordering the patient to place his heel on the opposite knee, by asking him to touch the tip of his nose with his finger or to pick up a needle or another small object. *Static ataxia* becomes evident by swaying in standing upright due to incoordinated tonus of synergistic and antagonistic muscle groups.

16. Traumatic lesions of the lung, perforation of an aneurysm or of an esophageal carcinoma, or hemorrhagic diathesis of various kinds may account for *hemoptysis*.

17. Multiple cartilaginous exostoses resulting from a disturbance of proliferation and ossification of the bone-forming cartilage are known to occur as a hereditary trait. Hereditary *chondro-dysplasia* is the most nearly correct although not officially accepted name for this condition.

18. Patients with prolonged *hyperthermia* are a common occurrence in medical practice. Search for possible infectious origin may fail to discover infected tonsils, teeth, or sinuses, endocarditis, mild chronic cholecystitis, regional ileitis, pyelitis, prostatitis, phlebitis, and the like.

D. Answer each of the following questions.

1. What are *neuroleptic* drugs?

2. What is *ptyalin*?

3. What is meant by an *aerogen*?

4. What is the purpose of a *gnathodynamometer*?

5. What type of articulation is a *syndesmosis*?

6. What is *diathermy*?[1]

7. What is *cytometaplasia*?

8. What is the meaning of *nosotropic*? *etiotropic*?[2]

9. What is *dipsomania*?

10. What is the meaning of *orthognathous*?

## DRILL AND REVIEW

E. The meaning of each of the following words can be determined from its etymology. Determine the meaning of each and verify your answer in the medical dictionary.

1. blennemesis
2. otoblennorrhea
3. blennogenic
4. maniacal
5. oreximania
6. myoischemia
7. ischidrosis
8. ectoparasite
9. endoparasite
10. sitology

---

[1]Greek *dia-*, through
[2]Greek *aitia*, cause, origin

11. sitotoxism
12. sitotherapy
13. sitomania
14. melalgia
15. symmelia
16. amelia
17. celiac
18. celitis
19. celiogastrotomy
20. celiogastrostomy
21. celiomyositis[1]
22. celioparacentesis
23. schistocelia
24. nephradenoma
25. adenomalacia
26. adenosclerosis
27. adenoncus
28. adenemphraxis
29. enteradenitis
30. hidradenitis
31. scleradenitis
32. adenoidectomy
33. omphalitis
34. omphalorrhexis
35. periomphalic
36. nephropexy
37. gastropexy
38. phrenocolopexy
39. amorphous
40. dimorphous[2]
41. isomorphous
42. paramorphia
43. gynandromorph
44. aerenterectasia
45. aerobic
46. aerogenic
47. aerophyte
48. aerosis
49. aerotherapy
50. aerobiosis
51. tenorrhaphy
52. enterorrhaphy
53. angiorrhaphy
54. myodynamometer
55. pediatry
56. pediatrician[3]
57. pedodontia
58. pedologist
59. pedicterus
60. ptyalolithiasis
61. ptyalorrhea

62. hypoptyalism
63. aptyalia
64. anerythroplasia
65. neuroplasty
66. myoplasty
67. arthroplasty
68. chiroplasty
69. stomatoplasty
70. enteroplasty
71. tenontoplasty
72. hemostasis
73. enterostasis
74. blennostasis
75. astasia
76. prostatectomy
77. prostatodynia
78. prostatomegaly
79. prostatorrhea
80. gnathitis
81. anisognathous
82. prognathism
83. atelognathia
84. gnathoplasty
85. gnathoschisis
86. agnathia
87. hemoclasis
88. lipoclasis
89. odontoclasis
90. osteoclasia
91. trichoclasia
92. lithoclasty
93. histoclastic
94. pachychilia
95. atelocheilia
96. cheiloplasty
97. microcheilia
98. synchilia
99. desmodynia
100. desmology
101. desmopathy
102. desmorrhexis
103. desmotomy
104. desmectasia
105. syndesmorrhaphy
106. tenodesis
107. hemotropic
108. enterotropic
109. sitotropism
110. phototropism
111. trophotropism
112. leiotrichous

---

[1]See page 44, footnote 1.

[2]derived from Greek *di(s)*-, twice, double

[3]The Latin suffix *-ian* often indicates a specialist in a certain field.

113. aerothermotherapy
114. thermoalgesia
115. thermanalgesia
116. thermhypesthesia
117. isothermal

118. cephalometry
119. algometer
120. hydropenia
121. acroataxia
122. epileptic

# LATIN NOUNS AND ADJECTIVES

*Just as agriculture promises nourishment to healthy bodies, so does the practice of medicine promise health to the sick.* [Celsus, *De Medicina*, Proemium 1]

Latin, like Greek, is an inflected language, and nouns, pronouns, and adjectives have different endings to indicate their grammatical function in a sentence. Latin nouns are divided into five classifications called declensions, and in each of these declensions the endings of the various grammatical cases is substantially different in both singular and plural. The first three of the declensions are most productive of English derivatives.

Nouns of the first declension, mostly feminine, have the ending *-a* in the nominative singular, the vocabulary form of the noun. The combining form of these nouns is found by dropping the final *-a*. Latin nouns of the first declension appear in English in either their vocabulary form, or with the final *-a* dropped or changed to silent *-e*.

| LATIN NOUN | MEANING | ENGLISH DERIVATIVE |
|---|---|---|
| *fistula* | pipe | **fistula** |
| *vagina* | sheath | **vagina** |
| *tibia* | shin bone | **tibia** |
| *axilla* | armpit | **axilla** |
| *larva* | ghost | **larva** |
| *lympha* | clear water | **lymph** |
| *forma* | shape | **form** |
| *palma* | palm | **palm** |
| *tunica* | garment | **tunic** |
| *membrana* | skin | **membrane** |
| *urina* | urine | **urine** |
| *sutura* | seam | **suture** |
| *tuba* | trumpet | **tube** |
| *valva* | folding door | **valve** |

The nominative plural of first-declension nouns is *-ae: antenna, antennae; larva, larvae; vertebra, vertebrae.* The genitive singular of first-declension nouns ends in *-ae.* This form is sometimes found in descriptive terminology and can be translated by the word "of": **os coxae** (*os*, bone, *coxa*, hip), the hip bone; **cervix vesicae** (*cervix*, neck, *vesica*, bladder), neck of the bladder.

Nouns of the second declension are either masculine or neuter. Masculine nouns in the nominative end in *-us*, and neuter nouns end in *-um*. The combining form of these nouns is found by dropping this ending. Nouns of the second declension are usually found in the vocabulary form, but sometimes the ending is dropped or changed to silent -e.

| LATIN NOUN | MEANING | ENGLISH DERIVATIVE |
|---|---|---|
| *bacillus* | small staff | **bacillus** |
| *cuneus* | wedge | **cuneus** |
| *fungus* | mushroom | **fungus** |
| *humerus* | upper arm | **humerus** |
| *globus* | sphere | **globe** |
| *digitus* | finger | **digit** |
| *ileum* | groin | **ileum** |
| *ovum* | egg | **ovum** |
| *cerebrum* | brain | **cerebrum** |
| *palatum* | palate | **palate** |
| *intestinum* | intestine | **intestine** |

The nominative plural of second-declension masculine nouns is -*ī*, and the plural of neuter nouns is -*a*: bacillus, bacillī; cilium, cilia; ovum, ova. The genitive singular of second-declension nouns ends in -*i*. This form is sometimes found in descriptive terminology: **cervix uteri** (*cervix*, neck, *uterus*, womb); **labium cerebelli** (*labium*, lip, margin, *cerebellum*, brain). The genitive plural of these nouns ends in -*orum*: **icterus neonatorum** (Greek *neos*, new, Latin *natus*, born).

Latin nouns of the third declension are like Greek third-declension nouns in that it is not always possible to determine the base of these nouns from a knowledge of the nominative singular, the dictionary form. To find the base, it is usually necessary to know the form of some case other than the nominative, and, for this reason, dictionaries and vocabularies cite, along with the nominative case, the genitive singular, which ends in -*is*. The base is found by dropping this ending. In the formation of English words, often the nominative case is used alone and sometimes suffixes are added directly to it. But more often it is the base of these nouns that is used in forming compound words. Third-declension nouns can be either masculine, feminine, or neuter. In this manual, if the base of a noun is the same as the dictionary form, or if the genitive case is the same as the nominative case, the genitive case will not be given in the vocabularies.

| LATIN NOUN | COMBINING FORM | MEANING | ENGLISH DERIVATIVE |
|---|---|---|---|
| *auris (auris)* | AUR- | *ear* | **auris, auricle** |
| *latus, lateris* | LATER- | *side* | **latus, lateral** |
| *os, ossis* | OSS- | *bone* | **os coxae, ossify** |
| *radix, radicis* | RADIC- | *root* | **radix, radicle** |
| *sopor (soporis)* | SOPOR- | *sleep* | **sopor, soporific** |
| *vas (vasis)* | VAS- | *vessel* | **vas deferens, vascular** |

The genitive singular of nouns of the third declension is sometimes found in descriptive terminology: **labia oris** (*labia*, lips, *ōs*, *ōris*, mouth); **corona capitis** (*corona*, crown, *caput*, *capitis*, head).

The nominative plural of masculine and feminine nouns of the third declension ends in -*ēs*, and the plural of neuter nouns ends in -*a*: *cervix, cervicis*, neck: **cervix** (plural, **cervices**); *naris, naris*, nostril: **naris** (plural, **nares**); *rēn, rēnis*, kidney: **ren** (plural, **renes**); *corpus, corporis*, body: **corpus** (plural, **corpora**); *genus, generis*, kind: **genus** (plural, **genera**); *viscus, visceris*, internal organ: **viscus** (plural, **viscera**).

There are a few nouns of the fourth and fifth declension in medical terminology. Most fourth-declension nouns are masculine and end in -*us* in the nominative singular, with the plural in -*ūs*: *meātus*, passage: **meatus** (plural, **meatus**), **meatoscopy, meatotomy**; *plexus*, a braid: **plexus** (plural, **plexus or plexuses**). Neuter nouns of the fourth declension end in -*ū* in the nominative singular: *genū*, knee: **genupectoral**, pertaining to the knees and chest (*pectus, pectoris*, chest). The nominative plural of fourth-declension neuter nouns ends in -*a*: *cornu*, horn: **cornu** (plural, cornua). The nominative singular of most fifth-declension nouns ends in *-iēs: cariēs*, decay; *ra-biēs*, madness; *scabiēs*, itch. Most fifth-declension nouns are feminine; the plural is identical to the singular in the nominative case.

## LATIN ADJECTIVES

Latin adjectives are of two classes; they are either of the first- and second-declension, with endings like those of masculine, feminine, and neuter nouns of the first and second declensions, or they are of the third declension. Latin dictionaries and grammars cite first- and second-declension adjectives by using the masculine singular in *-us* as the entry form, and following it with the feminine and neuter endings *-a* and *-um: bonus, -a, -um*, good; *magnus, -a, -um*, large; *medius, -a, -um*, middle. In this manual, adjectives of this class will be cited only in the form of the masculine nominative singular in *-us*, the dictionary form.[1]

Third-declension adjectives usually have two terminations: *-is* for the masculine and feminine, and *-e* for the neuter: *gravis, -e*, severe; *fortis, -e*, strong; *levis, -e*, light.[2] Some adjectives of the third declension have one form for the masculine, feminine, and neuter genders: *atrox*, genitive *atrocis*, fierce; *praegnans*, genitive *praegnantis*, pregnant; *sapiens*, genitive *sapientis*, knowing, wise. There are no adjectives of the fourth and fifth declensions.

Latin adjectives usually follow the nouns that they modify and agree with them in gender and number:

> myasthenia **gravis**
> meatus **acusticus externus**
> meatus **auditorius**
> genu **recurvatum**
> membrum **muliebre**
> membrum virile
> vena **cava**

## LATIN PREFIXES

Latin prefixes, like Greek, modify or qualify in some way the meaning of the word to which they are affixed. It is difficult to assign a single specific meaning to each prefix, and often it is necessary to adapt a meaning that will fit the particular use of a word. A word may have more than one prefix, and, in compound words, a prefix may follow a combining form. Latin prefixes (and suffixes) are frequently used with Greek combining forms.

**ab-** (a- rarely before certain consonants; **abs-** before *c* and *t*): away from:

| | |
|---|---|
| **ab**-ductor | **abs**-cess |
| **ab**-lation | **abs**-tract |
| **ab**-ortion | **a**-vulsion |

---

[1] There are some adjectives of the first and second declension whose masculine form ends in *-er*, but with the feminine and neuter in *-a*, and *-um: asper, aspera, asperum*, rough; *tener, tenera, tenerum*, tender. Some adjectives in *-er* drop the *-e-* in the feminine and neuter: *integer, integra, integrum*, whole; *ruber, rubra, rubrum*, red.

[2] There are some adjectives of the third declension whose masculine form ends in *-er*; these have *-ris* in the feminine, and *-re* in the neuter: *acer, acris, acre*, sharp; *saluber, salubris, salubre*, healthful; *volucer, volucris, volucre*, winged.

**ad-** (**ac-** before *c*; **af-** before *f*; **ag-** before *g*; **al-** before *l*; **an-** before *n*; **ap-** before *p*; **as-** before *s*; **a-** before *sp*; **at-** before *t*): to, toward:

ad-apt
ad-renaline
ac-cessory
af-fusion
ag-glomerate

al-literation
an-nectent
ap-pendix
as-sist
a-spirate
at-traction

**ambi-**: both:

ambi-dextrous
ambi-lateral

ambi-opia
ambi-valent

**ante-**: before, forward:

ante-febrile
ante-natal

ante-pyretic
ante-version

**bi-** (**bin-**, **bis-**): twice, double, both:

bi-furcate
bi-lateral
bi-para

bin-aural
bin-ocular
bis-acromial

**circum-**: around:

circum-articular
circum-duction

circum-ocular
circum-renal

**con-** (**co-** before *h*; **col-** before *l*; **com-** before *e*, *m*, and *p*; **cor-** before *r*): together, with; thoroughly, very

con-genital
co-habitation
co-hesive
col-lapse

com-edo
com-mensal
com-press
cor-rosive

**contra-**: against, opposite:

contra-ception
contra-fissura

contra-indication
contra-lateral

**de-**: down, away from, absent

de-generation
de-hydration

de-sensitize
de-toxify

**dis-** (**di-** before *g*, *v*, and usually before *l*; **dif-** before *f*): apart, away:

dis-infect
dis-locate
di-gest

di-vert
di-late
dif-fuse

ex- (e- before certain consonants; ef- before *f*): out of, away from:

ex-hale                          ef-ferent
ex-pectorate                     e-viscerate

extra- (rarely extro-): on the outside, beyond:

extra-sensory                    extro-spection
extra-vasation                   extro-vert

(1) in- (il- before *l*; im- before *b*, *m*, and *p*; ir- before *r*): in, into:

in-cubation                      im-bibe
in-farct                         im-merse
in-gestion                       im-pregnate
il-luminate                      ir-radiate

(2) in- (il- before *l*; im- before *b*, *m*, and *p*; ir- before *r*): not:

in-continence                    im-balance
in-firm                          im-mune
in-nominate                      im-potent
il-legal                         ir-reducible

(3) in-: very, thoroughly:

in-duration                      in-flammable
in-ebriation                     in-toxication

infra-: beneath, below:

infra-maxillary                  infra-vascular
infra-sternal                    infra-venous

inter-: between:

inter-costal                     inter-meningeal
inter-dental                     inter-renal

intra- (rarely intro-): within:

intra-gastric                    intra-venous
intra-muscular                   intro-version

non-: not:[1]

non-conductor                    non-toxic
non-protein                      non-viable

ob- (oc- before *c*; op- before *p*): against, toward; very, thoroughly:

ob-session                       oc-cult
oc-clusion                       op-pose

---

[1] *non* is not a prefix in Latin, but an adverb. Since it is used as a prefix in English, it is included here with prefixes.

**per-** (**pel-** before *l*): through; very, thoroughly:

| | |
|---|---|
| **per**-manent | **per**-spiration |
| **per**-meable | **pel**-lucid |

**post-**: after, following, behind:

| | |
|---|---|
| **post**-mortem | **post**-partum |
| **post**-nasal | **post**-uterine |

**pre-**: before, in front of:

| | |
|---|---|
| **pre**-dormition | **pre**-tibial |
| **pre**-gnant | **pre**-urethritis |

**pro-**: forward, in front:

| | |
|---|---|
| **pro**-cedure | **pro**-ject |
| **pro**-cess | **pro**-tect |

**re-**: back, again:

| | |
|---|---|
| **re**-cess | **re**-sonance |
| **re**-fraction | **re**-suscitation |

**retro-**: backward, in back, behind:

| | |
|---|---|
| **retro**-grade | **retro**-peritoneal |
| **retro**-nasal | **retro**-pharyngeal |

**se-**: apart, away from:

| | |
|---|---|
| **se**-crete | **se**-gregate |
| **se**-duce | **se**-paration |

**semi-**: half:

| | |
|---|---|
| **semi**-comatose | **semi**-permeable |
| **semi**-normal | **semi**-prone |

**sub-** (**suf-** before *f*; **sup-** before *p*): under:

| | |
|---|---|
| **sub**-costal | **suf**-fusion |
| **sub**-dural | **sup**-purate |

**super-** (often **supra-**): over, above; excess:

| | |
|---|---|
| **super**-lactation | **supra**-mastoid |
| **super**-secretion | **supra**-renal |

**trans-**: across, through:

| | |
|---|---|
| **trans**-parent | **trans**-thoracotomy |
| **trans**-plant | **trans**-vaginal |

# LATIN SUFFIXES

Suffixes are elements that are added to the combining forms of nouns, adjectives, and verbs to form new words. Nouns are either abstract or concrete. Abstract nouns indicate a state, quality, condition, procedure, or process, while concrete nouns give names to objects and agents. Adjectives impart qualities or characteristics to nouns. The Latin language was rich in suffixes, but only those that are in common use in modern medical terminology are presented here.

## NOUN-FORMING SUFFIXES

Most of the abstract noun-forming suffixes that were used in Latin were affixed to verbal stems and will be presented in Lesson 9. The suffixes given below are those that are attached to the combining forms of adjectives or nouns. In most instances, Latin suffixes have come into English in a form slightly changed from their original due to their transition through French.[1] The following list gives their English form. It should be noted that when the base of a noun or adjective ends in a consonant and the suffix begins with a consonant, a combining vowel, usually *i*, sometimes *o* or *u*, is inserted.

-**ia** forms abstract nouns: **somnolentia**, sleepiness (*somnolentus*, sleepy)
-**ty**[2] forms abstract nouns: **gravity**, heaviness (*gravis*, heavy, severe)
-**y**[3] forms abstract nouns: **memory**, mindfulness (*memor*, mindful)
-**arium** denotes a place for something: **aquarium**, a place for water (*aqua*, water)
-**ary**[4] denotes a place for something: **library**, a place for books (*liber*, book)

## DIMINUTIVE SUFFIXES

There was a group of suffixes in Latin that formed diminutive nouns from other nouns. These diminutives were nouns of the first or second declension, ending in *-us*, *-a*, or *-um*, dependent upon the gender of the noun to which they were affixed, and were all characterized by the presence of a single or double *l*. These diminutives usually appear in English in their original Latin form, but final *-us* is sometimes changed to -e, *-culus* to -cle, and *-illa* to -il.

| | |
|---|---|
| -**culus** | ventriculus, ventricle (*venter*, belly) |
| -**olus** | alveolus (*alveus*, cavity); arteriole (*arteria*, artery) |
| -**ulus** | calculus (*calx*, *calcis*, stone); globule (*globus*, ball) |
| -**illa** | fibrilla, fibril (*fibra*, fiber) |
| -**ellum** | cerebellum (*cerebrum*, brain) |

Such words as **rubella** (*ruber*, red) and **roseola** (*roseus*, rosy, reddish) are New Latin formations from Latin adjectives of the first and second declension. These particular words are neuter plural in form; thus, rubella, or German measles, is named for the "little red things," the eruptions that accompany this disease, and roseola, a skin condition marked by maculae or red spots, for the "little reddish things" that characterize this condition. **Variola** (*varius*, spotted), smallpox,

---

[1]See the Appendix for a brief history of the English language.

[2]The suffix *-ty* is from Latin *-tas*: Latin *gravitas*, French *gravité*.

[3]The suffix *-y* is from Latin *-ia*: Latin *memoria*, Old French *memorie*, *memoire*, *memore*, French *mémoire*.

[4]The suffix *-ary* is from Latin *-arium*: Latin *librarium*, French *librarie*.

and **varicella** (an irregularly formed diminutive from *varius*), chickenpox, are similar formations. Often a new genus of bacteria is named by adding the neuter plural suffix *-ella* to the surname of its discoverer: *Salmonella* (Daniel E. Salmon, 1850–1914), *Brucella* (Sir David Bruce, 1855–1931), *Shigella* (Kiyoshi Shiga, 1870–1957).

## ADJECTIVAL SUFFIXES

The Latin language was particularly rich in adjectival suffixes, but many of these are not in common use in the formation of medical terms. Only those suffixes that are frequently found are listed here; the less common ones will be identified as they occur. As with the noun-forming suffixes, adjectival suffixes usually come into English in a form slightly changed from their original. The following list gives their English form.[1]

**-al** pertaining to, located in: **dorsal** (*dorsum*, back)
**-an** pertaining to, located in: **median** (*medius*, middle)
**-ar** pertaining to, located in: **ocular** (*oculus*, eye)
**-ary** pertaining to: **salivary** (*salīva*, saliva)
**-ate** having the form of, possessing: **cordate** (*cor, cordis*, heart), **caudate** (*cauda*, tail)
**-ic** pertaining to: **pregravidic** (*gravidus*, pregnant)
**-id**[2] pertaining to: **morbid** (*morbus*, disease)
**-ile** pertaining to: **senile** (*senis*, old)
**-ine** pertaining to, located in: **uterine** (*uterus*, uterus)
**-ive** pertaining to: **tussive** (*tussis*, cough)
**-lent** full of: **somnolent** (*somnus*, sleep)
**-ose** full of: **adipose** (*adeps, adipis*, fat)
**-ous** full of, pertaining to: **bilious** (*bilis*, bile)

Note tha ⸻ than one suffix: **adiposity, morbidity.** Greek prefixes and suffixes may b ⸻ : **adipositis, periocular.** Greek and Latin words may be combined in ⸻ nonary (Greek *kardia*, heart, Latin *pulmo, pulmonis*, lung). Such w ⸻ s (Latin *hybrida*, mongrel).[3]

It should ⸻ ted that many Latin words and expressions are in use in medical terminology in their original form: **membrum virile** (*vir*, man, *virilis, -e*, belonging to a man), the male member, the penis; **membrum muliebre** (*mulier*, woman, *muliebris, -e*, belonging to a woman), the female member, the clitoris; **medulla oblongata** (*medulla*, marrow, *oblongata* [New Latin], elongated); **morbus caeruleus** (*morbus*, disease, *caeruleus*, blue), congenital cyanosis.

The English suffix **-ad** forms adverbs from nouns. These adverbs indicate direction toward a part of the body: **dextrad**, toward the right side (*dextra*, the right hand); **sinistrad**, toward the left side (*sinistra*, the left hand); **cephalad**, toward the head (Greek *kephalē*). (See the Etymological Notes to this lesson.)

# VOCABULARY

| LATIN WORD | COMBINING FORM(S) | MEANING |
|---|---|---|
| *adeps, adipis* | *ADIP-*[4] | fat |
| *auris* | *AUR-* | ear |

---

[1]Many Latin adjectives end in *-eus, -ea, -eum*; this explains the presence of -e- in many English words: esophageal, sanguineous, cesarean, and so forth.

[2]Note that there is a Greek-derived suffix *-id*, an alternate form of *-oid*, meaning "having the form of": hominid (*homō, hominis*, man).

[3]A child born of a Roman father and a foreign mother, or one born of a freeman and a slave was known as a *hybrida*. The word is probably a borrowing from Greek *hybris*, insolence.

[4]Commencing with this lesson, combining forms of Latin words will be printed in italics.

| | | |
|---|---|---|
| *bacillus* | *BACILL-* | [rod, staff] bacillus |
| *bursa* (Medieval Latin) | *BURS-* | [leather sack] bursa |
| *calx, calcis* | *CALC-* | stone, calcium, lime (salts) |
| *caput, capitis* | *CAPIT-* | head |
| *cerebrum* | *CEREBR-* | brain |
| *costa* | *COST-* | rib |
| *dorsum* | *DORS-* | back (of the body) |
| *externus, -a, -um* | *EXTERN-* | outer |
| *fibra* | *FIBR-* | fiber, filament |
| *fistula* | *FISTUL-* | [tube, pipe] fistula, an abnormal tubelike passage in the body |
| *insula* | *INSUL-* | island[1] |
| *internus, -a, -um* | *INTERN-* | inner |
| *meātus* | *MEAT-* | passage, opening, meatus[2] |
| *pus, puris* | *PUR-* | pus |
| *radix, radicis* | *RADIC-, RAD-, RADIX* | root |
| *rēn, rēnis* | *REN-* | kidney |
| *sanguis, sanguinis* | *SANGUI(N)-* | blood |
| *synovia*[3] (New Latin) | *SYNOV(I)-* | synovial fluid, synovial membrane *or* sac |
| *tussis* | *TUSS-* | cough |
| *vacca* | *VACC-* | cow[4] |
| *vīrus* | *VIR(U)-, VIRUS-* | [poison, venom] virus[5] |
| *viscus, visceris* (plural, *viscera*) | *VISCER-* | internal organ(s) |

## THE PRONUNCIATION OF LATIN

In Latin, all consonants and vowels are pronounced, with no silent letters. The sound of the consonants is the same as in English, except that *c* and *g* are always "hard"; thus, *cancer* is pronounced "kanker," and the *g* of *genus* is pronounced like the *g* of gate. *t* is always pronounced like the *t* in tin and never has the sound of the *t* in nation. It is customary to pronounce *j* like the *y* in yes, and *v* like the *w* in win. Vowels may be long or short and are pronounced as follows:

| SHORT VOWELS | LONG VOWELS | DIPHTHONGS |
|---|---|---|
| *a* as in adrift | *ā* as in father | *ae* as ie in tie |
| *e* as in bet | *ē* as in they | *au* as ou in house |
| *i* as in tin | *ī* as in machine | *ei* as ei in eight |
| *o* as in obey | *ō* as in tone | *oe* as oi in boil |
| *u* as oo in look | *ū* as in rude | |

---

[1]See the Etymological Notes to this lesson.

[2]Pronounced mee-ate'-us

[3]The word synovia has no etymology; it seems to have been the invention of Paracelsus. See the Etymological Notes to this lesson.

[4]Words in vaccin- have to do with vaccine.

[5]Words in virulent- are from the Latin adjective *vīrulentus*, strong, powerful (literally, full of poison).

Latin words are accentuated on the penult, the syllable next to last, if that syllable is long. A long syllable is one that contains a long vowel or a diphthong, or one in which the vowel, whether long or short, is followed by two consonants.[1] If the penult is short, the syllable before that, the antepenult, receives the accent.

## ETYMOLOGICAL NOTES

As Latin as a spoken language gradually became French, a number of sound changes took place. The sound of an initial Latin *c* when followed by *a* usually developed into *ch* in French: Latin *caballus*, horse, French *cheval*; Latin *caldus*, hot, French *chaud*; Latin *castus*, pure, French *chaste*. Latin *cancer*, crab, ulcer, became French *chancre* and was borrowed into English in that form. A **chancre** is a venereal ulcer, the first outward manifestation of syphilis. This disease takes its name from Syphilus, the hero of a kind of medical poem entitled *Syphilis sive Morbus Gallicus* (Syphilis, or the French Disease) by the Italian physician and poet Girolamo Fracastoro (1484–1553). In this poem, Syphilus suffered from an infectious disease which Fracastoro named syphilis, perhaps from the Greek verb *philein*, love.

**Insulin** (*insula*, island) takes its name from the islets of Langerhans, cell clusters in the pancreas. These cells are of three types: alpha, beta, and delta, and it is the beta cells that produce the protein hormone insulin, which regulates the metabolism of carbohydrates in the body. Deficient production or utilization of insulin causes **hyperglycemia** (Greek *glykys*, sweet), the characteristic of the disease **diabetes mellitus** (Latin *mel, mellis*, honey), commonly known as sugar diabetes. The islets of Langerhans were named after the German pathologist Paul Langerhans (1847–1888), who first realized their existence and function.

The words **vaccine** and **vaccination** come from the Latin *vacca*, cow. In 1789 Edward Jenner, an English country doctor, announced to the world his discovery that injection of the cowpox virus into humans, that is, vaccination, provided immunity against smallpox. It was known at that time that persons who were employed on dairy farms and who happened to contract the bovine disease cowpox became immune to smallpox. Jenner began his experimentation in 1796 by inoculating a healthy young boy with matter taken from an ulcerating sore on the hand of a milkmaid suffering from cowpox. Later, this boy was inoculated with the smallpox virus and resisted the disease. This was the first vaccination. Smallpox has now virtually disappeared from the United States, Great Britain, and Europe, and in recent years mass vaccinations in Africa and Asia have reduced the incidence of this disease to isolated areas in these continents.

The English words viscous and viscid bear no relationship to the internal organs, the viscera, but are derived from Latin *viscum*, mistletoe. The ancient Romans prepared a sticky substance from the berries of the mistletoe plant which they spread on branches of trees. Unfortunate birds that perched on those branches were caught and held fast by this glutinous substance which we call birdlime. The Roman poet Vergil writes of the olden days when men had to toil for their living and hunt for their food:

*It was then that men found a way to snare wild beasts in nets, to trap birds with birdlime* (viscum) *and to surround the huge groves of trees with hounds.* [*Georgics* 1.139–140]

The suffix **-ad**, which indicates direction toward a part of the body, as in the words **dextrad**, toward the right, **sinistrad**, toward the left, or **cephalad**, toward the head, entered the English language early in the nineteenth century following a proposal by the British scholar James Barclay in his work, *New Anatomical Nomenclature* (1803), that it be so used as an equivalent of -ward in English: homeward, forward, and so forth. The suffix -ad did not exist in Latin and seems to have been an adaptation of the prefix *ad-*, toward.

---

[1]However, if the second of two consonants is *l* or *r*, the syllable need not be considered long; *cerebrum* is accented on the antepenult.

Aureolus Theophrastus Bombastus von Hohenheim (1493–1541), better known as Paracelsus, a name which is supposed to have been bestowed upon him as an indication of his superiority to the Roman physician Celsus, has been called the "precursor of chemical pharmacology and therapeutics, and the most original medical thinker of the 16th century."[1] The son of a physician, he became professor of medicine at Basle in 1527. A pioneer in chemistry, he wrote extensively (in Latin) on medicine during a stormy career which was terminated by his death in a tavern brawl in Salzburg. The word **synovia** is first found in his writing and seems to have been coined by him, perhaps from the Latin *ovum*, egg, because of the viscous quality of this colorless fluid. Paracelsus considered that synovia was the nutritive fluid of the body, but its use by later physicians was restricted to the lubricating fluid secreted within synovial membranes of joints, bursae, and tendon sheaths.

The word **bursa** is first found in the Latin of the Medieval period and is a borrowing from Greek *byrsa*, skin, hide of an animal. The Medieval Latin word meant a leather bag or sack, and later the term *bursa mucosa* was applied to the sac or cavity found in connecting tissue and containing synovial fluid. One of the original senses of the word, that of a bag to hold money, is retained in the English words purse (where the initial p is unexplained), burse, a scholarship for school or university, bursar, disbursement, and so forth, and in the French *bourse*, purse, and *Bourse*, the stock exchange of Paris. The Burse was the original Royal Exchange in London.

The Latin words *occipitium* and *occiput, occipitis* are compounds of the prefix *ob-* and *caput, capitis*, head, and meant the back part of the head, the **occiput**. Latin *sinciput* was an abbreviated form of *semi-caput*, and in Latin meant half of a head, in particular the smoked cheek or jowl of a hog. **Sinciput** now means the fore and upper part of the cranium, or the upper half of the skull. The words *occiput* and *sinciput* show a reduction of the *a* of *caput* to *i* in the nominative case and of the *u* to *i* in the genitive case. This is thought of as being due to a strong stress-accent on the first syllable of Latin words that occurred during an early period of the development of the language. Other examples of this vowel reduction can be seen in *biceps*, two-headed, or *triceps*, three-headed, which are also from *caput*. This change can be seen more clearly in Latin verbs and in their derivatives in English; further examples will be seen in Lesson 9.

The word *fistula*, tube, pipe, was used by Ovid in the *Metamorphoses* in a simile to describe how the blood of the unhappy lover Pyramus spurted from his body when he took his own life with the sword. Pyramus and Thisbe were a young couple of Babylon who lived next door to one another. Soon they fell in love, but their parents forbade them to meet. However, they used to speak to one another through a chink in the common wall that separated their houses, and at length decided to creep out one night and meet at the nearby tomb of Ninus, an ancient king of Babylon, under a mulberry tree that was laden with snow-white berries. The young girl, Thisbe, arrived first at the appointed place that night, and, as she waited, a lioness came along, fresh from the kill, to quench her thirst at a nearby pool. Thisbe fled in terror, dropping the thin cloak that she had brought along; when the lioness had drunk her fill, the beast found the cloak and mangled it with her bloodied jaws. Pyramus arrived shortly after and, seeing the blood-stained cloak and thinking that Thisbe had met a cruel death, drew his sword and fell upon it. As he lay there dying,

*Cruor emicat alte,*
*non aliter quam cum vitiato fistula plumbo*
*scinditur et tenui stridente foramine longas*
*eiculatur aquas atque ictibus aera rumpit.*
[*Metamorphoses* 4.121–124]

The blood gushed forth, just as water bursts through a broken pipe (*fistula*) and, with a strident sound, spurts through the air.

---

[1] *An Introduction to the History of Medicine*, Fielding H. Garrison, WB Saunders Company, Philadelphia, 1929.

Ovid goes on to say that the fruit of the mulberry tree was stained with the crimson blood. Thisbe came out of her hiding place and found Pyramus with his life's blood ebbing. She fitted the point of the sword to her own breast and fell forward on the blade that was still warm from the blood of her lover. From that day on, the fruit of the mulberry tree reddens as it ripens, a remembrance of the lovers' blood that was shed there.

# EXERCISE 8

A. The following words have combining forms from Greek with Latin prefixes. Analyze and define each of these words, noting the force of the prefix in each.

1. abenteric _____

2. antepyretic _____

3. binotic _____

4. extracystic _____

5. extrahepatic _____

6. interchondral _____

7. intracranial _____

8. intracystic _____

9. intradermal _____

10. intragastric _____

11. nontoxic _____

12. postencephalitis _____

13. posticteric _____

14. postnecrotic _____

15. preantiseptic _____

16. prenarcosis _____

17. retrography _____

18. retromorphosis _____

19. retroperitoneal _____

20. subarachnoid _____

21. subdermal _____

22. subdiaphragmatic _____

23. subendocardial _____

24. subepidermal _____

25. submicron _____

26. subnarcotic _____

27. subphrenic _____

28. supradiaphragmatic _____

B. Analyze and define each of the following words.

1. auris externa[1] _____

2. subaural _____

3. auricula _____

4. retroauricular _____

5. adipose _____

6. adipopexia _____

7. bacillemia _____

8. diplobacillus[2] _____

_____

[1]Latin *auris* is a feminine noun.
[2]Greek *diploos*, double.

9. bursae _____

10. bursalogy _____

11. bursula _____

12. chancre[1] _____

13. chancroid _____

14. calcium[2] _____

15. calcipenia _____

16. calculus _____

17. capitulum _____

18. decapitation[3] _____

19. biceps[4] _____

20. occiput[4] _____

21. sinciput[4] _____

22. caudad[5] _____

23. cerebritis _____

24. cerebrophysiology _____

25. cerebellum _____

26. costalgia _____

27. costotome _____

28. chondrocostal _____

---

[1]Latin *cancer*, crab; see the Etymological Notes to this lesson.

[2]This word was coined by Sir Humphry Davy on the analogy of the names of other metals in -ium.

[3]Words in -ation are nouns formed from Latin verbs or on the analogy of Latin verbs. These will be discussed in Lesson 9.

[4]See the Etymological Notes to this lesson.

[5]Latin *cauda*, tail

29. dorsad _____

30. dorsocephalad _____

31. fistula _____

32. fibroid _____

33. fibroma _____

34. fibrosis _____

35. neurofibromatosis _____

36. fibromyoma _____

37. fibrilla _____

38. leiomyofibroma _____

39. myelofibrosis _____

40. myofibril _____

41. insulin _____

42. insuloma _____

43. meatus acusticus internus[1] _____

44. meatoscopy _____

45. purulent[2] _____

46. purulence[3] _____

47. suppurate[4] _____

48. radix[5] _____

---

[1] Latin *meātus* is a masculine noun.

[2] Note the use of -u- as a combining vowel before the suffix -lent: virulent, succulent, and so forth.

[3] This word is derived from purulent and the noun-forming suffix -ia; the termination -tia frequently becomes -ce.

[4] Many words in -ate have been formed on the analogy of Latin verbs. These are explained in Lesson 9.

[5] Note that the nominative singular, the vocabulary form, of some words is used in medical terminology.

49. radicle _____

50. polyradiculitis[1] _____

51. radiculomeningomyelitis _____

52. renogastric _____

53. adrenal _____

54. adrenalism _____

55. Adrenalin _____

56. sanguirenal _____

57. sanguicolous[2] _____

58. synovia _____

59. synovium _____

60. osteosynovitis _____

61. tussis[3] _____

62. pertussis _____

63. antitussive _____

64. vaccine _____

65. vaccination[4] _____

66. vaccinia _____

67. ventrad[5] _____

---

[1]Words in radic- and radicul- usually refer to roots of spinal nerves.
[2]Latin *colere*, inhabit
[3]See page 107, footnote 5.
[4]Words in -ation are nouns formed from Latin verbs or on the analogy of Latin verbs. These will be discussed in Lesson 9.
[5]Latin *venter, ventris*, belly, abdominal area

68. virus _____

69. neurotropic virus _____

70. viremia _____

71. virulent _____

72. viscus[1] _____

73. viscera _____

74. viscerotrophic _____

75. viscerotropic _____

C. The meaning of each of the following words can be determined from its etymology. Determine the meaning of each and verify your answer in the medical dictionary.

1. auris interna[2]
2. aural
3. auriscope
4. binaural
5. auricular
6. interauricular
7. adipoid
8. adipoma
9. adiposis
10. adiposis hepatica[3]
11. adipectomy
12. adipogenous
13. adiponecrosis
14. adiposity
15. adipocele
16. adipolysis
17. bursal
18. bursitis
19. bursopathy
20. bursectomy
21. bursolith
22. bacillar
23. bacillosis
24. bacillophobia

25. calculosis
26. hemic calculus
27. hypocalcemia
28. hypercalcemia
29. bicipital
30. occipital[4]
31. sincipital[4]
32. suboccipital
33. supraoccipital
34. caudate[5]
35. acaudal
36. cerebral
37. cerebromalacia
38. cerebromeningitis
39. cerebropathy
40. cerebrosclerosis
41. cerebrosis
42. cerebrotomy
43. cerebellar
44. cerebellitis
45. supracerebellar
46. costal
47. intercostal
48. infracostal

---

[1]See page 107, footnote 5.
[2]Latin *auris* is a feminine noun.
[3]The word adiposis, as well as most abstract nouns, is feminine.
[4]See the Etymological Notes to this lesson.
[5]Latin *cauda*, tail

49. subcostal
50. costochondral
51. dorsal
52. dorsodynia
53. fistulous
54. fistulatome
55. fistulectomy
56. fibroplasia
57. fibromatosis
58. fibromyomectomy
59. fibrillolysis
60. interfibrillar
61. insulinemia
62. insulinogenic
63. insulinoid
64. hypoinsulinism
65. meatal
66. meatus acusticus externus[1]
67. meatometer
68. meatotome
69. suprameatal
70. puruloid
71. suppuration[2]
72. suppurant[3]
73. suppurative[4]
74. purohepatitis
75. radicular
76. radiculalgia
77. radiculomyelopathy[5]
78. radiculoneuritis
79. myeloradiculitis
80. myeloradiculodysplasia
81. renal calculus
82. renography
83. renogram
84. circumrenal
85. interrenal
86. suprarenal
87. suprarenalopathy
88. hypoadrenalism
89. synovial
90. synovioma
91. purulent synovitis
92. parasynovitis
93. perisynovial
94. synovectomy
95. sanguinolent
96. sanguinopoietic
97. sanguineous
98. tussive
99. pertussoid
100. vaccinal
101. vaccinogenous
102. vaccinotherapeutics
103. viral
104. virology
105. virusemia
106. virustatic
107. avirulent
108. supervirulent
109. viscerad
110. visceralgia
111. viscerogenic
112. visceromegaly
113. visceroptosis
114. viscerosomatic
115. perivisceritis

[1]Latin *meātus* is a masculine noun.

[2]Words in -ation are nouns formed from Latin verbs or on the analogy of Latin verbs. These will be discussed in Lesson 9.

[3]Words in -ant are adjectives formed from verbs. These forms will be discussed in Lesson 9.

[4]*-ive* is an adjectival suffix attached to verbal stems.

[5]See page 108, footnote 1.

# LATIN VERBS

*I would have given the name* insectology *to that part of natural history which has insects as its object: that of* entomology *. . . would undoubtedly have been more suitable . . . but its barbarous sound terrify'd me.* [Bennet's *Contemporary Natural History*, London 1776]

There are four classes of Latin verbs, called conjugations. The difference among these is seen in the stem vowel of the verb, shown in the present infinitive. The ending of the present infinitive in the first conjugation is *-āre*, in the second it is *-ēre*, in the third, *-ere*, and in the fourth, *-īre*. Latin verbs have three stems on which the various tenses are formed: the present, the perfect active, and the perfect passive. Only the first and third of these have been fruitful in furnishing English derivatives, and these will be the only ones considered here. The first stem is that of the infinitive, and the third is that of the perfect passive participle, which is an adjective of the first and second declension, with the endings *-us*, *-a*, or *-um*, indicating masculine, feminine, or neuter gender. In this text the perfect passive participle will be given with the ending *-us*, the form in which all such adjectives are cited here.

Thus, Latin verbs have two combining forms; the first is found by dropping the ending of the infinitive, and the second by dropping the *-us* of the perfect passive participle. As with Greek verbs, Latin verbs are customarily cited in Latin dictionaries and grammars in the form of the first person singular (*duco*, I lead; *cado*, I fall); but English dictionaries usually cite them in the form of the present infinitive and this practice will be followed here.

Some verbs appear only in the passive form but with active meanings. These are known as *deponent* verbs. The infinitives of the four conjugations of deponent verbs end in *-ārī*, *-ērī*, *-ī*, and *-īrī*. The combining form is found by dropping these endings. The verb *ducere, ductus*, lead, bring, has the two combining forms DUC- and DUCT-, giving the stem of such English derivatives as induce, reduce, induction, and reduction. The deponent verb *patī, passus*, endure, suffer, gives us such words as patient, patience, and passion.[1]

## VERBAL SUFFIXES

Many suffixes are added only to the stems of verbs. Adjective- and noun-forming suffixes are listed below. Latin suffixes often undergo some changes in English words and are presented here in the form in which they appear in English.

---

[1] *patī, passus* is related to the Greek verb *paschein, epathon*; thus the English words compassion and sympathy are etymological equivalents.

# ADJECTIVAL SUFFIXES

| SUFFIX | MEANING | EXAMPLE |
|---|---|---|
| -able | capable of[1] | **tenable** (*tenēre*, hold) |
| -ible | capable of[1] | **audible** (*audīre*, hear) |
| -ile | capable of | **facile** (*facere*, make, do) |
| -id | in a state *or* condition of | **fluid** (*fluere*, flow) |
| -ive | pertaining to | **active** (*agere, actus*, do, drive) |
| -ory | pertaining to | **expository** (*ponere, positus*, place) |

# NOUN-FORMING SUFFIXES

| SUFFIX | MEANING | EXAMPLE |
|---|---|---|
| -ce | abstract noun | **patience** (*patī*, suffer, endure) |
| -cy | abstract noun | **constancy** (*stāre*, stand) |
| -or | agent *or* instrument | **abductor** (*ducere, ductus*, lead, bring) |
| -ment | agent *or* instrument | **ligament** (*ligāre*, tie, bind) |
| -ure, -ura | result of an action | **fissure, fissura** (*findere, fissus*, split) |
| -ion | the act of | **tension** (*tendere, tensus*, stretch) |
| -orium[2] | place for something | **auditorium** (*audīre, audītus*, hear) |
| -ory[2] | place for something | **dormitory** (*dormīre, dormītus*, sleep) |

Verbal prefixes are the same as those used with nouns. See Lesson 8. Note the use of the English suffix -e to form verbs from Latin infinitives: **reduce** (*ducere*, lead), **excite** (*excitāre*, rouse), **inspire** (*spirāre*, breathe) and so forth.

# PRESENT PARTICIPLES

The Latin present participle (translated into English with -ing added to the meaning of the verb) is an adjective of the third declension that is formed upon the stem of the present infinitive. The forms of the nominative and genitive singular are -*ans*, -*antis* for the first conjugation; *ens*, -*entis* for the second and third; and -*iens*, -*ientis* for some of the third and for the fourth conjugation. The combining form of participles is found by dropping the -*is* ending of the genitive case. In some instances this combining form becomes an English word:

> **sonant** (*sonāre*, sound) sounding
> **latent** (*latēre*, lie hidden) lying hidden
> **cadent** (*cadere*, fall) falling
> **incipient** (*incipere*, begin) beginning
> **sentient** (*sentīre*, feel) feeling

---

[1]The suffixes -able and -ible mean "capable of" usually in a passive sense. Thus, tenable means "capable of being held," not "capable of holding"; audible means "capable of being heard."

[2]The suffixes -arium and -ary, with the same meaning as -orium and -ory, are usually found with nouns: sanitarium (*sanitas*, health), library (*liber*, book).

Most English derivatives of Latin present participles are abstract nouns ending in -ce or -cy. These endings represent the *t* of the present participial stem plus the abstract noun-forming suffix *-ia*; the resultant *-tia* becomes either -ce or -cy in English:

> **redundancy** (*redundāre*, be superfluous; *redundant-ia*)
> **reverence** (*reverērī*, revere; *reverent-ia*)
> **fluency** (*fluere*, flow; *fluent-ia*)
> **sequence** (*sequī*, follow; *sequent-ia*)
> **science** (*scīre*, know; *scient-ia*)

Sometimes words have been formed in English as if from Latin present participles, although such verbs did not exist in Latin. Some of these words have been formed from Greek nouns and verbs: **intoxicant** (and **intoxicate**, as if from a Latin verb *intoxicāre, intoxicātus*), **deanesthesiant**, and so forth. Note that intoxicant and deanesthesiant, as well as other similar formations, although structurally adjectives, are now used as nouns.

## DENOMINATIVE VERBS

The Romans readily made verbs from nouns and adjectives. These are called *denominative* verbs and are mostly of the first conjugation. For example, *formāre, formātus*, shape, form, from the noun *forma*, form, gives the stems of English **reform, reformation, conform, conformation**; *gravāre, gravātus*, weigh down, from the adjective *gravis*, heavy, gives the stem of **aggravate** and **aggravation**, and *stillāre, stillātus*, from *stilla*, drop, drip, gives the stem of **instill, distill**, and **distillation**.

Many English verbs have been formed on the analogy of Latin denominative verbs—that is, as if such a verb had existed when, in fact, it never did. From the noun *sanguis*, blood, there was formed the English verb **exsanguinate**, deprive of blood; the word **decapitate** is formed as if from a denominative verb from *caput, capitis*, head.

## FREQUENTATIVE VERBS

There is a class of verbs known as *frequentative* verbs which originally had the force of a repeated or frequent action. These verbs are mostly all of the first conjugation and are formed upon the perfect passive participle of other verbs, regardless of their conjugation. *dictāre, dictātus* is a frequentative verb from *dicere, dictus*, speak, and means to declare repeatedly, to **dictate**. The frequentative verb of *gerere, gestus*, bear, carry, is *gestāre, gestātus*, from which was formed the noun *gestatio, gestationis*, a bearing or carrying. The Latin noun seems not to have been used in the sense of the period of time from conception to birth, but the English noun **gestation**, with that meaning, has been in use in the English language since the early seventeenth century.

## INCEPTIVE VERBS

There is a small group of verbs in Latin called *inceptive* or *inchoative* verbs. These are characterized by the presence of the letters *-sc-* between the stem and the ending of the infinitive. These are verbs of the third conjugation which have been formed from other verbs or, infrequently, from nouns or adjectives, and they all have the meaning of beginning an action. *candēre*, glow, *candēscere*, begin to glow: English **incandescent**. *valēre*, be well, *valēscere*, begin to get well: English **convalescence**. Some English words have been formed on the analogy of Latin denominative inceptive verbs: **luminescence**, as if from a verb *luminēscere* from the noun *lumen, luminis*, light. The noun existed in Latin but not the verb, although there was a verb *lumināre, luminātus*, light up, brighten.

## VOWEL WEAKENING

During the pre-historic period in the development of the Latin language there seems to have been a strong stress accent upon the first syllable of words, and, as a result of this, vowels in internal syllables became weakened, both quantitatively and qualitatively. The effects of this can be seen in both nouns and verbs. The *-u-* of *caput*, head, becomes weakened to *-i-* in cases other than the nominative singular: *caput, capitis*. *virgō*, maiden, loses the final *-n-* of the nominative singular, and the long *-o-* of the final syllable is reduced to short *-i-*: *virgō(n), virginis; pater*, father, and *mater*, mother, drop the *-e-* of the final syllable: *patris, matris*.

It is with verbs that this phenomenon is most apparent, especially when prefixes are added: *caedere, caesus*, cut: *incīdere, incīsus, dēcīdere, dēcīsus*. *capere, captus*, seize: *incipere, inceptus, recipere, receptus*. *facere, factus*, make: *efficere, effectus, inficere, infectus*. Sometimes the perfect passive participle was not affected by this change: *cadere, cāsus*, fall: *incidere, incāsus*. In the vocabularies in this manual, the verbal stems that undergo these changes will be indicated by a dash before the stem in question: *facere, factus*, make: FAC-, FIC-, -FECT, and so forth.

## VOCABULARY

| LATIN WORD | COMBINING FORM(S) | MEANING |
|---|---|---|
| *anterior* | ANTER- | front, in front |
| *bracchium* | BRACHI- | (upper) arm |
| *⸱⸱⸱⸱⸱⸱ntus* | -CIP-, -CEPT-[1] | take |
| *⸱⸱⸱⸱esus* | -CID-, -CIS- | cut, kill |
| *⸱⸱⸱⸱ētus* | CRESC-, -CRET- | (begin to) grow |
| *⸱⸱⸱⸱ctus* | DUC-, DUCT- | lead, bring, conduct |
| *⸱⸱⸱⸱tus* | FAC-, -FIC-, -FECT-[2] | make |
| | FACI-, -FICI-, FACIES | face, appearance, surface |
| *febris* | FEBR-, FEBRIS | fever |
| *ferre, lātus* | FER-, LAT- | carry, bear |
| *flectere, flexus* | FLECT-, FLEX- | bend |
| *fundere, fusus* | FUS-[3] | pour |
| *fungus* | FUNG- | [mushroom] fungus |
| *gerere, gestus*[4] | GER-, GEST- | carry, bear |
| *gignere, genitus* | GENIT-[5] | bring forth, give birth |

[1]It should be noted that many of these forms appear in medical terminology only following a prefix or another form.

[2]The combining form -FY- is found in many English verbs. This is an adaptation in English of the French *-fier*, from Latin verbs in *-ficāre*, a first-conjugation form of *facere* found in compound verbs: *magnificāre*, make great, magnify; *sanctificāre*, make holy, sanctify.

[3]Both principal parts of Latin verbs are not always productive of English derivatives.

[4]There was a Latin frequentative verb (see the text of this lesson) *gestāre, gestātus*, which meant, among other things, to carry young, referring to what we call the period of gestation. The Roman scientist Pliny, in the *Natural History* [8.10.10], writes: [*elephantos*] *decem annis gestare in utero vulgus existimat*: It is commonly thought that elephants carry their young in the womb for ten years.

[5]Many words in *genit-*, often with the adjectival suffix *-al*, refer to the organs of the reproductive system: genitoplasty, hypergenitalism, and so forth.

| | | |
|---|---|---|
| *inferior* | INFERIOR- | below |
| *labī, lapsus* | LAB-, LAPS- | slide, slip |
| *latus, lateris* | LATER- | side |
| *ōs, ōris* | OR-, OS | mouth, opening |
| *ossa* | OSS- | bone |
| *pediculus* | PEDICUL- | louse |
| *posterior* | POSTER-, -POSTERIOR | behind, in back |
| *secāre, sectus* | SECT- | cut |
| *somnus* | SOMN- | sleep |
| *superior* | SUPERIOR- | above |
| *tumēre*[1] | TUM(E)- | be swollen |

## NOMINA ANATOMICA

Nomina Anatomica is the designation for anatomical terminology that has been adopted as official by the International Congress of Anatomists at various meetings held since 1950. The Tenth International Congress was held in Tokyo in 1975. The decisions of these Congresses on anatomical terminology are published following each meeting. The latest publication, *Nomina Anatomica*, containing the most recent nomenclature adopted, was published in 1977.

All of this nomenclature is in Latin or is composed of Greek words in the form of Latin. These terms bear the designation NA, Nomina Anatomica, meaning that one or another of these International Congresses has officially adopted the term.

The Latin noun *facies* has two distinct meanings in NA. It can refer to the face or the expression on the face, or it can refer to the surface of an organ or part of the body. *Facies abdominalis*[2] is the pinched, anxious, and shrunken expression on the face of those suffering from abdominal disorders. *Facies hepatica* is the facies seen in liver disease, and *facies aortica* is the facial appearance of those with aortic valve insufficiency.

The *facies anterior brachii* is the front surface of the brachium, the upper arm. In these anatomical designations, the word for the organ or part of the body is usually found in the genitive case (*brachii*), and the location of the surface is in the form of an adjective (*anterior*) modifying the word *facies*. Note the following similar formations:

*facies anterior renis*: the front surface of the kidney
*facies posterior renis*: the back surface of the kidney
*facies inferior linguae*: the lower surface of the tongue
*facies lingualis dentis*: the lingual surface of a tooth—that is, the surface facing the tongue (*lingua*)
*facies labialis dentis*: the labial surface of a tooth—that is, the surface facing the lips (*labia*)
*facies lateralis brachii*: the lateral surface of the upper arm
*facies diaphragmatica hepatis*: the diaphragmatic surface of the liver—that is, the surface facing the diaphragm
*facies posterior antebrachii*: the back surface of the forearm

## PLANES OF THE BODY

A plane (Latin *planum*) of the body is a flat surface formed by making an imaginary cut through the body. Planes are used as points of reference by which positions of parts of the body are

---

[1]This verb does not have a perfect passive participle.

[2]Pronounced fay'-sha-eez; in such expressions as this, the terms assume the form of Latin words. *abdominalis* is the adjective meaning abdominal, from the noun *abdomen, abdominis*. This adjective agrees with the noun that it modifies (*facies*, in this instance) in gender (feminine) and number (singular).

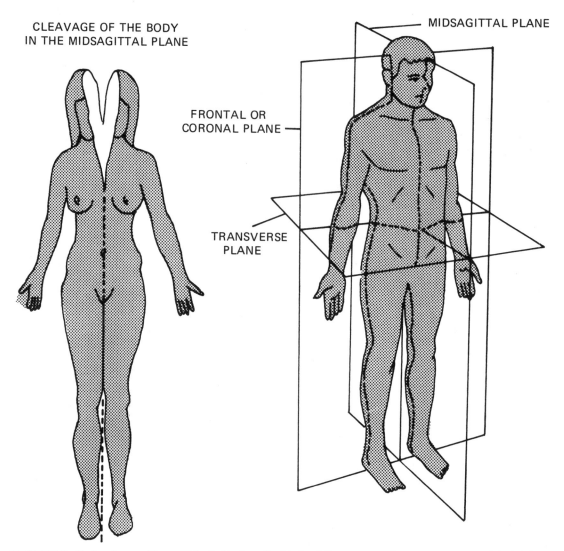

CLEAVAGE OF THE BODY
IN THE MIDSAGITTAL PLANE

MIDSAGITTAL PLANE

FRONTAL OR
CORONAL PLANE

TRANSVERSE
PLANE

FIGURE 1. Body planes. (From *Taber's Cyclopedic Medical Dictionary*, ed. 15. FA Davis, Philadelphia, 1985.)

indicated. There are three principal planes of the body, all based on the assumption that the body is in an upright position:

midsagittal plane (Latin *sagitta*, arrow), also called the sagittal or median plane: a vertical plane dividing the body into two equal and symmetrical right and left halves

frontal plane (Latin *frons, frontis*, front), also called the coronal plane (Latin *coróna*,[1] crown): a vertical plane at right angles to the midsagittal plane dividing the body into anterior and posterior portions

transverse plane (Latin *trans-*, across, *versus*, turned), also called the horizontal plane: a horizontal plane across the center of the body and at right angles to the midsagittal and frontal planes dividing the body into upper and lower portions.

Abduction of a limb is movement away from the median plane of the body, and adduction is movement toward the median plane. An abductor is a muscle which upon contraction

---

[1]borrowed from Greek *koróné*

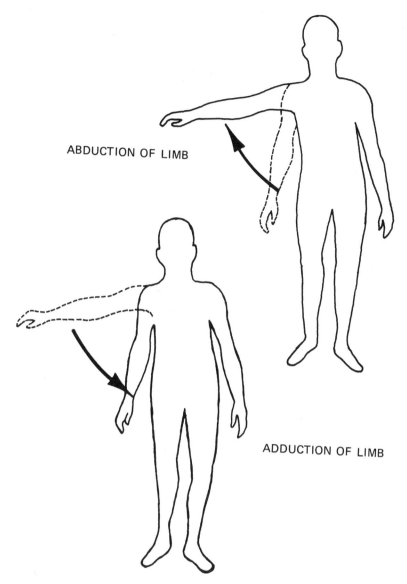

ABDUCTION OF LIMB

ADDUCTION OF LIMB

FIGURE 2. Abduction and adduction of a limb. (From *Taber's Cyclopedic Medical Dictionary*, ed 15. FA Davis, Philadelphia, 1985.)

draws a part away from the median plane, and an **adductor** is a muscle which draws a part toward the median plane.

# ETYMOLOGICAL NOTES

Aristotle and Pliny discuss insects:

*There are creatures called insects, as their name (entoma) indicates. They have incisions either on their upper or lower parts, or on both. They have neither separate bony parts (ostōdes) nor fleshy parts (sarkōdes) but consist of something intermediate, as their bodies, both inside and outside, are uniformly hard (skleron).* [Aristotle, *History of Animals* 4.523b 13–18]

*There are living creatures (animalia) of immeasurable minuteness which some people maintain do not breathe and are actually bloodless. There are great numbers and many kinds of these, some living on land and some in the air, some winged—bees, for example—some lacking wings—centipedes, for example—and some having the characteristics of both—ants, for example—and some lacking both wings and feet. All of these are correctly named insects (insecta), because of the incisions which encircle the necks of some, the chests or stomachs of others, and, in others, which separate their limbs from their bodies, these being connected by a slender tube (fistula). With some of these the incision does not encircle the entire body, but lies like a wrinkle on the belly or higher up. They have vertebrae that are flexible like gutter-tiles, displaying nature's craftsmanship in a more remarkable fashion than anywhere else. [Pliny, Natural History 11.1.1.1]*

## EXERCISE 9

*Earache and disorders of the ear are cured by the urine of a wild boar that has been kept in a glass jar, or by the gall of a wild boar or of a pig or an ox with equal portions of citrus and rose oil added. But the best cure of all is warm gall of a bull with leek juice. If there are suppurations, honey should be added, and if there is a foul odor the gall should be warmed with the rind of a pomegranate. [Pliny, Natural History 28.48.173]*

A. Analyze and define each of the following words.

1. anterolateral _____

2. posteroexternal _____

3. antebrachium _____

4. incipient[1] _____

5. inception _____

6. conception _____

7. contraception[2] _____

8. incisor _____

9. vermicide[3] _____

10. helminthicide _____

---

[1]Latin verbs often took on new and different meanings when compounded with prefixes. The verb *capere, captus,* meant to take; the compound verb *incipere, inceptus,* meant to take in hand, to undertake, and, thus, to begin. The word incipient is from the present participle of this verb.

[2]a shortened form of contra-conception

[3]Latin *vermis,* worm

11. virucidal _____

12. concretion _____

13. abduct _____

14. adduct _____

15. dorsiduction _____

16. ventriduct[1] _____

17. oviduct[2] _____

18. decalcify _____

19. infect[3] _____

20. infection _____

21. febrile _____

22. subfebrile _____

23. petrify[4] _____

24. petrifaction _____

25. olfactory[5] _____

26. dolorific[6] _____

27. calorific[7] _____

28. frigorific[8] _____

---

[1]Latin *venter, ventris*, belly, abdominal area

[2]Latin *ovum*, egg

[3]The Latin compound verb *inficere, infectus*, meant to stain, dye, spoil, corrupt.

[4]Greek *petra*, rock

[5]Latin *olēre*, smell

[6]Latin *dolor*, pain

[7]Latin *calor*, heat

[8]Latin *frigor*, cold

29. ossify _____

30. somnifacient _____

31. sanguifacient _____

32. faciocervical[1] _____

33. facioplegia _____

34. superficial _____

35. calciferous _____

36. odoriferous[2] _____

37. somnolent _____

38. ablate _____

39. ablation _____

40. introflexion _____

41. reflex _____

42. areflexia _____

43. dorsiflect _____

44. formication[3] _____

45. fulminant[4] _____

46. fulminating[5] _____

47. fungi[6] _____

---

[1]Latin *cervix*, *cervicis*, neck

[2]Latin *odor*, smell, scent, odor (often disagreeable)

[3]This word has been formed from the Latin denominative verb *formīcāre*, *formīcātus*, feel like the creeping of ants, from *formīca*, ant.

[4]This word has been formed from the Latin denominative verb *fulmināre*, *fulminātus*, strike with lightning, from *fulmen*, *fulminis*, lightning.

[5]Note the use of the English adjectival suffix -ing.

[6]Pronounced funj'-eye

48. fungistasis _____

49. ingesta[1] _____

50. egesta _____

51. digestion _____

52. digestant _____

53. congestion _____

54. gestation[2] _____

55. lactigerous[3] _____

56. genital _____

57. genitalia[4] _____

58. hypogenitalism _____

59. orad _____

60. aboral _____

61. orifice _____

62. os uteri externum[5] _____

63. insect _____

64. dissection _____

65. resect _____

66. venesection[6] _____

---

[1]The final -a of this word indicates the neuter plural, things.

[2]See the vocabulary note on *gerere, gestus* in this lesson.

[3]Latin *lac, lactis,* milk

[4]The final -ia of this word indicates the neuter plural, things. See page 114, footnote 5.

[5]The Latin noun *os* is neuter gender; this explains the neuter form of the adjective *externum. uterī* is the genitive singular of the Latin noun *uterus,* uterus.

[6]Latin *vēna,* vein

67. tumid _____

68. tumor _____

69. intumesce _____

70. intumescence _____

71. intumescent _____

72. Pediculus _____

73. Pediculus humanus[1] capitis _____

74. pediculosis _____

75. pediculosis capitis _____

76. stabile[2] _____

77. labile _____

78. frigostabile[3] _____

79. frigolabile _____

80. prolapsus _____

81. relapse _____

B. Using Latin prefixes, suffixes, and combining forms, form words meaning each of the following. Verify your answers in the medical dictionary.

1. (Passing from the) front to behind _____

2. (Located) behind and above (a part) _____

3. Pertaining to the arm _____

4. The act of cutting out _____

5. A cutting around _____

---

[1]Latin *humānus*, human
[2]pronounced stay′-bile; from Latin *stāre*, stand, and the adjectival suffix *-bile*, capable of
[3]Latin *frigor*, cold

6. An agent that kills a virus _____

7. (Occurring) after a fever _____

8. Carrying toward (a center) [use the present participle][1] _____

9. Carrying out from (a center) [use the present participle] _____

10. The act of bending backward _____

11. The act of pouring across _____

12. An agent that kills fungi _____

13. Pertaining to giving birth with _____

14. Around the mouth _____

15. Within the mouth _____

16. Through the mouth _____

17. Cut apart _____

18. The act of cutting back _____

C. Determine the meaning of each of the following words and terms.

1. adolescence[2] _____

2. concrescence _____

3. excrescence _____

4. fervescence[3] _____

5. defervescence _____

6. pubescence[4] _____

---

[1]For present participles see page 112 of the text.

[2]Latin *adolēscere*, *adultus*, come to maturity; see the section on Inceptive Verbs on page 113 of the text.

[3]Latin *fervēscere*, become hot, begin to boil, from *fervēre*, be hot, boil

[4]Latin *pūbēs*, *pūberis*, grown up

7. senescence[1] _____

8. tumescence _____

9. detumescence _____

10. procumbent[2] _____

11. recumbent _____

12. ventricumbent[3] _____

13. facies anterior renis[4] _____

14. facies inferior linguae _____

15. facies labialis dentis _____

16. facies lateralis brachii _____

D. Answer each of the following questions.

1. What is an *abductor* and what does it do?

2. What is an *adductor* and what does it do?

3. What is the meaning of the expression "to reduce a fracture"?[5]

4. What is *febris*[6] *enterica*?

---

[1]Latin *senex, senis,* old
[2]Latin *-cumbere* lie (down)
[3]See page 119, footnote 1.
[4]See the section Nomina Anatomica in this lesson.
[5]Latin *frangere, fractus,* break
[6]*febris* is a feminine noun.

5. What is *febris flava?*[1]

6. What is *facies hepatica?*

7. What is *myopathic facies?*

8. What is *adenoid facies?*

9. What is a *flexor* and what does it do?

10. What is a *pathologic reflex?*

11. What is meant by *effusion?*

12. What is an *intravenous infusion?*

13. What is *refusion?*

---

[1]Latin *flavus*, yellow

14. What is a *fungistat* used for?

15. What is *fungal septicemia*?

16. What is a *decongestant*?

17. What is the cause of *congestive* heart failure?

18. What is *adiposogenital dystrophy*?

19. What is *myatonia congenita*?

20. What is *pediculosis pubis*?[1]

21. What is the *sagittal plane*?[2]

22. What is the *transverse plane*?

---

[1]Latin *pūbēs*, *pūbis*, pubic area
[2]See the section on Planes of the Body in this lesson.

23. What is the *frontal plane*? 

24. What is meant by each of the following italicized terms?

    a. *referred* pain _____

    b. *ductus deferens* _____

    c. *remittent*[1] fever _____

    d. *remission*[1] of pain _____

    e. *resilience*[2] of muscle tissue _____

    f. *accretion* of purulent matter _____

    g. *exsanguination* _____

    h. *evisceration* _____

25. The Lattin verb *trahere, tractus* meant draw, drag. What is the meaning of each of the following terms?

    a. traction _____

    b. contractile _____

    c. extraction _____

    d. extractor _____

    e. retraction _____

    f. retractor _____

    g. retractile _____

[1]Latin *mittere, missus*, send
[2]Latin *salīre*, leap

26. The Latin verb *tenēre*, *tentus*, meant hold. What is the meaning of each of the following terms?

a. tenaculum _____

b. retinaculum _____

c. labiotenaculum[1] _____

## DRILL AND REVIEW

E. The meaning of each of the following words can be determined from its etymology. Determine the meaning of each and verify your answer in the medical dictionary.

1. anteroinferior
2. anterosuperior
3. posterointernal
4. brachialgia
5. brachiocephalic
6. contraceptive
7. excise
8. incise
9. incision
10. cytocide
11. cytocidal
12. microbicide
13. leukocidin
14. abduction
15. adduction
16. calcification
17. decalcification
18. recalcification
19. febrifacient
20. febrific
21. antefebrile
22. afebrile
23. somnific
24. detoxify
25. detoxification
26. ossification
27. deossification
28. sanguification
29. facial
30. faciobrachial
31. faciocephalalgia
32. hemifacial
33. sanguiferous
34. melaniferous
35. lipoferous
36. toxiferous
37. somniferous
38. somnipathy
39. reflexogenic
40. dorsiflexion
41. lateroflexion
42. fungistatic
43. fungoid[2]
44. ingestion
45. indigestible
46. calcigerous
47. cystigerous
48. genitoplasty
49. hypergenitalism
50. microgenitalism
51. adoral
52. aborad
53. os uteri[3]
54. os uteri internum[3]
55. prolapse
56. transection
57. resectable
58. vivisection[4]
59. revivification
60. tumefacient
61. tumefaction
62. Pediculus humanus corporis[5]
63. pediculosis corporis
64. pediculicide
65. pediculophobia
66. thermostabile
67. thermolabile
68. ductule

[1]Latin *labium*, lip
[2]pronounced fung'-oid
[3]See page 121, footnote 5.
[4]Latin *vīvus*, alive, living
[5]Latin *humānus*, human; *corpus*, *corporis*, body

# THE CARDIOVASCULAR SYSTEM

*If you kill a living animal by severing its great arteries, you will find that the veins become empty at the same time as the arteries. This could never happen unless there were anastomoses between them.* [Galen, *On the Natural Faculties* 3.15]

At the great institutions of learning in Alexandria, the Museum and the Library, which had been established in the early third century B.C. by Ptolemy I, a former Macedonian general of Alexander the Great, who founded the Ptolemaic dynasty in Egypt after Alexander's death, great advances were made in the field of medicine, and the medical school there (as well as the other institutes) became the focal point for men of learning for many centuries. In the middle of the second century A.D., the physician Galen went there from his native Pergamum in Asia Minor after studying at the Asclepium, the famed medical school in that city. Galen's theory of the movement of the blood in the human body was to influence and even rule medical thinking up to the seventeenth century, when the great discovery of William Harvey that the blood circulates—that is, all of the blood that leaves the heart, after passing to the organs and parts of the body, returns to its point of departure to begin the process all over again—revolutionized medical thought and formed the basis for modern scientific medicine.

Galen believed that food was converted in the intestines to a fluid which he called chyle[1] [*On the Use of the Parts* 4.3], which was then carried to the liver where it was transformed into blood and charged with a vapor or spirit. He, having no idea of what we know as circulation, thought that this supercharged blood was then carried from the liver through the veins to the various parts of the body in a forward and backward movement. One part of Galen's theory on the movement of the blood is of special interest. He believed that some of the blood which was carried by the veins to the right ventricle of the heart, instead of flowing back through the veins to the liver, passed through the septum into the left ventricle by means of small passages between the right and left heart.[2] It was, for the most part, the rigid adherence to this theory that the blood passed directly through the septum from the right to the left ventricle that prevented the realization of the true nature of the circulation of the blood for fifteen centuries.

One man did, however, dare to challenge the theories of Galen concerning the nature of the movements of the blood. This was a theologian, Michael Servetus, born in 1511 in Spain. Serve-

---

[1]Greek *chylos*, juice

[2]*The thinnest portion of the blood is drawn from the right cavity* (koilia) *of the heart into the left through passages in the septum* (diaphragma) *between these parts. These passages can be seen for the most part of their length; they are like pits with wide openings, but they keep getting narrower and it is not possible to see the end of them because of both their small size and the fact that the animal being dead, all of its parts are cold and shrunken.* [Galen, *On the Natural Faculties* 3.15]

tus studied theology at Toulouse in France and then went to Paris to study medicine. This was early in the period of the Reformation, and Servetus held some views that were considered almost heretical by both Catholics and Protestants. Along with his religious tracts, he wrote a work on physiology, the content of which, however, was clothed in the title *Christianismi restitutio* (Restitution of Christianity). The work was published in 1553 and in it Servetus challenged Galen's theory on the presence of a certain natural spirit that entered the blood in the liver. In addition, he maintained that the blood did not pass through the septum from the right to the left ventricle, but rather that it passed from the right ventricle to the lungs, where it was purified by inspired air, and then, lighter in color, conveyed to the left ventricle. Servetus was arrested, tried for heresy, found guilty, and burned alive at Geneva on October 27, 1553. Servetus' book was burned along with its writer. But a few copies survived, and his theories undoubtedly exerted some influence on later scientists. It would take three-quarters of a century before the actual circulation of the blood in the human body was perceived and made known.

In 1628 William Harvey, a fellow of the Royal College of Physicians in London, published his great work. It was written in Latin and was called *Exercitatio anatomica de motu cordis et sanguinis* (An Anatomical Treatise on the Motion of the Heart and Blood). Harvey's work was flawless as far as it went. It stopped short of completion only because in his time the microscope was not yet capable of revealing a clear image at high power. Harvey did not realize how the arterial blood passed into the veins via the capillaries. It was Marcello Malpighi who through his microscopic examination of the circulatory system of the frog revealed the action of the network of capillaries joining the arterioles to the venules. His work, *De Pulmonibus* (On the Lungs), was published at Bologna in 1661.

# THE CIRCULATION OF THE BLOOD

Blood commences its journey through the body as it is pumped from the upper end of the left ventricle into the great artery, the aorta. The aortic valve prevents the blood from flowing back into the ventricle (**aortic regurgitation**), and thus it can flow in but one direction, away from the heart, the direction in which the entire arterial network carries the blood. As the blood moves away from the heart, it enters the many branches of the arteries, two of which (the **coronary arteries**) supply blood to the muscle of the heart. A blood clot that lodges in one of the coronary arteries and obstructs the flow of blood through it can cause heart failure and sudden death (**coronary thrombosis**). As the arteries branch they become increasingly smaller and are now called arterioles, until at length they unite in a network of tiny vessels, the capillaries. From these microscopically small vessels, the blood passes into the venules, small veins, and then into the venous system, finally to enter the right atrium through the two venae cavae, the superior, which returns blood from the organs and parts above the diaphragm (except the lungs), and the inferior, which returns the blood from organs and tissues below the diaphragm.

From the right atrium the blood passes through the tricuspid valve into the right ventricle. Here the blood begins another journey, the pulmonary or lesser circulation. It passes into the pulmonary artery which branches out in the lungs, becoming smaller and smaller until these arterioles unite with capillaries which in turn unite with the pulmonary venules which carry the blood into the left atrium through the left superior and inferior pulmonary veins. From the left atrium the blood enters the left ventricle through the mitral or bicuspid valve to start its journey all over again. The contractions of the cardiac muscle which pumps about four quarts of blood a minute are governed by the vagus nerve, which slows the muscular action, and the sympathetic nervous system, which accelerates it. Regulation is achieved by a pacemaker, the sinoatrial node. If this natural pacemaker is defective, an electrical device called an artificial or electric pacemaker can be installed either externally or internally to control the heartbeat by rhythmic electrical discharges. Defects and malfunctions, either congenital or acquired, along this complicated network of vessels and valves can cause the numerous disorders, many often fatal, that we call heart disease.

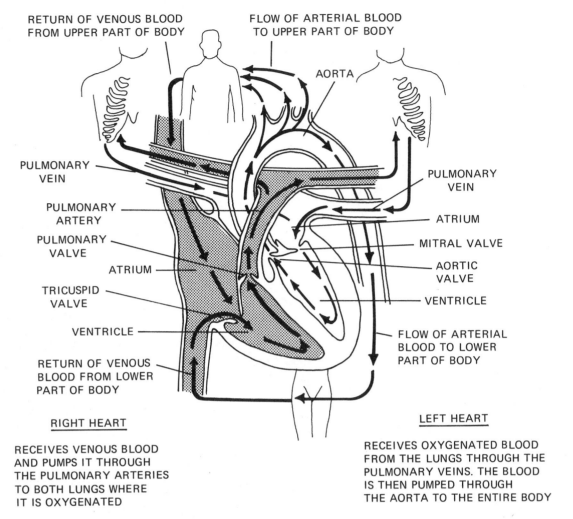

RETURN OF VENOUS BLOOD
FROM UPPER PART OF BODY

FLOW OF ARTERIAL BLOOD
TO UPPER PART OF BODY

AORTA

PULMONARY
VEIN

PULMONARY
VEIN

PULMONARY
ARTERY

ATRIUM

PULMONARY
VALVE

MITRAL VALVE

ATRIUM

AORTIC
VALVE

TRICUSPID
VALVE

VENTRICLE

VENTRICLE

FLOW OF ARTERIAL
BLOOD TO LOWER
PART OF BODY

RETURN OF VENOUS
BLOOD FROM LOWER
PART OF BODY

RIGHT HEART

LEFT HEART

RECEIVES VENOUS BLOOD
AND PUMPS IT THROUGH
THE PULMONARY ARTERIES
TO BOTH LUNGS WHERE
IT IS OXYGENATED

RECEIVES OXYGENATED BLOOD
FROM THE LUNGS THROUGH THE
PULMONARY VEINS. THE BLOOD
IS THEN PUMPED THROUGH
THE AORTA TO THE ENTIRE BODY

FIGURE 3. Circulation of blood through heart and major vessels. (From *Taber's Cyclopedic Medical Dictionary*, ed 15. FA Davis, Philadelphia, 1985.)

## VOCABULARY

*Life is short, the Art lasting, opportunity elusive, experiment perilous, judgment difficult. The physician must be ready not only to do what is necessary, but to see to it that his patient, the attendants, and all external arrangements are ready.* [Hippocrates, *Aphorisms* 1.1]

| GREEK OR LATIN WORD | COMBINING FORM(S) | MEANING |
|---|---|---|
| *amylon* | AMYL- | starch |
| *angina* | *ANGIN-* | choking pain; angina pectoris |
| *aortē* | AORT- | aorta |
| *arctāre, arctātus* | *ARCT(AT)-* | compress |
| *athērē* | ATHER- | [soup] fatty deposit |
| *atrium* | *ATRI-* | [entrance hall] atrium |
| *bolē* | BOL- | a throwing[1] |
| *capillus* | *CAPILL-* | [hair] capillary |
| *kirsos* | CIRS- | dilated and twisted vein, varix |

---

[1]See the Etymological Notes to this lesson.

131

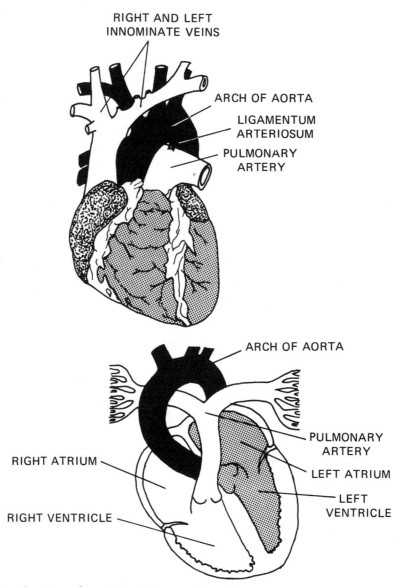

**FIGURE 4.** Anterior views of exterior and interior of heart and vessels. (From *Taber's Cyclopedic Medical Dictionary*, ed. 15. FA Davis, Philadelphia, 1985.)

| | | |
|---|---|---|
| *claudere, clausus* | *-CLUD-, -CLUS-* | close |
| *cor, cordis* | *COR, CORD-* | heart |
| *cuspis, cuspidis* | *CUSP, -CUSPID* | point |
| *dexter* | *DEXTR-* | right (side) |
| *forma* | *-FORM* | shape |
| *gurgitāre, gurgitātus* | *GURGITAT-* | flood, flow |
| *pectus, pectoris* | *PECTOR-* | breast, chest |
| *phleps, phlebos* | PHLEB- | vein |
| *pulmō, pulmōnis* | *PULM(ON)-* | lung, pulmonary artery |
| *rhythmos* | RHYTHM- | [steady motion] heartbeat |
| *saeptum* | *SEPT-* | wall, partition |
| *sinus* | *SIN-, SINUS-* | [curve, hollow] sinus |
| *sinister* | *SINISTR-* | left (side) |
| *sphygmos* | SPHYGM- | pulse |
| *stellein* | STAL-, STOL- | send |
| *thrombos* | THROMB- | blood clot |

| | | | |
|---|---|---|---|
| *topos* | TOP- | place |
| *vagus* | VAG- | [wandering] the vagus nerve |
| *varix, varicis* | VARIC-, VARIX | dilated and twisted vein, varix |
| *vas* | VAS- | (blood) vessel; vas deferens |
| *vēna* | VEN- | vein |
| *venter, ventris* | VENTR- | belly, abdomen, abdominal cavity |

## ETYMOLOGICAL NOTES

*I swear by Apollo the healer, by Asclepius, by Hygieia, by Panacea and by all the gods and goddesses as witnesses, that I will fulfill this oath and this covenant.* [The beginning of the Hippocratic Oath]

Among the many attributes of the god Apollo was the ability to heal the sick as well as to call down destruction and death upon the wicked. After the time of Homer he is often called Paean, whom Homer calls the physician of the gods. As a healer, Apollo was outstripped by his son Asclepius, born to the nymph Coronis. Asclepius, who received his medical education from the famed centaur Chiron, became so skilled that not only was he able to heal the sick but acquired the ability to bring the dead back to life. This unusual talent was said to have angered Hades, the ruler of the Home of the Dead, and he complained to his brother Zeus that his realms were becoming depopulated. Zeus struck Asclepius dead with one of his lightning bolts.

Asclepius was said to have learned how to bring the dead back to life when once, as he was pondering how to restore Glaucus, son of King Minos of Crete, to life, a snake coiled around his staff. He struck the creature and killed it. Later, a second snake came along carrying a leaf in its jaws and placed it upon the head of the dead snake. The serpent came to life, and Asclepius used the same medicament to restore Glaucus. And so two snakes curled around the staff of Asclepius became the symbol of this great healer. It is now the symbol of the American Medical Association, the Caduceus.

The words **systole** and **diastole** are from the Greek verb *stellein*, send. Systole refers to the period of contraction of the heart when the blood is sent through the aorta and the pulmonary artery. Diastole is the period of expansion when the heart dilates and the atria and ventricles fill with blood from the venae cavae and the pulmonary vein. Blood pressure is taken by means of an inflatable cloth cuff known as a **sphygmomanometer** (Greek *manos*, occurring at intervals) which is wound around the arm. As air is pumped into it and it expands, a column of mercury rises to indicate the pressure within the cuff. When the pressure is sufficient to stop the flow of blood through the brachial artery, which the doctor tells by listening to the heartbeat through his stethoscope pressed against the patient's arm, the pressure is released. When the doctor can once again hear the heartbeat, the level of the column of mercury indicates the systolic pressure. As more air is let out of the cuff, the pulse fades for a moment. The level of the mercury at this point indicates the diastolic pressure.

The **mitral** valve of the heart lies between the left atrium and the left ventricle and allows passage of the blood from the atrium into the ventricle. It is a one-way valve, and a mitral defect can cause **mitral regurgitation**, a back-flowing of the blood. It is also called the bicuspid valve because of its two cusps. The word mitral comes from Latin and was borrowed into that language from the Greek word meaning a type of turban worn by certain peoples of Asia. In Vergil's *Aeneid* the Moorish king Iarbas, scorned by Dido, the Phoenician princess who recently settled in North Africa, hearing that she and Aeneas, a wanderer from Troy, are openly flaunting their love, prays to Jupiter for vengeance, referring contemptuously to Aeneas as another Paris:

> *et nunc ille Paris cum semiviro comitatu,*
> *Maeonia mentum mitra crinemque madentem*
> *subnixus, rapto potitur.*

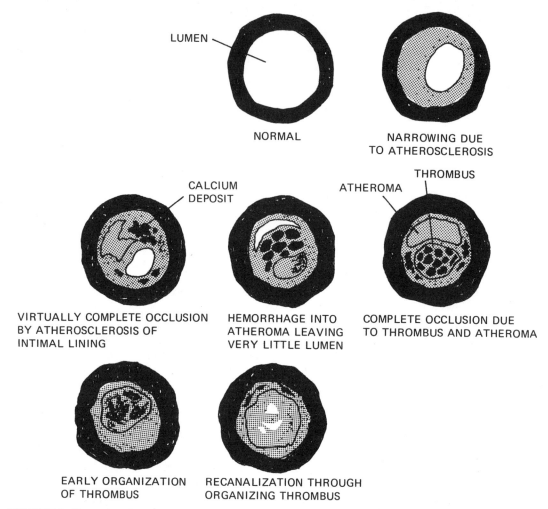

FIGURE 5. **Normal and diseased coronary arteries. (From** *Taber's Cyclopedic Medical Dictionary,* **ed. 15. FA Davis, Philadelphia, 1985.)**

> And now that Paris with his band of half-men,
> his chin and oiled hair bound with a
> Maeonian miter, possesses what he has stolen.
> [*Aeneid* 4.215–217]

The modern medical term comes directly from the miter or mitre, a tall, cleft, pointed hat worn by bishops of the Western church. The word valve comes from the Latin *valvae,* a plural word meaning a particular kind of door that folded within itself. **Facies mitralis** is the facial appearance of a person afflicted with mitral malfunction: distended capillaries and cyanosis.

The causes of what is often called simply a heart attack, or a stroke, are many and varied, the site of the initial attack usually being either a coronary artery, so called because these vessels form a crown over and around the heart, or the cerebrovascular system. Coronary artery disease results from the narrowing or closing of the coronary arteries, usually due to either **atherosclerosis** or the presence of a **thrombus** or an **embolus.** An embolus may be formed from clotted blood and thus is a form of thrombus, or it can be formed from a portion of a cardiac tumor, such as a myxoma, or from any foreign substance such as fibrous matter, fat, or gas. In any case, the artery is unable to carry the blood that is pumped into it by the cardiac muscle. The resultant condition, called **coronary occlusion** or **coronary thrombosis,** can and often does lead to **ischemia,** and this can be the cause of **myocardial infarction,** cardiac arrest, and sudden death.

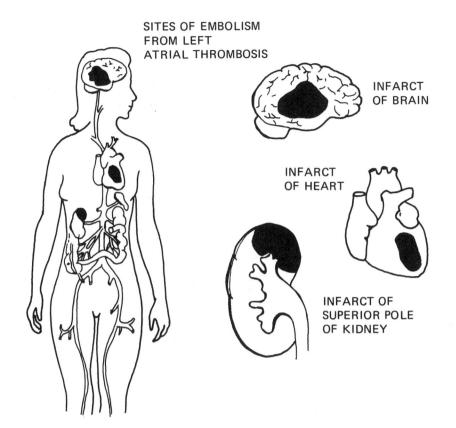

SITES OF EMBOLISM
FROM LEFT
ATRIAL THROMBOSIS

INFARCT
OF BRAIN

INFARCT
OF HEART

INFARCT OF
SUPERIOR POLE
OF KIDNEY

FIGURE 6. Embolism. (From *Taber's Cyclopedic Medical Dictionary*, ed. 14, FA Davis, Philadelphia, 1981.)

An **aneurysm**[1] is the local distention of the wall of a blood vessel, usually an artery, and often the aorta. The dilation is caused by a weakening of the vascular wall, often as a result of arteriosclerosis coupled with hypertension. Aneurysms of the aorta may occur anywhere along this great artery and often occur in the abdominal region or in the pulmonary arteries. Rupture of an aneurysm with subsequent massive hemorrhage is a frequent cause of death.

Cerebral **apoplexy**,[2] or stroke, is caused by intracerebral hemorrhage following the rupture of a vessel, often as the result of an aneurysm, or by thrombosis, embolism, or a reduction or loss of the blood supply to the brain (vascular insufficiency).

**Digitalis**,[3] a heart stimulant which acts by increasing the force of the muscular contractions, is made of the dried leaves of the plant *Digitalis purpurea*.[4] This plant is so called because of the fingerlike shape of its corolla.

The Greek verb *ballein*, throw, has many derivatives. The science of projectiles is *ballistics*. But it is in the form BOL-, from the noun *bolē*, a throwing, that it is most productive. An **embolism** is the blockage of a blood vessel by any mass of undissolved matter, a blood clot, or an air bubble. **Metabolism** is the sum of the processes of **anabolism**, the process by which the blood supplies the material for growth and repair of tissues, and **catabolism**,[5] the process by which complex compounds are reduced to simpler ones, usually accompanied by the release of energy.

---

[1]Greek *ana-*, up, *eurys*,, wide, *-m(a)*, noun-forming suffix

[2]Greek *apo-*, away

[3]Latin *digitus*, finger

[4]Latin *purpura*, purple

[5]Greek *kata-*, down

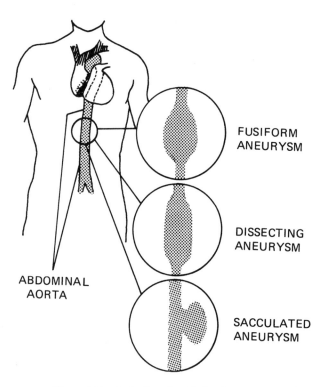

FIGURE 7. Types of aneurysms. (From *Taber's Cyclopedic Medical Dictionary*, ed 15. FA Davis, Philadelphia, 1985.)

The verb *diaballein*,[1] throw across, had a secondary meaning of slander, make a false accusation. From this meaning of the verb there was formed a noun *diabolē*, slander. The noun *diabolos* meant one who slanders, an evil person. This word is found in the Septuagint (*I Chron.*, 21.1) meaning the enemy, or Satan. Matthew (4.1) writes, "At that time Jesus was led into the wilderness by the Spirit, and there he was tempted by the devil (*diabolos*)."[2] When the Scriptures were translated into Old English, the Latin *diabolus* of the Vulgate was rendered by *deofol*, devil. *diabolos* remains in English in the word *diabolic*, devilish.

## EXERCISE 10

A. Analyze and define each of the following words.

1. amylase _____

2. amylolysis _____

3. anginoid _____

4. anisorhythmia _____

---

[1]Greek *dia-*, across
[2]King James version

5. aortoclasia _____

6. arctation _____

7. atheroma _____

8. atheronecrosis _____

9. atriotome _____

10. capillarectasia _____

11. cirsoid _____

12. cirsomphalos _____

13. cirsotome _____

14. cordate _____

15. corona[1] _____

16. corona capitis _____

17. corona dentis[2] _____

18. coronary arteries _____

19. cusp _____

20. tricuspid[3] _____

21. dextrocardia _____

22. dextrocardiogram _____

23. dextropedal[4] _____

24. ectopia cordis _____

----------

[1]Latin *corōna*, crown
[2]Latin *dens, dentis*, tooth
[3]Greek *treis*, three
[4]Latin *pēs, pedis*, foot

25. entopic _____

26. expectoration _____

27. extravasate _____

28. infarct[1] _____

29. mitral[2] stenosis _____

30. occlude _____

31. phlebemphraxis _____

32. phlebography _____

33. phlebomyomatosis _____

34. pulmometer _____

35. pulmonectomy _____

36. nonseptate _____

37. sinistrocardia _____

38. sinistrocerebral _____

39. sinogram _____

40. systole _____

41. thrombectomy _____

42. thromboclasis _____

43. thrombopathy _____

44. topognosia _____

45. topagnosis _____

_____

[1]Latin *farcīre, farctus*, stuff, cram
[2]Latin *mitra*, turban; see the Etymological Notes to this lesson.

138

46. toponarcosis _____

47. vagus _____

48. vagotropism _____

49. varices _____

50. varicography _____

51. vascular _____

52. vasectomy _____

53. vasodilator[1] _____

54. vena cava[2] inferior _____

55. venostasis _____

56. venostat _____

57. ventricle _____

B. Give the word derived from Greek and/or Latin elements meaning each of the following.
Verify your answer in the medical dictionary.

1. (The presence of) starch in the blood _____

2. Toward the right (side) _____

3. (The formation of) a blood clot in a vein (use Greek forms) _____

4. A little vein (use Latin forms) _____

5. The formation of calculi in the veins (use Greek forms) _____

6. Producing a blood clot _____

7. Muscle dislocation _____

8. A small varix _____

_____
[1]Latin *latus*, wide
[2]Latin *cavus*, hollow

9. An instrument to record the pulse _____

10. (Situated) between little vessels (use Latin forms) _____

11. Pain in the chest _____

12. (Having a) kidney shape (use Latin forms) _____

C. Give a clear, concise definition of each of the following italicized words.

1. Cardiomegaly is common, especially in older patients. Heart weight well over a kilogram has been reported. Advanced coronary *atherosclerosis* and systemic hypertension frequently coexist. Dyspnea, fatigue, marked edema, and *syncope*[1] are often the presenting symptoms.

2. *Coarctation* of the aorta raises the systolic blood pressure in the brachial artery, though not invariably, and lowers the blood pressure in the femoral artery.

3. With the onset of ventricular failure, it is usual to find sinus tachycardia, *arrhythmias*, evidences of *mitral*[2] *regurgitation*, or mural *thrombi*.

4. Regional ischemia can result in *myocardial infarction*[3] or a variety of physiologic abnormalities: anginal syndrome, arrhythmias, conduction disturbances, papillary muscle dysfunction, *ventricular asynergy*, and ventricular failure.

5. The sudden onset of pain, numbness, weakness, or paresthesias in the lower extremities, accompanied by coldness, pallor, mottled cyanosis, and absent pulsations in the same areas, is clinical evidence of an *embolus* lodged at the *aortic bifurcation*.[4]

---

[1] Greek *koptein*, strike
[2] See page 138, footnote 2.
[3] See page 138, footnote 1.
[4] Latin *furca*, fork

6. Intracardiac *thrombosis* may result from inflammation, injury, necrosis and fibrosis, and slowing and abnormal eddying of the blood stream.

7. Pulmonary hypertension can also result from anatomic curtailment of the capacity of the pulmonary vascular bed produced by massive embolization, recurrent multiple emboli, thrombosis, or occlusive *vascular lesions*[1] associated with sickle cell disease, or schistosomiasis.

8. Clinically, rapid occlusion of the lower portion of the aorta by thrombosis may be indistinguishable from occlusion due to embolism. *Aortography* may delineate irregular areas of narrowing.

9. Mitral stenosis may be revealed by a dome-shaped anterior bulging of the mitral valve into the left ventricle during *diastole*.[2]

10. Lesions of the aorta induced by syphilis, cystic medial necrosis, ankylosing spondylitis, or dissecting hematoma can also result in *aortic regurgitation*, as may severe systemic hypertension.

11. Atherosclerosis of the aorta produces no clinical symptoms unless there are complications of the process such as *aneurysm*,[3] embolization, thrombosis, or impingement upon the orifice of arteries, with reduction in regional blood flow.

---

[1]Latin *laedere*, *laesus*, injure

[2]Greek *dia-* through

[3]Greek *ana-*, up, *eurys*, wide

12. Auricular fibrillation or signs of recent cardiac infarction, confirmed by ECG, may accompany cerebral *embolism*.

13. Arrhythmias, especially extrastyoles, may cause palpitations. In the latter the skipped beats usually cause the frightening sensation of missing heart action in nervous apprehensive individuals. The more discomfort is caused by *ectopic* beats, the more probable is their innocuous character.

14. The pain in *angina pectoris* is described as a sensation of heaviness, pressure or tightness behind the sternum, usually in its upper part, sometimes in the precordial region or epigastrium. It may become excruciating, viselike (hence the term stenocardia derived from the Greek and meaning tightness in the chest), and may be accompanied by fear of impending death.

15. *Auscultation*[1] is the next and most important step of physical examination. It discloses whether the heart sounds are pure, replaced partially or completely by, or associated with, murmurs, and whether frequency and rhythm of the heart action are altered.

16. *Cor pulmonale*[2] is usually distinguished as the acute or the chronic variety. The first is caused by sudden massive obstruction of the pulmonary circulation by embolism or by perforation of an aortic aneurysm into the pulmonary artery.

17. *Atrial septal defect* occasionally is associated with rheumatic mitral stenosis, this association being known as Lutembacher's syndrome. For obvious reasons the septal defect is, in a certain way, a favorable complication of mitral stenosis because it relieves the pressure in the left atrium, and hence in the pulmonary circulation.

---

[1]Latin *auscultāre, auscultātus*, listen to

[2]*pulmonale* is New Latin, formed as the neuter singular of an adjective *pulmonalis*, of the lungs, a form that did not exist in Latin.

D. Answer each of the following questions.

1. What is meant by a *pyemic embolism? thromboembolism? pulmonary embolism?*

2. What is meant by *facies aortica? facies mitralis?*

3. The Latin noun *lumen, luminis* meant light, daylight. What is the meaning in anatomical terminology of the word *lumen? intraluminal?*

4. The Latin adjective *intimus* meant innermost. What is the meaning in anatomical terminology of the word *intima?*[1] What is *intimitis?*

5. What is the meaning of *ambidextrous? ambisinister? sinistrality?*

6. What is an *expectorant?*

7. What is the meaning of *peristalsis? bradystalsis?*

8. What is meant by *vasoligation?*[2]

---

[1]This is the feminine form of the adjective modifying a supposed feminine noun *tunica*, coat, covering (membrane).

[2]Latin *ligāre, ligātus*, tie, bind

9. What do the *vasomotor*[1] nerves control?

10. What is the meaning of the abbreviation CVA?

11. What is meant by *extravasation? intravasation?*

12. What is a *sphygmomanometer?*[2]

13. What is meant by *biological rhythm? circadian*[3] *rhythm?*

14. What are *ecchymoses?*[4]

15. In the terminology of dentistry the canines, or eyeteeth, are called *cuspids*. What is the reason for this name?

---

[1]Latin *movēre, motus*, move, set in motion
[2]Greek *manos*, occurring at intervals
[3]Latin *circā*, around, *diēs*, day
[4]Greek *chyma*, that which is poured, from *chein*, pour

144

16. The tetralogy[1] of Fallot[2] is a congenital condition characterized by four abnormalities: pulmonary stenosis, interventricular septal defect, dextroposition[3] of the aorta, and right ventricular hypertrophy. What does each of these terms mean?

17. What is meant by *intersystole*?

18. The Latin verb *tendere, tensus* meant stretch. What is the meaning of each of the following words?

   a. hypertension _____

   b. hypertensive _____

   c. hypotension _____

   d. hypotensive _____

## DRILL AND REVIEW

E. The meaning of each of the following words can be determined from its etymology. Determine the meaning of each and verify your answer in a medical dictionary.

| | |
|---|---|
| 1. cordiform | 16. aortorrhaphy |
| 2. variciform | 17. aortopathy |
| 3. vasiform | 18. aortarctia |
| 4. anginophobia | 19. atheromatous |
| 5. arteriarctia | 20. atheromatosis |
| 6. amylolytic | 21. interatrial |
| 7. amylogenic | 22. intra-atrial |
| 8. amylogenesis | 23. capillaritis |
| 9. amylophagia | 24. capillaropathy |
| 10. endaortitis | 25. capillaroscopy |
| 11. periaortitis | 26. cirsotome |
| 12. aortocoronary | 27. cirsotomy |
| 13. aortectomy | 28. cirsectomy |
| 14. aortectasia | 29. pectoral |
| 15. aortomalacia | 30. dextral |

---

[1]Greek *tettara*, four
[2]named for Etienne L.A. Fallot, French physician [1850–1911]
[3]Latin *ponere, positus*, place

31. dextrogastria
32. dextroversion[1]
33. endophlebitis
34. suppurative phlebitis
35. sclerosing phlebitis
36. osteophlebitis
37. varicophlebitis
38. septicophlebitis
39. phlebolith
40. phlebogram
41. phlebotome
42. phlebectomy
43. phleboplasty
44. phleborrhexis
45. intrapulmonary
46. subpulmonary
47. pulmonitis
48. pulmoaortic
49. pulmometry
50. septate
51. septulum
52. septotome
53. septotomy
54. septectomy
55. sinusitis
56. polysinusitis
57. sinusotomy
58. sinistral
59. sinistrad
60. sphygmic
61. presphygmic
62. sphygmoid
63. sphygmology
64. sphygmometer
65. sphygmocardiograph
66. sphygmocardiogram
67. bradysphygmia
68. bradyrhythmia
69. dysrhythmia
70. arrhythmic
71. tachyarrhythmia
72. peristaltic
73. systolic
74. prediastolic[2]
75. postdiastolic
76. asystolia
77. tachysystole
78. pulmonic regurgitation
79. tricuspid regurgitation
80. thromboid
81. thromboarteritis
82. thromboendocarditis
83. thromboclastic
84. thrombolytic
85. thrombolysis
86. thrombogenesis
87. osteothrombosis
88. topical
89. dystopic
90. adenectopia
91. osteectopia
92. splenectopia
93. ectopia renis
94. toponeurosis
95. vagal
96. vagitis
97. vagotomy
98. varicose
99. varicotomy
100. vasal
101. vasalgia
102. vasography
103. vasorrhaphy
104. vasotrophic
105. vasculitis[3]
106. intravascular
107. circumvascular
108. cerebrovascular
109. meningovascular
110. vena cava superior
111. intravenous
112. venosclerosis
113. venogram
114. venography
115. venovenostomy
116. ventrocystorrhaphy
117. ventroscopy
118. ventrotomy
119. intraventricular
120. ventriculography

---

[1]Latin *vertere, versus*, turn

[2]Greek *dia-*, through

[3]Latin *vasculum*, diminutive of *vas*, vessel. The force of the diminutive has been lost in derivatives of this word.

# THE RESPIRATORY SYSTEM

*It is through the veins that we take in most of our breath, for they are the vents of the body, taking in the air and bringing it to the smaller vessels where it is cooled and then released.* [Hippocrates, *The Sacred Disease* 7]

All organs, parts, tissues, and cells of the body require oxygen in order to function, and it is the respiratory system that furnishes oxygen to the circulating blood to carry it to the parts of the body. In all of the cells of the body the oxygen is exchanged for carbon dioxide, a waste material of the cells, and the veins return this carbon dioxide in the blood stream to the lungs to be discharged into the atmosphere. The sum of the inspiration of oxygen and the expiration of carbon dioxide is called respiration, and this is one of the vital processes of life.

Air enters the body through the nose and mouth and travels downward through the pharynx, the larynx, past the vocal cords, and into the trachea, or windpipe. The trachea branches into two tubes, the right and the left bronchi, which enter the lungs. After these bronchial tubes enter the lungs they branch off into smaller and smaller tubes called bronchioles until they finally reach a dead end. The inner surface of the lungs is lined with innumerable tiny sacs called alveoli, which become filled with air at each inspiration. The pulmonary arteries from the heart branch off into arterioles in the lungs, and then into capillaries, and it is the blood in the capillaries that receives the oxygen from the alveoli as the hemoglobin molecules become saturated with oxygen. Hemoglobin thus saturated is called oxyhemoglobin. As the blood becomes oxygenated, it discharges its carbon dioxide which is then exhaled. The oxygenated blood now passes from the capillaries into the pulmonary veins to be carried back to the heart and pumped to all parts of the body to exchange its oxygen for carbon dioxide, and the process commences all over again. This exchange, the crucial part of the process of respiration, normally takes place about eighteen times a minute in the human body from the moment of birth to the instant of death.

Each lung is enclosed within a sac called the pleura, which has two layers, the inner or visceral, and the outer or parietal.[1] Normally there is no space within these two layers except for a thin film of lubricating fluid. But in certain diseases of the lungs a space may be forced between these layers by the accumulation of fluid, a condition called **hydrothorax**, or by the accumulation of blood, **hemothorax**, caused by the rupture of small blood vessels in pulmonary disorders, or by the accumulation of air, **pneumothorax**, due to perforation of the pleura.

The lungs, with their pleural sacs, are separated from one another by a cavity called the mediastinum.[2] Beneath the lungs lies a muscular membrane, the diaphragm, which flattens and

---

[1]pronounced par-eye'-et-al, from Latin *pariēs, parietis*, wall.

[2]The word mediastinum is a New Latin formation meaning in the middle, from Medieval Latin *mediastinus*, intermedial, from Latin *medius*, middle.

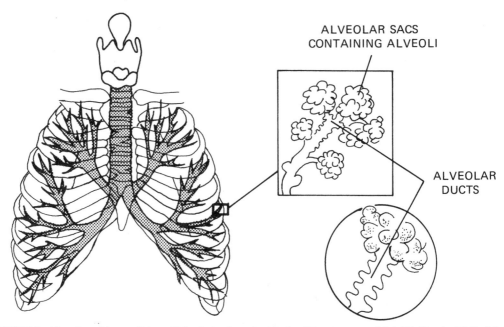

ALVEOLAR SACS
CONTAINING ALVEOLI

ALVEOLAR
DUCTS

FIGURE 8. Alveolus of lung. (From *Taber's Cyclopedic Medical Dictionary*, ed 14. FA Davis, Philadelphia, 1981.)

contracts during inspiration. It also exerts a downward pressure upon the abdominal viscera during the expulsion of feces from the bowel. The entire area between the diaphragm and the base of the neck is called the thorax, and the thoracic cavity contains the heart, lungs, and the origins of the great blood vessels.

Any interference with the flow of air into and out of the lungs is a potential cause of pulmonary disease, and any interference with the exchange of oxygen and carbon dioxide is a potential cause of respiratory failure. Opportunities for such interference are many and include disorders of the central nervous system, chemical changes in the blood, bacterial and viral invasion, and physical changes in the organs of respiration, often caused by the inhalation of material irritating to the lungs, bronchial tubes, and pleurae.

# VOCABULARY

*I especially approve of a physician who in the acute diseases, those which are fatal to the majority of the people, shows a certain amount of superiority over the others. These acute diseases are those which the ancients have named pleurisy, pneumonia, phrenitis, intense fever, and other diseases in which fever is generally unremitting.* [Hippocrates, *Regimen in Acute Diseases* 5]

| GREEK OR LATIN WORD | COMBINING FORM(S) | MEANING |
|---|---|---|
| | *ALVE-* | hollow, cavity[1] |
| | AMYGDAL- | [almond] tonsil |
| *thrakos* | ANTHRAX, ANTHRAC- | coal; anthrax |
| | AUX-, -AUXE,[2] -AUXIS[2] | increase, grow |
| | BACTER(I)- | [small staff] bacterium |
| *bronchos* | BRONCH(I)-[4] | [windpipe] bronchus |
| *kapnos* | CAPN- | [smoke] carbon dioxide |
| *kokkos* | COCC-, -COCCUS | [berry] coccus (a type of bacterium spherical in form) |

---

[1]Words in the diminutive form alveol- refer to alveoli of the lungs or to dental alveoli.

[2]These forms indicate nouns meaning increase in size, abnormal growth of a part.

[3]*bacterium* (plural, *bacteria*) is the Latinized form of this word.

[4]Words in bronchi- are from *bronchia*, the bronchial tubes.

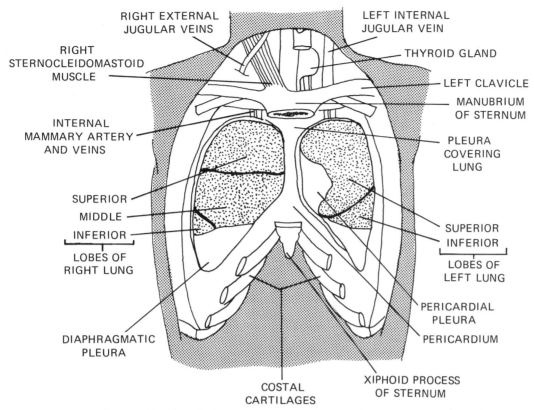

RIGHT EXTERNAL JUGULAR VEINS

LEFT INTERNAL JUGULAR VEIN

RIGHT STERNOCLEIDOMASTOID MUSCLE

THYROID GLAND

LEFT CLAVICLE

MANUBRIUM OF STERNUM

INTERNAL MAMMARY ARTERY AND VEINS

PLEURA COVERING LUNG

SUPERIOR
MIDDLE
INFERIOR
LOBES OF RIGHT LUNG

SUPERIOR
INFERIOR
LOBES OF LEFT LUNG

PERICARDIAL PLEURA

PERICARDIUM

DIAPHRAGMATIC PLEURA

COSTAL CARTILAGES

XIPHOID PROCESS OF STERNUM

FIGURE 9. Anterior view of lungs and adjacent structures. (From *Taber's Cyclopedic Medical Dictionary*, ed 14. FA Davis, Philadelphia, 1981.)

| *konis* | CONI-, KONI- | dust |
|---|---|---|
| *diploos* | DIPLO- | double |
| *labium* | *LABI-* | lip |
| *larynx, laryngos* | LARYNX, LARYNG- | larynx |
| *paresis*[1] | PARESIS | slackening of strength, paralysis |
| *pharynx, pharyngos* | PHARYNX, PHARYNG- | [throat] pharynx |
| *physa* | PHYS- | air, gas |
| *pleura* | PLEUR- | [side] pleura |
| *pnein* | PNE- | breathe |
| *pneuma, pneumatos* | PNEUM(AT)- | [breath[2]] air, gas |
| *pneumōn* | PNEUM(ON)- | lung |
| *sidēros* | SIDER- | iron |
| *spīrāre, spīrātus* | *SPIR(AT)-* | breathe |
| *staphylē* | STAPHYL- | [bunch of grapes] uvula, palate; staphylococci (microorganisms that cluster together like a bunch of grapes) |
| *streptos* | STREPT- | [twisted] streptococci (microorganisms that form twisted chains) |

[1]The Greek noun *paresis* is formed from the preposition *para* and the verb *hienai*, send, throw. The compound verb *parienai* meant to let fall, and, thus, the noun *paresis* meant a falling *or* slackening (of strength).

[2]Cf. The Gospel According to Mark 3:29: Whoever blasphemes the Holy Spirit *(Pneuma Hagion)* can never be forgiven. [King James version]

| | | |
|---|---|---|
| *sudor* | SUD(OR)- | sweat[1] |
| *thōrax, thōrakos* | THORAX, THORAC- | chest cavity, pleural cavity, thorax |
| *trachys*[2] | TRACH(E)-, TRACHY- | [rough] trachea |

## ETYMOLOGICAL NOTES

*In the winter occur pleurisy, pneumonia, colds, sore throat, coughs, pains in the side, chest, and hip, headache, dizziness, and apoplexy.* [Hippocrates, *Aphorisms* 23]

*Those with hemorrhoids do not get pleurisy or pneumonia.* [Hippocrates, *Humors* 20]

**Diphtheria** (Greek *diphthera*, leather) takes its name from a leatherlike false membrane composed of pus and dead cells that forms on the mucous surfaces of the air passages, a characteristic manifestation of this disease. It is caused by the diphtheria bacterium (*Corynebacterium diphtheriae*, named from the Greek *korynē*, club, from the clublike shape of these bacteria), which lodges in the throat and trachea, producing exotoxins that are lethal to the cells of the adjacent tissues. As the disease progresses, the leatherlike false membrane that is formed causes difficulty in swallowing. If the air passages become sufficiently swollen, **tracheostomy** or **intubation**[3] may be necessary to provide a respiratory passage.

**Emphysema**, a condition often resulting from constant exposure to a cold, damp environment, cigarette smoking, or the polluted air of cities, takes its name from the Greek *emphysēma*, a swelling or inflation, from the verb *emphysan*, inflate. The significance of the name is that the disease is characterized by a morbid excess of air in the lungs and lung tissue. The lung loses its normal elasticity, and inspiration and expiration require muscular effort. **Alveolar hypoventilation** then results in impaired gas exchange leading to **hypoxia** and **hypercapnia**. Cardiac function may become disturbed, and death is not infrequent.

**Influenza**, or grippe, is a contagious respiratory viral infection, symptoms of which are **coryza** (inflammation of the nasal mucous membrane with profuse discharge from the nostrils, that is, cold in the head), cough, sore throat, myalgia, and general weakness. It takes its name from the Italian *influenza*, influence (literally, a flowing upon). In the sixteenth century and later, the name was applied to various epidemic diseases which were afflicting the people of Italy and which were thought of as descending from the heavens. In 1743 it was applied specifically to the disease that we know as influenza, then called *la grippe*, which was ravaging western Europe.

**Pneumonia** is an inflammatory disease of the lungs causing acute infection of the alveolar tissues. There are many causes of pneumonia, some bacterial and some nonbacterial. The most common of the bacterial agents are **pneumococci**, **staphylococci**, and certain of the **streptococci**. The disease can also be caused by certain other bacilli, as well as by viruses and fungi. The type that is called pneumococcal or lobar pneumonia usually invades one or more entire lobes of the lung. Signs of pneumococcal pneumonia include chill, cough, chest pain, and expectoration of rust-colored sputum, and, as the disease progresses, tachypnea, tachycardia, and cyanosis. Prompt treatment with antibiotics, usually one of the penicillins, generally insures early recovery.

**Penicillin** was the term applied by Sir Alexander Fleming (1881–1955), the British bacteriologist, to a culture of certain molds that he observed to inhibit the growth of bacteria. These

---

[1]In some few words the form -sud- means fluid: exude, exudate, transudate.

[2]The word trachea is from Greek *tracheia*, the feminine form of this adjective, originally modifying the feminine noun *artēria*, artery. The ancient Greek anatomists thought that the arteries carried air (*aēr*, air, *tērein*, guard); the windpipe, the trachea, was called the "rough artery" because of the rings of cartilage that surround it.

[3]Latin *tubus*, pipe, tube.

molds were two of the genus *Penicillium*, named from the Latin *penicillum*, brush, because of the brush- or broomlike appearance of the mold under microscopy. The Latin *penicillum* is a diminutive of *penis*, the original meaning of which was tail.

**Anthrax** is a highly infectious disease caused by *Bacillus anthracis* that attacks animals, particularly cattle, horses, sheep, and goats, and it is transmitted directly to man from exposure to infected animals, their hair, hides, or waste matter. One manifestation of the disease in humans in its cutaneous (Latin *cutis*, skin) form is the eruption of reddish carbuncles (Latin *carbunculus*, diminutive of *carbō*, *carbōnis*, coal) called anthrax boils, accompanied by localized erythema, and it is from the color of this inflammation, like that of burning coal or charcoal, that the disease takes its name. Another form of this disease is inhalation anthrax, which attacks the mediastinum, causing hemorrhage and pulmonary edema.

There are a number of respiratory diseases caused by exposure to pulmonary irritants in one's occupation. Among these are **anthracosis**, a disease often suffered by coal miners, sometimes known as black lung. **Byssinosis** affects those who work in cotton mills. **Silicosis** affects those who work in granite and sandstone industries. Bronchial carcinoma can result from **asbestosis** in those who are exposed for any length of time to the fibers of asbestos. **Siderosis** affects iron and steel workers and welders.

**Tuberculosis** is a disease caused by *Mycobacterium tuberculosis*. It usually affects the respiratory system but may attack other body systems. In pulmonary tuberculosis, the commonest form of this disease, early signs are the development of lesions of the lung tissues. These lesions, collections of giant cells, are called **tubercles** (little swellings), and it is from this that the disease takes its name. Pulmonary tuberculosis is also known as **phthisis**, the name by which it was known to the ancient Greek physicians, and as **consumption**, a term used today.[1]

**Pertussis** and **streptococcal pharyngitis** are the names of the diseases commonly known as whooping cough and scarlet fever. The former is caused by the bacillus *Bordetella pertussis*, first isolated and identified by Jules Bordet, a Belgian physician and bacteriologist (1870-1961), and Octave Gengou, a French bacteriologist, and named after Bordet.

The Greek word *sphygmos*, pulse, had an alternate form *sphyxis*, most commonly found in the word **asphyxia**, lack of a pulse. This word has now come to mean a condition caused by insufficient intake of oxygen. Its adjectival form, **asphyctic**, means either pertaining to, affected with, asphyxia, *or* without a pulse. Modern derivatives of Greek *asphyxia* include **asphyxiate**, **asphyxiated**, and **asphyxiation**, all having to do with suffocation—lack of oxygen.

# EXERCISE 11

A. Analyze and define each of the following words.

1. alveolar _____

2. amygdaline _____

3. amygdalopathy _____

4. anthrax _____

5. anthracosis _____

---

[1]*In the case of those who are afflicted with phthisis, if the sputum that is coughed up has an offensive smell when poured upon hot coals, and if the hair falls from the head, the disease will be fatal.* [Hippocrates, *Aphorisms* 5.11]

6. auxesis _____

7. auxin _____

8. myelauxe _____

9. bacterioclasis _____

10. bacteriolysin _____

11. bacteriophage _____

12. bacteriostasis _____

13. bronchiarctia _____

14. bronchiolectasis _____

15. bronchostaxis _____

16. coccus _____

17. meningococcemia _____

18. coccobacilli _____

19. diplococcemia _____

20. diplosomia _____

21. coniosis _____

22. dermatoconiosis _____

23. hypocapnia _____

24. labiomycosis _____

25. laryngismus _____

26. otorhinolaryngology _____

27. paresis[1] _____

_____

[1]pronounced par'-e-sis

152

28. vasoparesis _____

29. pharyngismus _____

30. glossopharyngeal[1] _____

31. rhinopharynx _____

32. oropharynx _____

33. nasopharynx[2] _____

34. physocele _____

35. physometra[3] _____

36. peripleuritis _____

37. pneometer _____

38. apnea _____

39. pneumatocardia _____

40. pneumatosis _____

41. pneumocentesis _____

42. pneumoencephalography _____

43. pneumoventriculography _____

44. pneumonocele _____

45. pneumocephalus _____

46. pneumonolysis _____

47. sideroderma _____

48. siderofibrosis _____

_____

[1]Greek *glōssa*, tongue

[2]Latin *nasus*, nose

[3]Greek *mētra*, uterus

49. spirogram _____

50. aspirate _____

51. expiration _____

52. perspiration _____

53. respiration _____

54. staphyle _____

55. staphylococcus _____

56. staphylolysin _____

57. staphylotoxin _____

58. peristaphyline _____

59. streptococci _____

60. streptococcicosis _____

61. streptococcolysin _____

62. sudor _____

63. exude _____

64. transudate _____

65. antisudorific _____

66. thoracalgia _____

67. thoracoceloschisis _____

68. thoracentesis _____

69. pyohemothorax _____

70. tracheocele _____

71. tracheotome _____

154

72. tuberculostatic[1] _____

B. Give the word derived from Greek elements that means each of the following. Verify your answer in the medical dictionary.

1. Suture of a lung _____

2. The presence of staphylococci in the blood _____

3. Deficiency of iron (in the body) _____

4. A specialist in the study of the ear and larynx _____

5. Bronchial hemorrhage _____

6. Any disease of the thorax _____

7. Hernia of the pharynx _____

8. Increased carbon dioxide (in the blood) _____

9. Fissure of the uvula _____

10. Resembling bacteria _____

11. Across (use the Latin form) the thorax _____

12. Behind (use the Latin form) the pharynx _____

13. (Surgical) puncture of the pleural cavity _____

14. Paralysis (of the muscles of the walls) of the bronchial tubes _____

15. Instrument for cutting (out) a tonsil _____

C. Give a clear, concise definition of each of the following italicized words.

1. *Silicosis*[2] must be differentiated from the following conditions which may present a nodular pattern by chest x-ray: miliary tuberculosis, *siderosis* of welders and grinders, hemosiderosis as in mitral stenosis, carcinomatosis, sarcoidosis, beryllosis, Hodgkin's disease, lipoid *pneumonitis*, fungus infections such as histoplasmosis and disseminated pulmonary actinomycosis, and miliary calcifications of undetermined origin.

---

[1]Latin *tūber*, lump, swelling; words in tubercul- are from the Latin diminutive noun *tuberculum* and usually refer to either the disease tuberculosis or to tubercles, the characteristic lesions resulting from infection by tubercle bacilli. See the Etymological Notes to this lesson.

[2]Latin *silex, silicis*, any hard stone; flint

2. *Byssinosis*[1] exists in both acute and *chronic*[2] forms.

3. Asbestosis is a diffuse fibrous *pneumoconiosis* resulting from the inhalation of asbestos dust. The fibrosis, which is due to direct mechanical irritation, appears first peribronchially and in the alveolar septa and then becomes diffuse.

4. Congenital *bronchiectasis* arises from agenesis of the *alveoli*, with resultant cystic dilation of the terminal *bronchi*.

5. In bronchiectasis, hemoptysis is frequent and may appear early before purulent *exudate* is manifest or may occur repeatedly during the chronic course of the disease.

6. *Pneumococcal pneumonia* should be suspected in any patient with a history of acute febrile illness associated with chill, chest pain, and cough, especially with expectoration of viscid, rusty sputum.

7. Hemolytic *streptococcal pneumonia* is usually a fulminant infection, especially when accompanied by *bacteremia* and/or empyema.

8. Many serious disorders (including measles, *diphtheria*,[3] streptococcal *pharyngitis*, meningitis, and whooping cough) cause catarrhal upper respiratory symptoms at their onset and therefore may be confused with *coryza*.[4]

---

[1]Greek *byssinos*, made of cotton, from *byssos*, cotton
[2]Greek *chronos*, time
[3]Greek *diphthera*, leather; see the Etymological Notes to this lesson.
[4]Greek *koryza*, mucous discharge from the nostrils

9. Diagnosis of *influenza*[1] may be confirmed by isolation of virus from garglings during early stages of the disease, or by serologic tests during the acute and convalescent phases.

10. Severe dyspnea, always the most obvious symptom, should immediately warn the physician of the possibility of laryngotracheobronchitis. Laryngeal diphtheria should be excluded by direct *laryngoscopy* and culture of secretions.

11. Intercostal neuritis may be confused with *pleurisy*,[2] but rarely is the pain related to respiration and there is no friction rub.

12. The infectious agents of *psittacosis*[3] of birds and man and pneumonitis of mice and cats have been placed in a group that one designates as mycoplasmas. The clinical picture of psittacosis is strikingly similar to that of influenza, atypical pneumonia, or typhoid fever.

13. *Staphylococcal* pneumonia should be suspected in patients with influenza who develop recurrence of fever, dyspnea, or cyanosis.

14. *Tracheostomy* rather than laryngeal *intubation*[4] is indicated when respiratory obstruction is imminent or when the dyspnea is so great as to exhaust the patient.

15. The *tubercle*[5] bacillus enters the body by inhalation, ingestion, or direct inoculation.

---

[1]Latin *fluere*, flow; see the Etymological Notes to this lesson.

[2]The word pleurisy takes its form from French *pleurésie*, which was derived from Latin *pleurisis*, which, in turn, was borrowed from Greek *pleuritis*.

[3]Greek *psittakos*, parrot

[4]Latin *tubus*, pipe, tube

[5]Latin *tūber*, lump, swelling; see the Etymological Notes to this lesson.

16. The diagnosis of *emphysema* can be inferred from the barrel-shaped chest with its increased dimensions, especially the anteroposterior diameter, the elevation of the ribs, and the wide epigastric angle.

17. Chronic *bronchitis* frequently accompanies *pulmonary fibrosis*, obstructive emphysema, chronic asthma,[1] pulmonary tuberculosis, bronchiectasis, chronic sinusitis, and kyphoscoliosis, and also bronchial constriction, compression, or narrowing from any cause.

18. *Mediastinitis*[2] may produce pain and swelling of the neck, crepitation[3] of soft tissues, or chest pain. There is usually leukocytosis, change in the voice, fever that rapidly rises to high levels, and sometimes dysphagia. Severe cardiovascular collapse is common.

19. A sudden sharp pain on one side of the chest followed immediately by dyspnea, particularly if it occurs during physical exercise or straining at the toilet, must arouse the suspicion of a *pneumothorax*. If there was no previous tuberculosis, a so-called spontaneous pneumothorax with good prognosis but the possibility of recurrence has to be considered. Respiratory lagging of the affected side of the chest, less depressed intercostal spaces on this side, distant, absent, or *amphoric*[4] breath sounds make the diagnosis certain even before x-ray.

20. Vital capacity is defined as the largest volume of air which the patient can exhale voluntarily, beginning with the lungs fully inflated. In practice this is most conveniently measured by having the patient exhale fully into a *spirometer.*

---

[1]*There is a condition in the region of the throat for which the Greeks have different names, depending upon its intensity. In all, it consists in difficulty of breathing, which when moderate and without any choking is called* dyspnea. *When it is more severe, so that one cannot breathe without a noisy gasping, it is called* asthma. [Celsus, *De Medicina* 4.8.1]

[2]See page 147, footnote 2 for the etymology of mediastinum.

[3]Latin *crepitāre, crepitātus,* crackle

[4]New Latin *amphoricus,* an adjective formed from Latin *amphora* from Greek *amphoreus,* a shortened form of *amphiphoreus,* a jar with two handles (*amphi- + pherein*)

21. *Atelectases* by bronchial obstruction are the most common cause of physical signs in bronchogenic carcinoma. Atelectases of different origin, however, must be borne in mind, although they will hardly be confused with those of malignant nature. Aspiration of foreign bodies, but also injuries to the chest and general anesthesia, especially in abdominal surgery, may cause pulmonary atelectases.

22. The common cause of *hypoventilation*[1] is referred to as obstructive lung disease. This includes asthma, emphysema, and restriction of lung expansion or recoil by pleural effusion, *pneumothorax*, extreme obesity, or loss of elasticity in chronic cardiac congestion or varying degrees of pulmonary fibrosis such as forms of *pneumoconiosis*.

23. Dizziness may be the complaint of patients who are merely experiencing the effects of chronic alkalosis due to over-breathing. *Hyperventilation* associated with metabolic acidosis may also cause lightheadedness as an early symptom.

D. Answer each of the following questions.

1. What is *dentoalveolitis*?[2]

2. What is the meaning of *anthracemia*?

3. What are *trichobacteria*?

4. What is the meaning of *orthopnea*?

---

[1]Latin *ventilāre, ventilātus*, expose to air
[2]Latin *dens, dentis*, tooth

5. What are *hemokonia?* *otoconia?* What is a *koniometer?*

6. What is the *Diplococcus pneumoniae?*

7. What is the *labium inferius[1] oris?* the *labium superius oris?*

8. What is a *sudatorium?*[2]

9. What is *trachyphonia?*

10. What is *streptoleukocidin?*

11. What is *asphyxia?*[3]

12. What is a *binaural stethoscope?*[4]

---

[1]The neuter nominative singular of Latin adjectives in *-ior* ends in *-ius.*
[2]from the Latin verb *sudāre, sudātus,* sweat
[3]See the Etymological Notes to this lesson.
[4]Greek *stethos,* chest

13. Why is the disease *tuberculosis* so named?[1]

14. What is the *laryngeal reflex*?

15. What is *myxadenitis labialis*?

16. What is *Staphylococcus pyogenes aureus*?[2]

17. What is meant by *tachyauxesis*?

## DRILL AND REVIEW

E. The meaning of each of the following words can be determined from its etymology. Determine the meaning of each and verify your answer in the medical dictionary.

1. alveolitis
2. alveolobronchiolitis
3. amygdaloid
4. amygdalolith
5. periamygdalitis
6. onychauxis
7. trichauxis
8. dermatauxe
9. hepatauxe
10. nephrauxe
11. bactericidal
12. bacteriolysis
13. bacteriostatic
14. bacteriotoxin
15. bacteriophagia

16. bronchadenitis
17. bronchorrhea
18. bronchoblennorrhea
19. bronchomycosis
20. bronchoscopy
21. bronchiostenosis
22. bronchiogenic
23. bronchiolitis
24. peribronchiolitis
25. acapnia
26. eucapnia
27. diplobacterium
28. diplococcus
29. diplocephaly
30. antistaphylococcic

---

[1] See the Etymological Notes to this lesson.
[2] Latin *aureus*, golden (colored), from *aurum*, gold; *pyogenes* has been formed on the analogy of Greek adjectives in -*ēs*.

31. antistreptococcic
32. pneumococcemia
33. coniology
34. labioplasty
35. macrolabia
36. laryngalgia[1]
37. laryngectomy[2]
38. laryngopharyngectomy
39. laryngitic
40. laryngocentesis
41. endolaryngeal
42. perilaryngitis
43. laryngoplasty
44. laryngostenosis
45. angioparesis
46. hemiparesis
47. myoparesis
48. pharyngomycosis
49. pharyngoamygdalitis
50. pharyngotome
51. pharyngemphraxis
52. retropharyngitis
53. rhinopharyngitis
54. nasopharyngitis[3]
55. physocele
56. emphysematous
57. pleuralgia
58. pleurectomy
59. pleuritic
60. pachypleuritis
61. pleuropericarditis
62. pneograph
63. dyspnea
64. hyperpnea
65. oligopnea
66. bradypnea
67. tachypnea
68. polypnea
69. eupnea
70. pneumatorachis
71. pneumatotherapy
72. hydropneumopericardium
73. pyopneumopericardium
74. pneumarthrosis
75. pneumohypoderma
76. pneumonectomy
77. pneumomalacia
78. pneumonomelanosis
79. pneumonomycosis
80. pneumonopexy
81. pneumonectasia
82. siderogenous
83. sideropenia
84. sideropenic
85. spirograph
86. spirometry
87. aspiration
88. inspiration
89. staphylectomy
90. staphyledema
91. staphylitis
92. staphyloncus
93. staphylodermatitis
94. streptodermatitis
95. streptococcemia
96. streptosepticemia
97. sudoresis
98. sudation
99. sudoriferous
100. sudorific
101. antisudoral
102. hydrosudotherapy
103. stethoscopy[4]
104. thoracodynia
105. thoracobronchotomy
106. thoracocentesis
107. thoracomyodynia
108. thoracoplasty
109. thoracoschisis
110. hemothorax
111. cholohemothorax
112. pneumopyothorax
113. hydropneumothorax
114. schistothorax
115. stenothorax
116. tracheobronchoscopy
117. tracheoaerocele
118. tracheomalacia
119. tracheopyosis
120. tracheoschisis
121. tracheoscopy
122. trachitis
123. endotracheitis
124. laryngotracheitis
125. laryngotracheotomy

---

[1]Pronounced lar-in-gal′ gee-a

[2]Pronounced lar-in-jek′ toe-me

[3]Latin *nasus*, nose

[4]Greek *stethos*, chest

# THE DIGESTIVE SYSTEM

*There is but one entrance, the mouth, for the various kinds of food. But what is nourished is not one single part, but many, and they are widely separated. And so, do not be surprised at the great number of organs which Nature has created for the purpose of nutrition.* [Galen, *On the Natural Faculties* 1.10.23]

Every part of the body needs nutrition in order to maintain its ability to function and to repair and replace damaged cellular tissue. The cells receive their nutrition from the circulating blood which carries the utilizable material from digested food in the intestine to all parts of the body. When the cells receive this digested food, it is changed into other compounds for use by the body. This is called **metabolism** and involves two processes: **anabolism**[1] and **catabolism**.[2] **Anabolism**, the constructive phase of metabolism, is the process by which simple substances are converted into complex substances and then into protoplasm—that is, the conversion of nonliving material into living cellular material. **Catabolism**, the destructive phase of metabolism, is the process by which complex substances are converted into simpler substances, usually accompanied by the release of energy. It is the sum of anabolism and catabolism that maintains, builds up, and repairs the cellular structure of the body and provides the energy for the body to function properly. All of this is dependent upon nutrition.

Nutrition is achieved in the body through the various processes of ingestion, digestion, absorption, and metabolism. The first three of these processes take place in the alimentary tract. This passage begins at the mouth and ends at the anus, where undigested, unabsorbed, and inutilizable wastes are eliminated from the body. Ingested food is softened by mastication and by the addition of saliva. There are three pairs of glands which secrete and supply saliva: the parotid, the submandibular, and the sublingual. The masticated, moistened, and softened food, called a bolus, is swallowed, a process called **deglutition**, and passes through the pharynx into the esophagus. A thin structure of membranous cartilage called the epiglottis folds over the larynx during deglutition to prevent food from entering the larynx and into the respiratory passage. The esophagus, also called the gullet, is a tube about ten inches long whose only function is to convey food to the stomach. At the juncture of the esophagus and the stomach is a muscle called the cardiac sphincter or constrictor, as it lies at the entrance to the upper orifice of the stomach called the cardia, so named because of its proximity to the heart. The purpose of this sphincter muscle is to prevent the reflux of food into the esophagus. Failure of this muscle to relax and allow the passage of food into the cardia of the stomach creates a condition known as **achalasia**, also called cardiospasm. If the cardiac sphincter malfunctions and food does regurgitate into the esophagus, the irritation to the esophageal mucosa from the gastric acid causes the distress that we call heartburn or **pyrosis**.

---

[1]Greek *ana-*, up

[2]Greek *kata-*, down

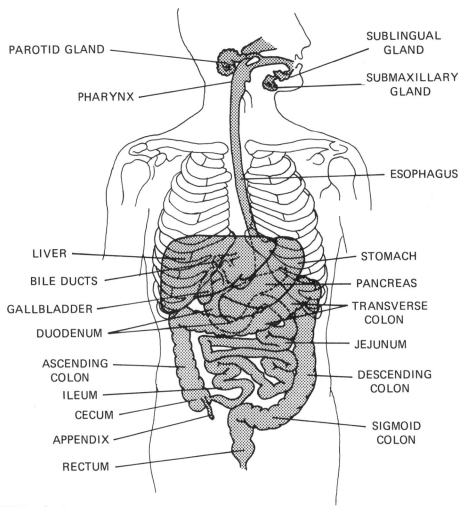

FIGURE 10. **The digestive system. (From** *Taber's Cyclopedic Medical Dictionary,* **ed 14. FA Davis, Philadel-phia, 1981.)**

Most of the organs of the alimentary tract lie in the area known as the abdominopelvic cavity, which is lined with a serous membrane called the peritoneum. The outer surface of this membrane is called the **parietal**[1] peritoneum, and the inner surface covering the visceral organs is called the **visceral** peritoneum. Inflammation of this membrane is the condition known as peritonitis. Each portion of the alimentary canal lying within the enclosure of the peritoneum is attached to the posterior wall of the body by a double fold of peritoneal membrane known as the **mesentery.** Individual mesenteries are named from the specific organ to which each is attached, as, for example, the **mesogastrium,** the **mesoduodenum,** and so forth. Two other double folds of the peritoneum, called the omenta (plural of omentum), lie between the stomach and two other of the abdominal viscera: one, the greater omentum, or *omentum majus,* is attached to the colon, and the other, the lesser, or *omentum minus,* is attached to the liver. Organs of the abdominal cavity that are not held in position by mesenteries but lie behind the peritoneum are called retroperitoneal organs, as, for example, the kidneys.

Food, still undigested, enters the stomach through the cardiac sphincter, and it is here that proteins are digested as the food is attacked by pepsin, the chief enzyme of gastric juice, and by hydrochloric acid. The mass of digesting food, called **chyme,** is propelled forward to the lower end of the stomach, the pylorus. The force that propels food through the digestive tract from the esophagus to the anus is **peristalsis,** an involuntary wavelike series of contracting and relaxing

---

[1]See page 147, footnote 1.

164

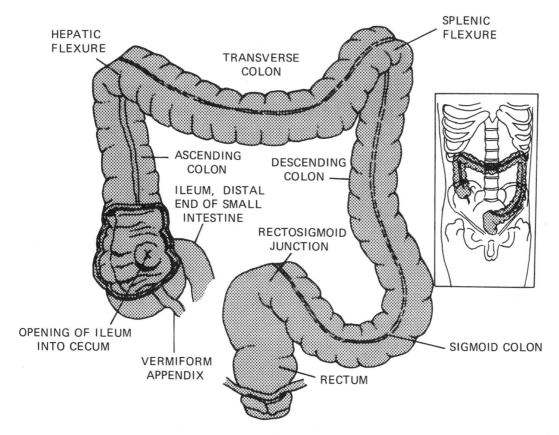

FIGURE 11. The colon. (From *Taber's Cyclopedic Medical Dictionary,* ed 15. FA Davis, Philadelphia, 1985.)

motions of the walls of the organs through which the digesting and digested food pass. At the juncture of the stomach and the duodenum is the pyloric sphincter which is normally closed, but which relaxes and opens to allow partially digested food to pass through when it is ready to leave the stomach and when the duodenum is ready to receive it.

The duodenum is the first of three divisions of the small intestine. The other two are the jejunum and the ileum. It is here that the process of digestion is completed. When fats enter the duodenum, the gallbladder sends bile through the bile duct to emulsify the fat. Bile has been manufactured in the liver and sent through the hepatic duct to the gallbladder to be stored until fatty substances enter the duodenum, when it is released. Bile and other juices, including pancreatic juice and juice from the intestine itself, *succus entericus,* complete the process of digestion. It is in the small intestine that the nutrients of digested food pass into the blood stream. The mucous lining of the small intestine contains thousands of minutely small projections called villi (plural of villus), and these villi contain a network of capillaries which carry the nutrients from the digested food to the arterial capillaries which then unite with the venous capillaries to join the venules and venous system. The lymphatic vessels also receive their lymph fluid within these tiny villi.

The residue of the digested food passes through the ileocecal sphincter into the large intestine, which consists of the cecum, the colon, and the rectum, which ends at the anal opening. The colon itself consists of four segments: the ascending colon, the transverse colon, the descending colon, and the sigmoid colon. In addition to these organs is the appendix, a dead-end tube which extends from the cecum. It has no known function and makes itself known only when it becomes inflamed, a condition that we call appendicitis. The large intestine functions to form fecal matter from the waste food after digestion, lubricate it with mucus, absorb water from it, and carry it to the colon and the anal area. There are two anal sphincters: the first, or internal, is involuntary, while the second, or external, is voluntary.

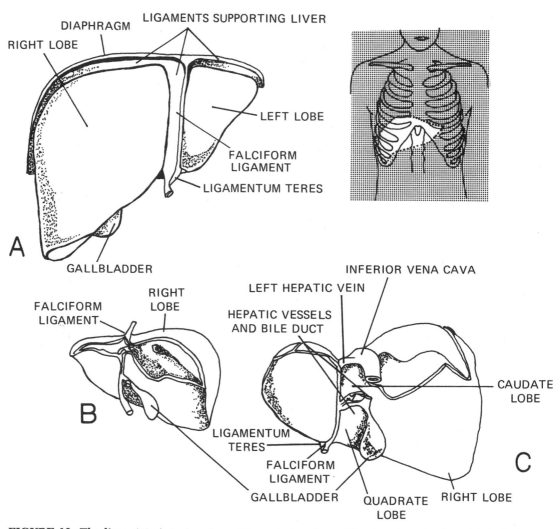

FIGURE 12. The liver. *(A)*, Anterior view; *(B)*, posterior view; *(C)*, view from back and below. (From *Taber's Cyclopedic Medical Dictionary*, ed 15. FA Davis, Philadelphia, 1985.)

The liver is one of the vital organs of the body, and one of its essential services is to produce bile which is carried through the hepatic ducts to the gallbladder for storage. Bile is not only stored in the gallbladder but becomes concentrated by absorption of water. If the bile becomes too concentrated, minerals in the bile may precipitate and form gallstones. If one or more of these concretions is carried into the bile duct and blocks that passage, preventing bile from entering the small intestine, the excess bile may enter the blood stream and cause the condition known as **jaundice**.[1]

Bile is carried from the liver by the left and the right hepatic ducts which unite to form the common hepatic duct. This vessel branches off into the cystic duct which carries bile to the gallbladder to be concentrated and stored until needed for digestion, and then carries it off to the small intestine. Inflammation of any of these ducts, the left or right hepatic ducts and the cystic duct, is known as **cholangitis**. X-ray examination of any of these ducts is known as **cholangiography**; surgery on these ducts is called **cholangiotomy**.

When leaving the gallbladder enters the common hepatic duct; as it descends into the duodenum this vessel is now called the common bile duct, and the Greek word *dochos*, receptacle, is used in naming it. Thus, inflammation of the common bile duct is called **choledochitis**. As this duct is about to enter the duodenum it is joined by the pancreatic duct carrying pancreatic

---

[1]For the etymology of this word, see the Etymological Notes to Lesson 3.

digestive enzymes. Control over the entry of bile and the pancreatic juices is exercised by a muscle called the sphincter of Oddi, named after Ruggero Oddi, a nineteenth-century Italian physician. If concretions form in the gallbladder (gallstones), the condition is known as **cholelithiasis**. If one or more of these gallstones becomes lodged in the common bile duct, the condition is known as **choledocholithiasis**. If it becomes necessary to create a passage between the common bile duct and the small intestine, the surgical procedure called **choledochoenterostomy** is used.

The entire alimentary tract is lined with a mucus-secreting membrane called the mucosa. Inflammation or erosion of the gastric mucosa causes the condition known as **gastritis**. If the erosion is deep enough to penetrate to the outer, muscular wall of the canal, the circumscribed area of erosion is known as a peptic ulcer. The cause of peptic ulcers is obscure, but **hyperchlorhydria**, an excess of hydrochloric acid in the gastric juices, may be a contributing factor. Peptic ulcers generally occur in the stomach or duodenum but are occasionally found at the lower end of the esophagus or at the juncture of an anastomosis following a gastrectomy.

## VOCABULARY

*When the more lax intestine, which is named the colon, tends to be painful, and when the pain is nothing more than flatulence, one should endeavor to promote digestion by reading aloud and other exercises. Hot baths and hot food and drinks are helpful, but all cold foods, all manner of cold, all sweets, all kinds of beans and whatever else contributes to flatulence should be avoided.* [Celsus, *De Medicina* 1.6.7]

| GREEK OR LATIN WORD | COMBINING FORM(S) | MEANING |
|---|---|---|
| bilis | BILI- | bile |
| kardia[1] | CARDI- | cardia: (upper orifice of the stomach) |
| caecus | CEC- | [blind] cecum |
| klyzein | CLY(S)- | rinse out, inject fluid |
| kopros | COPR- | excrement |
| kreas, kreatos | CREAT- | flesh |
| dochos | -DOCH- | duct |
| duodēnī | DUODEN- | [twelve] duodenum |
| oisophagos | ESOPHAG- | esophagus |
| faex, faecis | FEC- | [sediment] excrement |
| geuein | GEUS(T)- | taste |
| gingiva | GINGIV- | gum (of the mouth) |
| glōssa | GLOSS- | tongue |
| ileum | ILE- | ileum |
| jejunus | JEJUN- | [empty] jejunum |
| liēn | LIEN-[2] | spleen |
| lingua | LINGU- | tongue |
| mesos | MES- | [middle[3]] mesentery |
| osmē | OSM- | sense of smell; odor |
| osphrēsis | OSPHR- | sense of smell |
| peptein | PEPS-, PEPT- | digest |
| proktos | PROCT- | anus |
| pylē | PYLE- | [gate] portal vein |
| pylōrus | PYLOR- | [gatekeeper] pylorus |
| rectus | RECT- | [straight] rectum |

[1]This is the Greek word for heart; it is also used to designate the upper orifice of the stomach connecting with the esophagus. It is so named because of its proximity to the heart.

[2]pronounced in two syllables: lie'-en

[3]There are some words in medical terminology in which MES- means middle: mesad, mesosternum, mesobronchitis, and so forth. Such words are not included in this text.

| | | |
|---|---|---|
| *skōr, skatos* | SCAT- | excrement |
| *sialon* | SIAL- | saliva, salivary duct |
| *sigma* | SIGM- | [sigma, the Greek letter *s*] sigmoid colon |
| *sphinctēr* | SPHINCTER- | sphincter muscle |
| *splanchnon* | SPLANCHN- | internal organ, viscus |
| *typhlos* | TYPHL- | [blind] cecum |
| *zymē* | ZYM- | [leaven] ferment, enzyme, fermentation |

## ETYMOLOGICAL NOTES

Celsus, the Roman physician of the first century A.D., had a good idea of the arrangements of the internal organs, acquired, undoubtedly, by dissection. In his discussion of these organs, after a description of the liver, he turns his attention to the digestive tract.

*These are the locations of the visceral organs. The gullet* (stomachus), *which is the beginning of the intestines, is sinewy and begins at the seventh vertebra of the spine. It joins the stomach* (ventriculum) *in the region of the precordia. The stomach, which is the receptacle of food, is comprised of two coats, and it is located between the spleen and the liver, with both of these organs overlapping it a little. There are also thin membranes by which the stomach, the spleen, and the liver are connected, and they are joined to that membrane which I have described above as the transverse septum.*

*The lowest part of the stomach turns a little to the right and narrows as it enters the top of the intestine. This entry is called by the Greeks* pylōrus *because, like a gateway, it allows through to the lower parts whatever is to be excreted.*

*From this point begins the* jejunum intestinum, *which is not folded upon itself as much. It is called the empty intestine because it does not retain what it has received, but immediately passes it along to the lower parts.*

*After that comes the thinner intestine, folded into many loops, which are connected to the more internal parts with membranes. These loops are turned toward the right, ending in the region of the hip, occupying, however, mostly the upper parts.*

*Then this intestine joins crosswise with another, which, beginning on the right side, is long, and on the left it is pervious but on the right it is not and so it is called* caecum intestinum.

*But that one which is pervious . . . bending backward and to the right, descends straight downwards to the place of excretion, and for this reason is called the* rectum intestinum.

*The omentum, which lies over all these organs, is smooth and compact at its lower part, but at the top is softer. It produces fat, which, like the brain and bone marrow, is without feeling.* [De Medicina 4.1.6–10]

The duodenum is so named because it is about the length of twelve fingerbreadths. Actually, it varies in length from 8 to 11 inches, the average being 10 inches.

**Salmonella** is a form of gastroenteritis that is produced by the ingestion of food containing one or more of the Salmonella organisms. The disease was named after the American pathologist Daniel E. Salmon (1850–1914), who first isolated the genus of these organisms.

Diverticula (Latin *di-*, apart, aside, *vertere*, turn, and *-cula*, the plural of *-culum*, the diminutive suffix) are small pouches or sacs formed by herniation of the wall of a canal or organ, occurring most frequently in the colon. The condition is known as **diverticulosis** and may present no complications. However, these pouches can become filled with digested wastes and inflamed. This condition is known as **diverticulitis**. It is often accompanied by pain and fever, and if treatment (usually with antibiotics) does not alleviate the condition, and, especially, if the inflammation spreads, surgery may be necessary, sometimes resulting in a **colostomy**.

The pancreas gland was so named because it is entirely constituted of flesh without muscular tissues. John Banister (1540–1610) in *The History of Man*, London, John Daye 1578, says of the pancreas: "This body is called Panchreas, that is, all carnous or fleshy, for that it is made and contexted of Glandulous flesh." Both Aristotle and Galen used the word *pankreas* to refer to this organ.

The word hiatus means an opening. A hernia is the protrusion of an organ or part of it through the wall of the canal or cavity in which it is normally contained. A **hiatus hernia** is the protrusion of any organ, usually the stomach, upward through the esophageal hiatus of the diaphragm, that is, the opening of the diaphragm through which the esophagus passes. More common types of hernia are umbilical, femoral, and inguinal.

The Greek noun *zymē* meant leaven (Latin *levāre*, raise), any substance which causes fermentation in bread dough, fruit juice, and so forth. Words in our terminology in zym- refer to fermentation or to the presence of enzymes. **Enzymes**, complex proteins, are catalysts (Greek *kata-*, down, *lyein*, break), agents which induce chemical changes in other substances without being altered themselves. Enzymes are found in digestive juices and act upon the mass of ingested food as it passes along the alimentary tract, causing it to be broken down into simpler compounds. Each enzyme has a more or less specific function: *ptyalin*, secreted in the salivary glands, hydrolyzes starch; *pepsin* and *rennin*, in the gastric juice, act upon proteins, and *steapsin*, an enzyme present in pancreatic juice, hydrolyzes fat. Thus, ptyalin is an amylase, or amylolytic enzyme, and steapsin is a lipase, or lipolytic enzyme. A list of the principal enzymes can be found in your medical dictionary.

A **zymogen** is a substance that develops into an enzyme or ferment. **Zymology** is the science of fermentation; **azymic** denotes the absence of an enzyme or of fermentation, and a **zymophyte** is a microorganism that causes fermentation. We read in the Scriptures of the Festival of Passover and Unleavened Bread. In the Septuagint,[1] reference is made in Exodus 29.2 to loaves of unleavened bread, *artous*[2] *azymous*, and unleavened cakes, *lagana*[3] *azyma*.

The Greek noun *sphinctēr*, from which the sphincter muscles take their name, is related to the verb *sphingein*, bind tight. Also related to this verb is the noun *sphinx*, strangler, destroyer. In Greek mythology, a dreadful calamity befell the kingdom of Thebes. A monster, the Sphinx, was sent by Hera, queen of the gods, to ravage the land. Apollodorus, the mythographer and author of *The Library*, an encyclopedic work on what we call Greek mythology—his dates are unknown, probably either first century B.C. or first A.D.—has described the Sphinx for us: She had the face of a woman, the breast, feet, and tail of a lion, and the wings of a bird. She propounded her riddle (which she had learned from the Muses) to the Thebans: What has one voice and becomes four-footed, two-footed, and three-footed? While the Thebans were pondering the riddle, she would snatch them one by one and devour them. Finally Oedipus came along and found the answer, declaring that man as an infant is four-footed, as an adult is two-footed, and as an old man gains a third foot in a staff. The Sphinx killed herself, and Oedipus was asked to wed the late king's widow Jocasta and become the ruler of the land. She, of course, unknown to both at the time, was his mother. And so begins the tragic tale of Oedipus the King.

The portal vein is formed by the union of several veins of the visceral area, and this vessel carries blood to the liver. It enters the liver at the porta hepatis, a fissure on the undersurface of the liver where the hepatic artery also enters this organ, and where the right and left hepatic

---

[1] the Greek translation of the Old Testament

[2] accusative plural of *artos*, bread

[3] plural of *laganon*, a thin broad cake

ducts leave it. In medical terminology the portal vein is referred to by the Greek word *pylē*, gate, entrance. Thus, **pylemphraxis** means an occlusion of the portal vein; if the occlusion is caused by a blood clot, the condition is called **pylethrombosis**. The word *pylē* is generally found in the plural form *pylai* in Greek, and in this form it meant the gates of a city or the entrance to an area. Perhaps the most famous of these gates in Greek history was a narrow mountain pass in the northern part of Greece, Thermopylae, the "hot gate" (*thermos*, hot), so called because of the hot sulphur springs there. It was thought of as being the northern entry into Greece and it was here that the famous battle was fought in 480 B.C. The Greek forces, after holding the pass for two days against the huge Persian army that was invading Greece from the north, were forced to abandon their position when a Greek traitor showed Xerxes, the Persian king, a way around the pass. Leonidas, the Spartan king, and 300 of his men, together with 700 Thespians, are said to have perished here while making a symbolic stand against the barbarian army.

**Botulism**, a form of food poisoning caused by eating foods contaminated with the *Bacillus botulinus*, especially prevalent in preserved meats, takes its name from the Latin word for preserved meat, *botulus*, stuffed intestine, or sausage.


# EXERCISE 12


A. Analyze and define each of the following words.

1. bilirubin[1] _____

2. bilifuscin[2] _____

3. biliverdin[3] _____

4. cardia _____

5. cardiospasm _____

6. cecopexy _____

7. cecostomy _____

8. clysis _____

9. hypodermoclysis _____

10. coprolith _____

11. coprophobia _____

---

[1]Latin *rubēre*, be red
[2]Latin *fuscus*, dark, dusky
[3]Old French *vert, verd*, from Latin *viridis*, green

12. choledochal _____

13. choledochoduodenostomy _____

14. duodenojejunostomy _____

15. esophagismus _____

16. periesophagitis _____

17. hemafecia _____

18. defecation _____

19. amblygeustia[1] _____

20. oxygeusia _____

21. gingivoglossitis _____

22. labioglossopharyngeal _____

23. baryglossia[2] _____

24. melanoglossia _____

25. ileocolic _____

26. ileocolostomy _____

27. jejunostomy _____

28. lienocele _____

29. lienomalacia _____

30. retrolingual _____

31. lingula _____

32. mesentery _____

---

[1]Greek *amblys*, dull
[2]Greek *barys*, heavy

33. mesojejunum _____

34. osmidrosis _____

35. osmodysphoria _____

36. dysosmia _____

37. hyposphresia _____

38. parosphresia _____

39. pancreatic[1] _____

40. pancreaticoduodenostomy _____

41. pepsin _____

42. eupepsia _____

43. hypopepsia _____

44. proctoclysis _____

45. proctoscopy _____

46. procteurynter[2] _____

47. pylephlebectasia _____

48. pylethrombosis _____

49. pylorus _____

50. pyloromyotomy _____

51. pylorostenosis _____

52. rectorrhaphy _____

53. colorectostomy _____

_____

[1]Greek *kreas, kreatos*, flesh; see the Etymological Notes to this lesson.
[2]Greek *eurynein*, widen; the suffix -ter indicates an instrument.

54. scatology _____

55. sialadenoncus _____

56. sialodochitis _____

57. sigmoiditis _____

58. sigmoidopexy _____

59. sphincter ani[1] _____

60. ileocecal sphincter _____

61. splanchnography _____

62. splanchnoscopy _____

63. splanchnemphraxis _____

64. typhlectasis _____

65. typhloempyema _____

66. zymogen _____

67. zymohydrolysis _____

68. zymology _____

69. zymophyte _____

70. zymosthenic _____

B. Give the word derived from Latin and/or Greek elements that means each of the following. Verify your answer in the medical dictionary.

1. Behind the cecum _____

2. X-ray examination of the bile duct _____

---

[1]Latin *anus*, anus

3. Formation of a passage between the duodenum and the (small) intestine _____

_____

4. Hernia of the esophagus _____

5. Absence of (the sense of) taste _____

6. Under the tongue (use Latin forms) _____

7. Abdominal incision into the ileum _____

8. Formation of a passage between two parts of the jejunum _____

9. Related to the spleen and kidney (use Latin forms) _____

10. Prolapse of the viscera (use Greek forms) _____

C. Give a clear, concise definition of each of the following italicized words.

1. Periodontitis is the result of the same etiologic factors (both local and systemic) as *gingivitis*, but the rate of osseous resorption is modified by the duration and severity of these factors as well as by the resistance and repair potential of the patient.

2. New techniques of *hyperalimentation*[1] by continuous IV infusion into the superior vena cava permit the use of concentrated nutrient solutions that are not tolerated by peripheral veins. Intravenous hyperalimentation, which allows achievement of the anabolic state, is used in special circumstances when prolonged parenteral feeding is needed or when the patient who cannot eat is unable to tolerate a catabolic state.

3. In addition to the peristaltic contraction, *deglutition*[2] appears to initiate an inhibitory process, which results in relaxation of the tonically contracted superior sphincter permitting a bolus of food to enter the esophagus. Primary peristalsis then closes the sphincter and moves down the esophagus, stripping it of its contents.

_____

[1]Latin *alimentum*, nourishment, from *alere*, nourish
[2]Latin *glutīre*, *glutītus*, swallow

4. Operations carried out in various gastroduodenal disorders include sections of the vagus nerve, *pyloroplasties*, gastroenterostomies, and resections of the stomach ranging from antrectomy to total removal. When a partial distal gastrectomy is performed, continuity is reestablished by anastomosing the gastric stump to the duodenum, or to a loop of upper jejunum.

5. Numerous operations have been devised to improve the drainage of pancreatic juice and thus alleviate pain and pancreatic insufficiency. Procedures advocated include *sphincterotomy*, sphincteroplasty, partial to total pancreatectomy with recent emphasis on a 95 percent resection, distal pancreatectomy with pancreaticojejunostomy, and longitudinal splitting of the pancreas with side-to-side pancreaticojejunostomy.

6. *Choledocholithiasis* is one of the three major causes of jaundice in the adult. When it follows biliary colic, is associated with fever, chills, and leukocytosis, and presents a transient, fluctuating, or recurrent jaundice with laboratory findings of biliary tract obstruction, the differential diagnosis from hepatic and pancreatic disease is usually easy.

7. Chronic diverticulitis with active perisigmoiditis or a perisigmoidal abscess may involve the urinary bladder, leading at first to dysuria and later to a sigmoidovesical fistula with pneumaturia. Occasionally, the infection spreads into the portal venous system, with the production of *pylephlebitis*, multiple liver abscesses, or both.

8. *Hiatus hernia*[1] is accepted as a common cause of dyspepsia, but little attempt has been made to examine the symptoms of hiatus hernia in physiologic terms.

---

[1]Latin *hiātus*, an opening; *hernia*, rupture

9. Esophageal obstruction may occur with carcinoma; with *strictures*[1] due to esophagitis associated with hiatal hernia or following ingestion of corrosive chemicals or foreign bodies (bones, teeth), pressure from adjacent masses (tumors, thyroid enlargement, aortic aneurysms, enlarged lymph nodes); and from mucosal webs of the esophagus, *achalasia*,[2] benign smooth muscle tumors of the esophagus, and pulsion diverticulitis.

10. Although *peptic ulcer*[3] is the most common organic cause of dyspepsia, it can be mimicked more or less accurately by a variety of disorders. Since the symptoms of these disorders are probably caused in part by a disordered motor function of the gastroduodenal segment, it is not surprising that they are at times so similar.

11. If the distinction between mechanical and paralytic *ileus*[4] is to be made accurately, the stage of the illness at which observations are being made must be kept clearly in mind. In paralytic ileus the bowel sounds are absent from onset.

12. *Macroglossia* is seen in infantile myxedema, cretinism, acromegaly, or primary amyloidosis.

13. Bisthmus may produce slate-gray deposits in the gingiva similar to the lead line in chronic plumbism. Cadmium used in electrotechnical industry may cause a similar yellow line besides chronic impairment of the respiratory tract, *anosmia*, and proteinuria.

14. *Proctosigmoidoscopy* is the method of choice for the diagnosis of diseases of the rectum and lower sigmoid. It discloses tumors, inflammatory conditions, ulcers, strictures, varicosities, hemorrhages, and even foreign bodies. Carcinoma appears as a nodular, often cauliflower-like growth with superficial ulceration, and polyps are easily recognized by their pedicle. In doubtful cases, biopsy of the growth must be done.

---

[1]Latin *stringere*, *strictus*, draw tight, press together
[2]Greek *chalan*, slacken, loosen
[3]Latin *ulcus*, *ulceris*, sore, ulcer
[4]Greek *ileos*, intestinal obstruction, from *eilein*, squeeze, twist

15. *Inspissated*[1] fecal masses are sometimes mistaken for tumors. They disappear, however, at a later examination.

16. The clinical presentation of *pancreatitis* is as variable as the setting in which it occurs, ranging from a sudden acute abdominal catastrophe with shock and cyanosis to mild episodes of deep epigastric pain and vomiting.

17. Although no direct proof can be given, it seems likely that *dyspepsia* is caused by a disturbance of gastroduodenal motility, regardless of whether the associated disorder is an ulcer in the mucosa, a malfunctioning gallbladder, coronary insufficiency, or an emotional problem.

18. *Hyperosmia* may occur in some hysterias and has been observed following drug addiction.

19. Adverse reactions to this drug include anorexia, gastric irritation, nausea, vomiting, cramping, diarrhea, constipation, intrahepatic cholestatic jaundice, and *sialadenitis*.

20. According to the medical report, the patient was suffering from an increasingly common phenomenon known as *bulimia*.[2]

21. Some victims of Gilles de la Tourette's syndrome begin to experience attacks of *coprolalia* at the time of puberty.

---

[1]Latin *spissāre, spissātus*, thicken, condense

[2]Latin *būlīmāre*, have an insatiable appetite, from Greek *bous*, bull, ox, and *limos*, hunger; that is, the hunger of an ox

D. Answer each of the following questions.

1. What is the meaning of *biliary colic*?[1] *renal colic*?

2. What is *botulism*?[2]

3. What is *salmonellosis*?[2]

4. *Clysma* and *clyster* are both names for the same procedure. What is this commonly called?

5. What is meant by the procedure called *cholelithotripsy*?[3]

6. *Fecaloma* and *scatoma* are names for the same thing. What do they mean?

7. What is the meaning of *idiopathic hypogeusia*?

8. What is the meaning of *ankyloglossia*?

---

[1]Greek *kōlikos*, painful spasm
[2]See the Etymological Notes to this lesson.
[3]Greek *tripsis*, friction, rubbing

9. What is the meaning of *phantosmia*?[1]




10. What is the *splanchnocoele*?




11. What does an *antizymotic* do?




12. The Latin verb *plicāre, plicātus* meant fold. What is the meaning of each of the following terms?

    a. plication _____

    b. gastroplication _____

    c. coloplication _____

13. The Latin verb *terere, trītus* meant rub, grind, crush. What is the meaning of each of the following terms?

    a. lithotrite _____

    b. osteotrite _____

14. The Greek verb *tribein* meant rub, grind, crush. What is the meaning of each of the following terms?

    a. histotribe _____

    b. angiotribe _____

15. What is the significance of the name of the part of the intestine called the *cecum*? _____

    _____


16. What is obcecation? _____

17. What is the meaning of *excreta*?[2] _____

---
[1]Greek *phantazein*, become visible
[2]Latin *cernere, crētus*, sift, separate

# DRILL AND REVIEW

E. The meaning of each of the following words can be determined from its etymology. Determine the meaning of each and verify your answers in the medical dictionary.

1. biligenesis
2. biligenic
3. biliary calculus
4. enterobiliary
5. bilirachia
6. cecotomy
7. cecitis
8. cecoptosis
9. cecosigmoidostomy
10. pericecitis
11. mesocecum
12. mesorrhapy
13. coloclysis
14. pleuroclysis
15. venoclysis
16. enteroclysis
17. copremesis
18. coprology
19. intraduodenal
20. coprophagy
21. choledochectasia
22. choledochoenterostomy
23. choledochoplasty
24. choledochorrhaphy
25. duodenectasis
26. duodenocholecystostomy
27. duodenogram
28. duodenohepatic
29. mesoduodenum
30. esophagalgia
31. esophagomalacia
32. esophagomycosis
33. esophagotome
34. esophagogastrostomy
35. retroesophageal
36. fecal
37. fecalith
38. fecaloid
39. pyofecia
40. hypergeusesthesia
41. parageusia
42. dysgeusia
43. hemigeusia
44. gingiva
45. labial gingiva
46. lingual gingiva
47. gingivalgia
48. gingivectomy
49. glossal

50. glossodynia
51. glossolabial
52. glossopathy
53. aglossia
54. hypoglossal
55. labioglossolaryngeal
56. megaloglossia
57. microglossia
58. pachyglossia
59. schistoglossia
60. ateloglossia
61. glossopyrosis
62. orolingual
63. faciolingual
64. melanotrichia linguae
65. lienal
66. lienitis
67. lienomyelogenous
68. ileac
69. ileitis
70. ileocolitis
71. ileostomy
72. ileoproctostomy
73. jejunoileostomy
74. jejunoileitis
75. jejunocolostomy
76. cholecystojejunostomy
77. osmesis
78. osmics
79. osmology
80. osmonosology
81. parosmia
82. hemianosmia
83. osmodysphoria
84. osphresis
85. osphresiology
86. oxyosphresia
87. anosphrasia
88. osphresiometer
89. pancreatalgia
90. pancreatoncus
91. pancreatopathy
92. pancreaticocholecystostomy
93. pancreatolithectomy
94. apepsia
95. autopepsia
96. dyspeptic
97. eupeptic
98. antipepsin

99. proctalgia
100. proctectasia
101. proctocolonoscopy
102. proctodynia
103. proctology
104. proctologist
105. proctopexy
106. proctosigmoiditis
107. periproctitis
108. proctostasis
109. ankyloproctia
110. proctorrhaphy
111. pylemphraxis
112. peripylephlebitis
113. pyloralgia
114. pylorectomy
115. pyloric stenosis
116. pyloroschesis
117. pyloroscopy
118. pylorotomy
119. cardiopyloric
120. peripyloric
121. rectostomy
122. rectoclysis
123. rectoplasty
124. rectoscope
125. rectostenosis
126. mesorectum
127. ileorectostomy
128. scatophagy
129. scatoscopy
130. sialaden
131. sialolith
132. sialoschesis
133. sialostenosis
134. angiosialitis
135. antisialic
136. asialia
137. oligosialia
138. sialoaerophagy
139. sialorrhea
140. sialemesis
141. sialogenous
142. sialine
143. sigmoidoscope
144. sigmoidoproctostomy
145. ileosigmoidostomy
146. mesosigmoid
147. perisigmoiditis
148. sphincter pancreaticus
149. sphincter choledochus
150. pyloric sphincter
151. sphincteralgia
152. sphincteroplasty
153. sphincteritis
154. sphincterismus
155. splanchnectopia
156. splanchnopathia
157. splanchnosclerosis
158. splanchnodynia
159. splanchnography
160. splanchnoscopy
161. perisplanchnitis
162. typhlitis
163. paratyphlitis
164. typhlectomy
165. typhlostenosis
166. typhloenteritis
167. typhlolithiasis
168. typhlopexy
169. typhlostomy
170. laparotyphlotomy
171. zymogenic
172. zymologic
173. zymologist
174. azymic
175. zymolysis

# OPHTHALMOLOGY

*There is a certain weakness of the eyes in which people see well in the daytime but not at all at night. This condition does not exist in women whose menstruation is regular. Those who suffer with this disability should anoint their eyeballs with the drippings from a liver while it is roasting—preferably that of a he-goat; if that is not possible, one from a she-goat; and the liver itself should be eaten.* [Celsus, *De Medicina* 6.6.38]

The globe of the eye is surrounded by three layers of tissue called tunics. The exterior tunic, the sclera, is a tough, fibrous coat forming a protective covering for the delicate nerves and membranes beneath. The anterior, visible, and transparent portion of the sclera forming about one-sixth of its total surface is called the cornea. The sclera and the cornea form one continuous coat. The anterior portion of the sclera is covered with a transparent mucous membrane, the conjunctiva, an extension of the lining of the eyelids. The portion of this membrane lining the lids is called the palpebral conjunctiva, and that covering the sclera is the bulbar conjunctiva; the loose fold connecting the two is the fornix conjunctivae (Latin *fornix*, arch).

The middle layer, a dark brown tissue, is called the uvea from its resemblance to a grape (Latin *uva*). The uvea possesses three parts: the choroid, the posterior portion extending to the point opposite the lens; the ciliary body, a thickened triangular-shaped tissue, an extension of the choroid to the base of the iris; the iris, the anterior extension of the ciliary body.

The innermost tunic of the ocular globe is the retina, an outgrowth of the optic nerve extending as far as the ciliary body where it terminates.

The exterior surface of the sclera is covered with a thin layer of tissue called the episclera which contains blood vessels to nourish the sclera. The most common of the diseases of the sclera is episcleritis. Its cause is unknown, and the inflammation usually subsides after a few days of treatment. The cornea, exposed as it is, is subject to bacterial, viral, and fungal infection, as well as to injury by a foreign body. Ulceration of the cornea is a major cause of blindness. Bacterial corneal ulcers are caused usually by either the pneumococci or the streptococci bacilli. The commonest of the viral agents to cause corneal ulcers is the herpes simplex virus. This condition is known as **herpetic keratitis.** (The herpes virus will be discussed in the Etymological Notes to this lesson.) Hypopyon, the formation of pus in the anterior chamber of the eye, is a complication of both bacterial and viral ulceration. Corneal ulceration can be caused also by avitaminosis A. Lack of vitamin A (due either to dietary deficiency or to impaired absorption and utilization from the gastrointestinal tract) can cause a hardening and drying of the epithelium throughout the body, a condition known as **xerosis.** Xerosis of the conjunctiva and cornea is called **xerophthalmia.** In corneal ulcer due to avitaminosis A, the cornea becomes soft, a condition called **keratomalacia,** and often necrotic.

The ciliary body secretes a fluid called the aqueous humor into the posterior chamber, the area behind the sides of the lens behind the iris. The aqueous humor flows into the anterior chamber and leaves the eye through one of three routes, the most important being a canal which

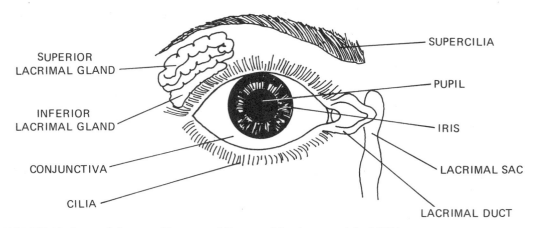

FIGURE 13. Parts of the eye. (Courtesy of Rosanne Martin, copyright 1977.)

opens at the inner corner of the anterior chamber, between the cornea and the iris, Schlemm's canal, named for Friedrich Schlemm, a German anatomist (1795–1858). Channels leading from Schlemm's canal carry the aqueous humor into the venous system. The combining form pertaining to the ciliary body of the eye is CYCL-, as in **cyclokeratitis**, inflammation of the ciliary body and the cornea. Intraocular pressure is controlled by the rate at which the aqueous humor leaves the eye through the canal of Schlemm. When, for whatever reason, the aqueous humor fails to drain normally, intraocular pressure increases. If this is allowed to go unchecked, pressure can rise high enough to cause blindness. This condition is called **glaucoma**. Infection or inflammation can cause blockage of the canal of Schlemm, but often normal drainage is impaired without infection or inflammation and for unknown causes. Glaucoma can be detected by the use of an instrument called a tonometer, which measures intraocular pressure, and can be treated with drugs and/or surgery. But extremely high pressure can cause blindness in a short time by damaging the optic nerve or by compression of the blood vessels of the retina to the point where the supply of blood is cut off.

The retina is the essential portion of the eye, as it receives visual images through the lens and transmits these images through the optic nerve to the proper receptors in the brain. The retina is composed of ten layers of cells. The first of these, the inner coating, consists of pigmented epithelial cells. The second layer consists of rods and cones, and it is these nerve receptors that respond to light. The rods control night vision (**scotopia**), and their function is dependent upon a supply of vitamin A. Thus, deficiency in this vitamin can cause night blindness (**nyctalopia**). The cones are sensitive to color, and any interference with their normal transmission of visual images can result in one or more forms of color blindness. It is thought that all colors result from mixtures of the three primary colors, red, green, and blue, and it is also thought that there are three types of cones, each sensitive to one of these primary colors. If there is a lack of sensitivity in the cones that are influenced by red, the person is said to have **protanopia**,[1] as red is the first of the primary colors. Green blindness is called **deuteranopia**.[2] Color blindness in which blue and yellow appear gray is called **tritanopia**.[3] The opposite of these conditions, the oversensitivity of the cones of either of these color groups, is thought to be the cause of visual defects in which the person sees everything either through a red haze (**erythropia**), a green haze (**chloropia**), or a blue haze (**cyanopia**). When all objects appear yellow, the condition is called **xanthopsia**.

The condition known as detached retina occurs when the rod and cone layer of the retina becomes partially separated from the pigmented epithelial layer of the retina. The upper exterior portion of the retina is the area most commonly affected, but any part may become detached. Among the causes of detachment of the retina are choroiditis, retinitis, trauma, and malignant melanoma of the choroid. But the majority of retinal detachments are due to degeneration of the

[1]Greek *prōtos*, first

[2]Greek *deuteros*, second

[3]Greek *tritos*, third

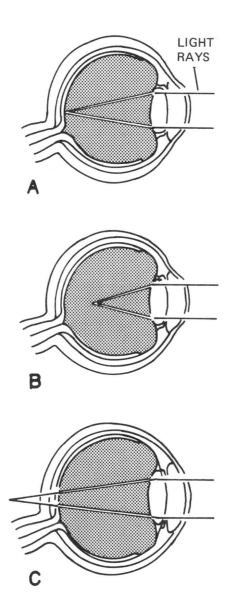

LIGHT
RAYS

A

B

C

FIGURE 14. (A), Emmetropia, light rays focus on retina; (B), myopia; and (C), hyperopia. (From *Taber's Cyclopedic Medical Dictionary,* ed. 15. F.A. Davis, Philadelphia, 1985.)

vitreous humor, the jellylike semifluid that fills the eyeball. Some cases of retinal detachment are idiopathic—that is, without any apparent cause. Correction of this condition can usually be carried out only by surgery, although minor detachments are being treated by photocoagulation, a process in which laser beams are directed through the pupil to cause a fusion of protein material from the choroid and the retina.

The lens of the eye is held in place by bands of ligament (zonula ciliaris) connecting it to the ciliary body on either side. It lies between the aqueous humor in front and the vitreous humor behind. Its purpose is to focus the light rays upon the retina by refracting them to the proper degree. When the focusing is normal, the condition is called **emmetropia**. There are three fairly common abnormalities, however, which interfere with normal focusing: **hyperopia** (hypermetropia), **myopia**, and **astigmatism**.

**Hyperopia**, or farsightedness, results from the failure of light rays to focus directly on the retina. Instead, they are diffuse when they strike the retina, focusing theoretically at some point to the rear of it. The common cause of this condition is a smaller than normal eye—that is, a shorter than normal distance between lens and retina. Hyperopia can be corrected by the use of eyeglasses with convex lenses.

**Myopia**, or nearsightedness, is caused by an eye larger than normal causing light rays to focus in front of the retina. This condition is corrected by the use of eyeglasses with concave lenses.

**Astigmatism** results when the lens or the cornea is egg-shaped rather than spherical, causing some of the light rays to focus behind the retina and some to focus in front of it. The condition is so named because those who suffer from it have difficulty in focusing their sight upon a point (Greek *stigma*).

# VOCABULARY

*It is a bad sign if hiccough and redness of the eyes follow vomiting.* [Hippocrates, *Aphorisms* 7.2]

| GREEK OR LATIN WORD | COMBINING FORM(S) | MEANING |
|---|---|---|
| *blepharon* | BLEPHAR- | eyelid |
| *chorioeidēs* | CHOROID- | [skinlike] choroid[1] |
| *korē* | COR(E)- | [girl] pupil (of the eye) |
| *kyklos* | CYCL- | circle; the ciliary body[2] |
| *dakryon* | DACRY- | tear; lacrimal sac *or* duct[3] |
| *herpēs, herpētos* | HERPES, HERPET- | [shingles] herpes, a creeping skin disease |
| *īris, iridos* | IR(ID)- | [rainbow] iris |
| *keras, keratos* | KERAT- | [horn][4] cornea |
| *oculus* | OCUL- | eye |
| *ōps* | OP(S)- | vision |
| *ophthalmos* | OPHTHALM- | eye |
| *optos* | OPT- | [seen] vision; eye |
| *phakos* | PHAC-, PHAK- | [lentil] lens |
| *xēros* | XER- | dry |

# ETYMOLOGICAL NOTES

*If the winter is dry and the winds are from the north, and if the spring is rainy and the winds are from the south, the summer will be laden with fever and will cause ophthalmia and dysenteries.* [Hippocrates, *Airs, Waters, and Places* 10]

The word *glaukōma*[5] was used by Aristotle, Galen, and others to indicate the condition of opacity of the lens of the eye that we call cataract. The earliest examples of the word glaucoma in English mean cataract, and it was not until 1705 that the difference between a true glaucoma and ordinary cataract was recognized in dissection by the French physician Pierre Brisseau. The term **glaucoma**, as now used, refers to the condition of increased intraocular pressure and takes its name from the fact that the optic disk, the area of the retina where the optic nerve enters,

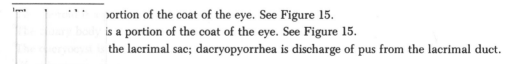

portion of the coat of the eye. See Figure 15.

is a portion of the coat of the eye. See Figure 15.

the lacrimal sac; dacryopyorrhea is discharge of pus from the lacrimal duct.

[5]Greek *glaukos*, gleaming, gray

186

changes its hue from its natural pink to a light gray color on account of atrophy caused by the increased pressure. It is this progressive atrophy of the optic disk that causes blindness in absolute glaucoma, the final stage of this disease.

The ultimate etymology of the medical term **cataract** is uncertain. The Greek *kataraktēs*, borrowed by Latin as *cataracta*, meant a waterfall, particularly a cataract of the Nile or Euphrates river. Later it came to mean a floodgate, as in the description of the Flood in Genesis 7.11: "In the six hundredth year of Noah's life, in the second month, the seventeenth day of the month, the same day were all the fountains of the great deep broken up, and the windows [or floodgates] of heaven were opened" [King James version]. The Hebrew word for the "windows of heaven" is *'arubot* and was translated in the Septuagint by *kataraktai*, and in the Vulgate by *cataractae*. These *'arubot* are also the "windows from on high" in Isaiah 24.18:

> *And it shall come to pass, that he who*
> *fleeth from the noise of the fear shall fall*
> *into the pit; and he that cometh up out of*
> *the midst of the pit shall be taken in the*
> *snare: for the windows from on high are*
> *open, and the foundations of the earth do*
> *shake.* [King James version]

It is uncertain whether the Greek *kataraktēs* is from *katarassein*, dash down, or from *katarrhēgnynai*, break in pieces. The first use of the word in its modern medical sense seems to have been by the French physician Ambroïse Paré (1510–1590) in a treatise in which he refers to a *cataracte* of the eye. Perhaps Paré had in mind the idea of a cataract being a sort of gate that shut out the light. The modern surgical method for treatment of cataract by removal of the lens was introduced by the French surgeon Jacques Daviel (1696–1762). His method was explained in an article in the Annals of the Royal Academy of Surgery (Paris), *Sur une nouvelle methode de guérir la cataracte par l'extraction du cristallin*, in 1753.

The herpes virus takes its name from the Greek *herpēs*, shingles, an acute inflammatory eruption of the skin or mucous membrane, a term that was used by Hippocrates in this sense. The noun *herpēs* is derived from the verb *herpein*, move slowly, creep, probably from the slow advance of the inflammation on the body. Pliny, in writing of ulcers and their treatment, says, "There is an animal which the Greeks call *herpes* by means of which all creeping ulcers are healed" [*Natural History* 30. 39.116]. It is not known what Pliny is referring to here, as the Greek word meant only the inflammatory disease. He may have meant some sort of snake, as the Latin noun *serpens, serpentis* (from the verb *serpere*, creep) meant a serpent or snake. The etymological identity between the Latin and Greek verbs *serpere* and *herpein*, both meaning creep, would not have been lost on Pliny. Cognate[1] words in Latin and Greek, if they show an initial *s-* in Latin show an initial "h" sound (the so-called rough breathing) in Greek; compare Latin *sēmi-* and Greek *hēmi-*, half; Latin *sex* and Greek *hex*, six; Latin *sudor*, sweat, and Greek *hydor*, water, and so forth. The name for the acute infectious skin disease herpes zoster comes from the Greek noun *herpēs*, plus the Greek *zōstēr*, belt. Herpes zoster is more commonly called shingles, from the Latin verb *cingere*, to gird, with a noun *cingulum*, a belt, formed from this verb. The word entered English through Old French *chengle*, with the alternate forms *cengle* and *sangle*. This skin infection was named by the ancient Greek physician Hippocrates because of the serpentlike scaly eruption and inflammation that generally encircles the trunk of the body. The virus that causes herpes zoster is a parasite and can affect one at any age, although it generally makes its unwelcome appearance in adulthood. It is a refractory disease, one that resists treatment.

There would seem to be no relationship between the trachea and trachoma, the eye disease that has blinded millions of people, particularly in Asia and Africa; but both terms are from the

---

[1]Just as the vocabularies of modern French, Spanish, Italian, and the other Romance languages are derived from Latin, so the vocabularies of Latin, ancient Greek, Sanskrit, and other related ancient languages were derived from an earlier parent language, which we call Indo-European. Words in two (or more) Indo-European languages, each derived from the same presumed Indo-European word, are called cognates.

Greek adjective *trachys*, rough. The trachea is so named because of the rings of cartilage that surround it, giving that organ its characteristic rough surface. Trachoma is caused by the micro-organism *Chlamydia trachomatis* (Greek *chlamys*, cloak) and is a form of conjunctivitis. It manifests itself by the presence of follicles (diminutive of Latin *follis*, bag), small secretory sacs, which become hypertrophic and cause scarring of the palpebral conjunctiva. Ulceration of the cornea often ensues from secondary bacterial infection, and it is this that ultimately causes blindness.

Myopia, nearsightedness, does not take its name from Greek *mys*, muscle (with the combining form MY-), but from the verb *myein* meaning close *or* shut, from the characteristic squinting of those affected with myopia in an attempt to see more clearly.

The pupil of the eye was so called by the ancient Romans because the reflection seen by one looking at the pupil of another's eye appeared like a little doll (Latin *pupilla*). The Greek word *korē*, girl, doll, was used by both Hippocrates and Galen to name the pupil of the eye, and it is from this word that we get the combining form CORE-: coreometry, coreoplasty.

Galen used the word *iris* to refer to the iris of the eye, and Pliny used it to refer to a precious stone. But to the ancient Greeks and Romans, Iris was the many-hued goddess of the rainbow, the goddess who acted as a special messenger for both the king and the queen of the gods. We meet her in Vergil's *Aeneid* at the end of the fourth Book. Dido, the Phoenician queen, who, exiled from her homeland, has founded the city of Carthage in North Africa, has been deserted by Aeneas after a year of intimacy. She, in despair, attempted to take her own life by falling upon her sword. But her spirit would not leave her because Proserpina, the queen of the Underworld, had not taken a lock of hair from her head in order to permit her to enter the realms of the dead, since she was a suicide. Juno, the queen of the immortals, took pity upon her and sent Iris down to release her struggling soul from her body.

*Ergo Iris croceis per caelum roscida pinnis,*
*mille trahens varios adverso sole colores,*
*devolat et supra caput adstitit. "Hunc ego Diti*
*sacrum iussa fero teque isto corpore solvo":*
*sic ait et dextra crinem secat; omnis et una*
*dilapsus calor atque in ventos vita recessit.*

And Iris, all covered with dew, flew down
from heaven on saffron wings, trailing
a thousand colors reflected in the
rays of the sun, and stood above her head.
"As I have been ordered, I take this
offering sacred to Dis[1] and free you
from your body." So Iris spoke, and
with her hand cut the lock of hair.
All of a sudden the warmth left her,
and life faded into the winds.

(*Aeneid* 4.700–705)

# EXERCISE 13

A. Analyze and define each of the following words.

1. amaurosis[2] _____ blindness; blindness that originates with a brain problem._____

---

[1] *Dis* is another name for Pluto, the king of the underworld.
[2] Greek *amauros*, blind

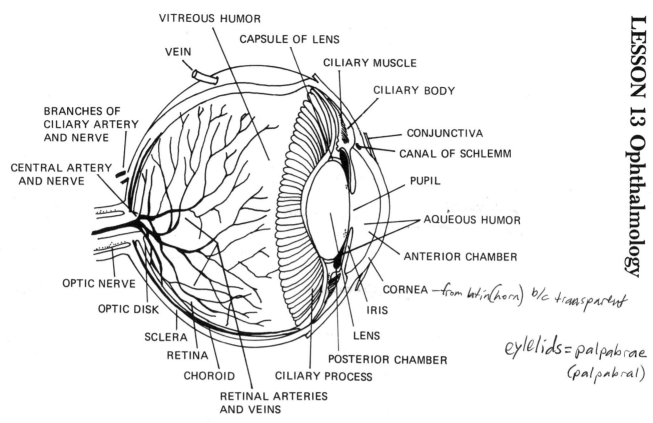

VITREOUS HUMOR
CAPSULE OF LENS
VEIN
CILIARY MUSCLE
CILIARY BODY
BRANCHES OF
CILIARY ARTERY
AND NERVE
CONJUNCTIVA
CANAL OF SCHLEMM
CENTRAL ARTERY
AND NERVE
PUPIL
AQUEOUS HUMOR
ANTERIOR CHAMBER
OPTIC NERVE
CORNEA —from latin (horn) b/c transparent
OPTIC DISK
IRIS
SCLERA
LENS
eylelids = palpabrae
(palpabral)
RETINA
POSTERIOR CHAMBER
CHOROID
CILIARY PROCESS
RETINAL ARTERIES
AND VEINS

FIGURE 15. Anatomy of the eye. (From *Taber's Cyclopedic Medical Dictionary*, ed. 15. F.A. Davis, Philadelphia, 1985.)

2. blepharism _____

3. ankyloblepharon _____*adhesion of eylids to each other.*_____

4. choroid _____

*discharging pus*
5. suppurative choroiditis _____*inflam. of the choroid membrane, discharging pus.*_____

6. corestenoma[1] _____

7. diplocoria _____

8. polycoria _____

*pus is present*
9. purulent conjunctivitis[2] _____*inflam. of the conjunctiva, with pus present.*_____

10. vernal[3] conjunctivitis _____*inflamation of the conjunctiva during the spring (season).*_____

---

[1]Note that, in the terminology of ophthalmology, many words in -oma do not designate tumors, but abnormal conditions of one kind or another.

[2]Latin *jungere, junctus*, join

[3]Latin *vernālis*, belonging to spring, from *ver*, spring

11. cyclokeratitis _____

12. iridocyclectomy _____

13. choroidocyclitis _____

14. dacryadenitis _____

15. dacryelcosis _ulceration of lacrimal sac + duct._____

16. dacryocystoblennorrhea *lacrimal sac/duct* _flow of mucous from the lacrimal sac / duct._

17. dacryohemorrhea _flow of blood in tears. (from the lacrimal sac)_

18. herpes simplex[1] _~~disease~~ dissease caused by herpes simplex 1 virus._

19. herpes facialis _facial herpes._____

20. herpes labialis _genital herpes._____

21. iridauxesis _____

22. iridectome _____

23. heterochromia[2] iridis _____

24. iridadenosis _____

25. keratorrhexis _____

26. keratoconjunctivitis _____

27. keratoleukoma _____

*how does it relate to meiosis ? → lessening of # chromosomes in a cell when it spl.ts.*

28. miosis[3] _abatement of symptoms in a dissease_____

29. binocular _____

30. monocular[4] _____

_____

[1]Latin *simplex*, simple

[2]Greek *heteros*, other

[3]Greek *meiōn*, the comparative degree of the adjective *mikros*, small

[4]Greek *monos*, single, one

31. oculogyration[1] _____

32. sinistrocularity _____

33. anisometropia _____

34. chromoptometer _____

35. orthoptic _____

36. myopia[2] _____

37. macropsia _____

38. micropsia _____

39. achromatopsia _____

40. presbyopia[3] _____

41. hypermetropia _____

42. ametropia _____

43. photopia _____

44. scotopia[4] _____

45. acyanopsia _____

46. ophthalmia neonatorum[5] _eye condition of newborns_____

47. ophthalmatrophy _____

48. ophthalmiatrics _____

49. ophthalmodesmitis _____

50. microphthalmia _____

_____

[1]Greek *gyros*, circle
[2]Greek *myein*, close, shut
[3]Greek *presbys*, old man
[4]Greek *skotos*, darkness
[5]-*ōrum* is the ending of the genitive plural for Latin second-declension nouns.

51. ophthalmostat _____

52. blepharostat _____

53. enophthalmos _____

54. optometer _____

55. optometrist _____

56. phacolysis _____

57. phacocystitis _____

58. aphakia _____

59. microphakia _____

60. xeroma _____


B. Give the word derived from Greek elements that means each of the following. Verify your answer in the medical dictionary.

1. Glandular tumor of the eyelid ~~blepharodep~~ *blepharoadenoma*

2. Measurement of the pupil (of the eye) _____

3. Pain in a lacrimal ~~gland~~ *aden* *dacryoadenalgia* _____

4. Absence of the iris *iridfreemia* (*aniridia*) _____

5. (Located) around the cornea _____

6. Fungal growth on the cornea _____

7. Vision in which all objects appear to be blue *cyanopia* _____

8. Paralysis of the eye (muscles) _____

9. Instrument for observing the lens _____

10. Ocular hemorrhage _____

C. Give a clear, concise definition of each of the following italicized words.

1. When a *scotoma*[1] appears in front of one eye, it must be due to pathologic change in the nerve or retina, most commonly hemorrhage or choroiditis.

2. Adverse reactions to this drug: anorexia, nausea, vomiting, diarrhea, dizziness, paresthesias, headache, *xanthopsia*.

3. *Dacryostenosis* with *epiphora* occurs in adults from chronic nasal infection with inflammatory obstruction of the duct. Fracture of the nose and facial bones may cause mechanical obstruction.

4. Pain, redness, and edema about the lacrimal sac, epiphora, conjunctivitis, *blepharitis*, fever, and leukocytosis are associated with acute *dacryocystitis*.

5. Photophobia, pain, *lacrimation*,[2] and gradual loss of vision are common in interstitial (parenchymatous) keratitis.

6. External *hordeolum*[3] begins with lacrimation and photophobia, a "foreign body" sensation, and pain and redness of the lid margin with a small, round, tender area of induration. Though usually localized, edema may be diffuse.

[1]Greek *skotos*, darkness
[2]Latin *lacrima*, tear
[3]Latin *hordeolus*, hordeolum, diminutive of *hordeum*, barley

7. Symptoms and signs of *iridocyclitis:* Edema of the upper lid and eye pain radiating to the temple are common symptoms. Photophobia and lacrimation may be present. Blurring of vision and transient myopia occur. The iris appears dull and swollen; brown irides become muddy, blue and gray ones greenish. The pupil may be irregular or *miotic,*[1] with adhesions between the posterior surface of the iris and the capsule of the lens (posterior synechiae).

8. Surgical exploration of orbit is indicated in unilateral *exophthalmos* if there is a palpable mass that can be biopsied; if there are x-ray changes of bone; or if progressive visual loss occurs. If there is no palpable mass, no x-ray changes, and no visual loss or corneal changes, conservative management is indicated. *Diplopia* alone is not a sufficient indication for exploration of the orbit.

9. Nutritional *amblyopia*[2] is the preferred term for the entity sometimes referred to as tobacco-alcohol amblyopia, tobacco amblyopia, or alcohol amblyopia, since they are all the same entity. Persons with poor dietary habits, particularly if the diet is deficient in vitamin B complex, may develop scotomas that are usually of constant density.

10. The management of *glaucoma*[3] is best left in the hands of the ophthalmologist, but all physicians should participate in diagnosis by making tonometry and ophthalmoscopy a part of the routine physical examination of all patients over 20 years of age.

11. When the nasociliary nerve is involved in facial *herpes zoster,*[4] as indicated by a lesion on the tip of the nose, invariably the cornea will become involved. Marked lid edema, ciliary and conjunctival injection, corneal infiltration, and pain are all present. The conjunctivitis and lid edema without keratitis are not important. Keratitis accompanied by uveitis may be severe and is followed by scarring. Glaucoma, often developing much later, is a common *sequela*[5] of ophthalmic herpes zoster.

---

[1]See page 190, footnote 3.
[2]Greek *amblys,* dull
[3]See the Etymological Notes to this lesson.
[4]See the Etymological Notes to this lesson.
[5]Latin *sequela,* that which follows, from *sequī, secūtus,* follow

12. A great deal is known about the dynamics of *aqueous humor*,[1] but the exact mechanism of production and elimination of aqueous humor is not completely understood.

13. In young patients, the danger of precipitating an attack of glaucoma by the use of *mydriatics*[2] is negligible. Before instilling mydriatics into the eyes of older people it is a wise precaution to estimate the depth of the anterior chamber by oblique illumination with a flashlight. If the anterior chamber is shallow, mydriatics can precipitate acute-angle-closure glaucoma (an ophthalmic emergency).

14. *Emmetropia* is best thought of as an ideal rather than a normal condition, since almost all adults have some degree of refractive error.

15. *Hyperopia* may be caused by shortness of the eyeball or weakness of the refractive power of the cornea or lens. Physiologic hyperopia is present at birth in about 80 percent of children. This is due to the shortness of the eye, partially compensated for by the fact that the infant lens is more convex than the adult lens. About 5 percent of children are born *myopic*,[3] and about 15 percent emmetropic. During the years from about age 2 to about age 25, there is a slight gradual decrease in hyperopia. Most persons remain slightly hyperopic during adulthood.

16. Cyclopentolate hydrochloride produces *cycloplegia* almost as profound as can be achieved with homatropine.

17. *Exotropia* is less common than esotropia, particularly in infancy and childhood. Its incidence increases gradually with age. Not infrequently, a tendency to divergent strabismus beginning as exophoria progresses to intermittent exotropia and finally to constant exotropia if no treatment is given.

[1]Latin *aqua*, water; *humor*, fluid
[2]Greek *mydriasis*, dilation of the pupil
[3]Greek *myein*, close

18. The cause of migraine is unknown, but evidence indicates a functional disturbance of cranial circulation. Prodromal symptoms (for example, flashes of light, *hemianopsia*, paresthesias) are probably due to intracerebral vasoconstriction, and the head pain to dilation of extracerebral cranial arteries; that is, those of the dura or scalp.

19. With mild degrees of astigmatism there may be no symptoms, or merely *asthenopia* with prolonged use of the eyes. The person with astigmatism tries to achieve a clearer image by rapidly changing focus, with resultant fatigue. With greater degrees of astigmatism, clear visual acuity may not be possible at any distance.

20. Correction of errors of refraction and other causes of eyestrain will relieve the simple forms of *nystagmus*.[1] Certain forms of nystagmus can be corrected by surgical transplantation of eye muscles.

21. *Mydriasis*[2] may be part of a more extended oculomotor paralysis, central or peripheral, or it may indicate an *ophthalmoplegia interna* without involvement of external eye muscles.

22. *Trachoma*[3] is the most common human disease of any kind; approximately 500,000,000 people suffer from it.

D. Answer each of the following questions.

1. What is the meaning of *isoiconia*?[4]

2. What is *astigmatism*?[5]

---

[1] Greek *nystagmos*, drowsiness
[2] See page 195, footnote 2.
[3] See the Etymological Notes to this lesson.
[4] Greek *eikon*, image
[5] Greek *stigma, stigmatos*, mark, point

3. What is a *cataract* of the eye?[1]

4. What is *strabismus*?[2] *convergent strabismus*?[3] *divergent strabismus*?

   *named after Strabo, who squinted.*

5. What is the *vitreous humor*?[4]

6. The following terms are formed from Greek words found in previous lessons. What is the meaning of each of these as it is used in ophthalmology?

   (a) esophoria _____

   (b) exophoria _____

   (c) hyperphoria _____

   (d) hypophoria _____

   (e) cyclophoria _____

   (f) orthophoria *(= isophoria)* _____

   (g) esotropia _____

   (h) entropion[5] _____

   (i) ectropion[5] _____

   (j) tonometer _____

---

[1] See the Etymological Notes to this lesson.

[2] Greek *strabismos*, deviation of the visual axis

[3] Latin *vergere*, turn

[4] Latin *vitreus*, of glass, from *vitrum*, glass; *humor*, fluid

[5] The Greek suffix *-ion* in this word indicates a condition.

7. The abbreviations O.D. and O.S. are often seen on prescriptions for eyeglasses. What Latin words do these letters represent, and what do they mean?

8. What is *herpesvirus simiae*[1] *encephalomyelitis?*

## DRILL AND REVIEW

E. The meaning of each of the following words can be determined from its etymology. Determine the meaning of each and verify your answer in the medical dictionary.

1. astigmatic[2]
2. astigmatometer
3. blepharedema
4. blepharectomy
5. blepharoncus
6. blepharoplasty
7. blepharoplegia
8. blepharoptosis
9. blepharorrhaphy
10. blepharadenitis
11. ablepharia
12. macroblepharia
13. microblepharism
14. pachyblepharosis
15. schizoblepharia
16. varicoblepharon
17. iridochoroiditis
18. corectasia
19. coreometer
20. corectopia
21. coreoplasty
22. isocoria
23. anisocoria
24. dyscoria
25. dacryoma
26. stenocoriasis
27. anisoiconia[3]
28. cyclochoroiditis
29. cyclectomy
30. dacryocele
31. dacryolith
32. dacryopyorrhea
33. dacryocystalgia
34. dacryocystectomy
35. dacryocystotome
36. dacryocystorrhinostomy
37. dacryopyosis
38. herpetic
39. herpetic neuralgia
40. herpetiform
41. herpes genitalis
42. iridology
43. iridalgia
44. iridectomy
45. iridocele
46. iridomalacia
47. iridoncus
48. iridotasis
49. iridodesis
50. iridoplegia
51. iridorrhexis
52. iridemia
53. iridectropium[4]
54. iridentropium[4]
55. iralgia
56. iritis
57. keratomalacia
58. keratometer
59. keratoplasty
60. keratoscope
61. keratoscopy
62. keratotome
63. iridokeratitis
64. oculomycosis

[1]Latin *simia*, ape, monkey
[2]Greek *stigma*, *stigmatos*, mark, point
[3]See page 196, footnote 4.
[4]The Latin suffix *-ium* in this word indicates a condition.

198

65. circumocular
66. intraocular
67. retroocular
68. dextrocularity
69. hypermetropic
70. hypometropia
71. orthoptics
72. anisopia
73. chloropia
74. erythropia
75. oxyopia
76. dysopia
77. achloropsia
78. anerythropsia
79. axanthopsia
80. hyperchromatopsia
81. ophthalmology
82. ophthalmomycosis
83. ophthalmomyitis
84. ophthalmomyotomy
85. ophthalmorrhexis
86. exophthalmic
87. macrophthalmia
88. megophthalmos
89. microphthalmus
90. pyophthalmitis
91. panophthalmitis
92. ophthalmovascular
93. ophthalmography
94. hydrophthalmos
95. ophthalmophlebotomy
96. optic
97. optometry
98. optomyometer
99. phacitis
100. phacocele
101. phacoid
102. phacomalacia
103. phacometer
104. phacosclerosis
105. iridoperiphacitis
106. xerophthalmia
107. xerostomia
108. xerocheilia
109. xeroderma
110. laryngoxerosis
111. xerotic

*It is not easy for large creatures, whether animal or anything else, to reach full development in a short time. For this reason horses and similar animals, although their life span is shorter than that of humans, have a longer period of gestation. The birth of horses occurs after a year; but in humans it is about ten months. For the same reason, birth takes a long time in elephants, whose gestation period is two years because of their great size.* [Aristotle, *Generation of Animals* 777b]

## THE FEMALE REPRODUCTIVE SYSTEM

The principal organs of the female reproductive system are the ovaries, the fallopian tubes, the uterus, and the vagina. The ovaries are two almond-shaped glands lying on either side of the cavity of the pelvis whose function is the production of ova and of hormones. These hormones, among which are estrogen and progesterone, are responsible for the development and maintenance of female secondary sexual characteristics. Within each ovary are hundreds of thousands of structures called follicles (Latin *folliculus*, diminutive of *follis*, bag), each consisting of epithelial cells surrounding a primitive ovum, the oogonium, which develops into an oocyte and then into an ovum. During the normal sexual life of each woman, on an average of once every 28 days a *single* ovum matures and is released from the ovaries, a process called ovulation, occurring approximately 14 days before the next menstrual period begins. The mature ovum enters the fallopian tube and is transported toward the uterus. If sperm are present, it may become fertilized; if not, the ovum degenerates and is passed out of the body with the next period of menstruation. Shortly after the follicle expels its ovum, the mass of cells of the follicle changes into a yellowish body called the corpus luteum (Latin *corpus*, body, and *luteus*, yellow). The corpus luteum grows for about a week following ovulation, and then, if the ovum is not fertilized, it degenerates. If fertilization has taken place, the corpus luteum continues to grow for the next several weeks and then is gradually replaced by connective tissue.

The two fallopian tubes, also called oviducts (often with the combining form OOPHOR- or SALPING-, from Greek *salpinx*, tube), extend from the uterus to each ovary. Their purpose is to convey the mature ovum each month from the ovary to the uterus and spermatozoa from the uterus toward the ovary. Fertilization of the ovum normally occurs in the fallopian tube. The fertilized ovum, or zygote (Greek *zygōtos*, yoked, from *zygon*, yoke), is then lodged in the uterus and develops there into the embryo. Occasionally the zygote remains in the fallopian tube, resulting in tubal, or ectopic, pregnancy.

The uterus, or womb, is a hollow, muscular, pear-shaped and pear-sized organ. It consists of three parts: the upper, or innermost portion, the isthmus, or central area, and the lowermost, the cervix uteri opening into the upper end of the vagina. The rounded upper end above the openings of the fallopian tubes is called the fundus (Latin *fundus*, base, foundation). The mucous membrane lining the inner surface of the uterus is called the endometrium (Greek *mētra*, uterus); the muscular wall of the endometrium forming its main mass is called the myometrium. During the child-producing years of a woman, from the beginning of menstruation (menarche) to the end (menopause), the uterine endometrium passes through the cyclic changes of menstruation each month. For a period of about 10 to 13 days before ovulation, the endometrium becomes swollen from the increased supply of blood that it has received to nourish the fertilized ovum. If fertilization does not take place, this excess blood is discharged in menstruation along with epithelial cells from the enlarged uterus, and the cycle starts over again. If the ovum is fertilized, the endometrium serves as its nesting place during the period of gestation. At birth the inner lining of the endometrium, the decidua (Latin *deciduus*, falling down, from *cadere*, fall), is shed. During pregnancy the decidua basilis (New Latin, from Greek *basis*, base), the portion of the endometrium lying between the chorionic membrane enclosing the fetus and the myometrium, develops into the maternal portion of the placenta. Uterine contractions assist in expelling the fetus at birth.

The vagina (Greek *kolpos, koleon,* or *elytron*) is a muscular, membranous sheath extending from the cervix uteri to the vulva, the external genitalia. It serves as a passage for the entrance of the penis in coitus, for receiving semen, and for the discharge of the menstrual flow, and it is the passageway as well for the fetus at birth.

# VOCABULARY

*If a woman is going to have a male child her complexion will be good; if a female child, her complexion will be bad.* [Hippocrates, *Aphorisms* 42]

*The embryo of a male child is usually on the right and that of a female usually on the left.* [Hippocrates, *Aphorisms* 48]

| GREEK OR LATIN WORD | COMBINING FORM(S) | MEANING |
|---|---|---|
| *agōgos* | AGOG-[1] | leading, drawing forth |
| *archē* | ARCH(I)-, -ARCHE | beginning, origin |
| *brōmos* | BROM- | stench, offensive odor |
| *cervix, cervicis* | *CERVIC-, CERVIX* | neck (of the uterus), cervix uteri |
| *kolpos* | COLP- | vagina |
| *kyein* | CYE- | be pregnant |
| *eurynein* | EURY(N)- | widen, dilate |
| *gala, galaktos* | GAL-, GALACT- | milk |
| *(g)nascī, natus* | -GN-, *NAT-* | be born |
| *gonad*[2] | GONAD- | sex glands |
| *gravidus*[3] | *GRAVID-* | pregnant |
| *hymēn* | HYMEN- | membrane; hymen |
| *hystera* | HYSTER- | uterus |
| *lac, lactis* | *LACT-* | milk |
| *mamma* | *MAMM-* | breast |
| *mastos* | MAST-, MAZ-[4] | breast |
| *mēn* | MEN- | [month] menstruation |
| *mētra* | METR-, -METRA | uterus |

---

[1]The form -agogue is from the French. Words in -agogue usually refer to agents used to promote the flow or secretion of fluids within the body. An exception to this is lithagogue, an agent used to expel calculi. See the Etymological Notes to this lesson.

[2]This word did not exist in either Greek or Latin; it is a modern formation as if from a Greek *gonas, gonados,* probably derived from the noun *gonē*, birth.

[3]This adjective, in the feminine singular form, *gravida*, was used as a noun to mean a pregnant woman.

[4]There was an alternate form of this word, *mazos,* in Greek: micromazia.

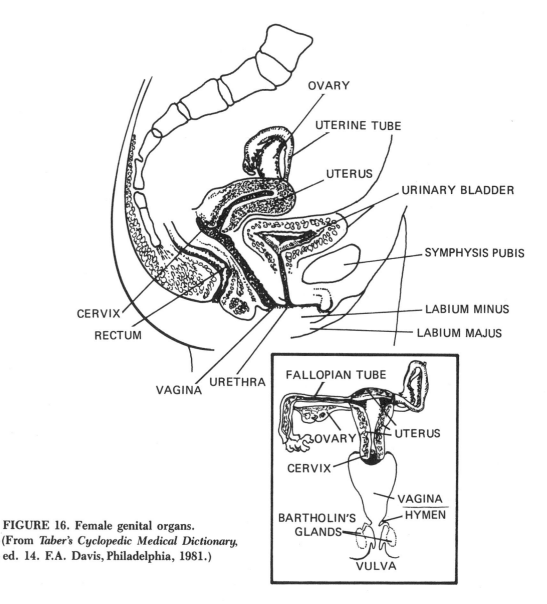

FIGURE 16. Female genital organs.
(From *Taber's Cyclopedic Medical Dictionary*,
ed. 14. F.A. Davis, Philadelphia, 1981.)

| | | |
|---|---|---|
| *oophoron*[1] | OOPHOR- | ovary |
| *ōvarium*[2] | OVARI- | ovary |
| *parere, partus* | PART-, -PARA[3] | give birth |
| *salpinx, salpingos* | SALPING-, -SALPINX | [war trumpet] fallopian tube[4] |
| *syrinx, syringos* | SYRING-, -SYRINX | [pipe] fistula, cavity, oviduct, sweat glands, syringe[5] |

[1]This compound word did not exist in Greek. It is a modern formation from Greek *ōon*, egg, and PHOR-, from *pherein*, bear, carry.

[2]This word did not exist in Latin, although there is a rare word, *ovarius*, found only in an inscription, meaning an egg-keeper, that is, one who takes charge of newly laid eggs (Latin *ōvum*). The Latin suffix *-arium* meant "a place (for something)"; thus, *ovarium*, "a place for the ovum," is a valid formation. Such formations are called New Latin.

[3]Words in -para indicate a woman who has given birth: primipara (Latin *primus*, first); nullipara (Latin *nullus*, none).

[4]The combining forms of this word are also used to indicate the eustachian tube of the ear. These words are not found in this textbook.

[5]The meaning of words in syring- and -syrinx must be determined from the dictionary.

| | | |
|---|---|---|
| *thēlē* | THEL(E)- | nipple |
| *tokos* | TOC- | childbirth, labor |
| SUFFIX | MEANING | EXAMPLE |
| **-ter** | instrument, device | colpeuryn-**ter**, metreuryn-**ter**, rhineuryn-**ter** |

## ETYMOLOGICAL NOTES

The Amazons, those legendary warrior-women of Asia Minor, were said to have one breast removed so as not to interfere with the use of the bow; thus their name: *a-mazon*. The Amazon River was discovered in 1500 by the Spanish explorer Vincente Pinzon, who named it *Rio Santa Maria de la Mar Dulce*. The first descent of the river from the Andes mountains to the sea was made in 1541 by Francisco de Orellano who renamed it the *Amazonas* from a battle that he and his followers had with a fierce tribe whose women fought alongside the men. De Orellano may have thought that these were indeed the Amazons described by the Greek writers.

The word *hymen* meant any of a variety of membranes; various writers used it to designate the pericardium, the peritoneum, the membrane that enclosed the brain, the nictitating (Late Latin[1] *nictitāre, nictitātus*, blink, wink) membrane (a third eyelid present in birds and some reptiles), parchment, and so forth. The ancients seem not to have used this word in its modern anatomical meaning.

In Greek mythology, Hymen was the god of marriage and weddings, often invoked in a wedding song *Hymenaeus*, the Hymeneal. Ovid tells us in his great poem the *Metamorphoses* of a wedding that was attended by this god, but one to which he failed to bring his customary auspices. The bridegroom and bride were Orpheus and Eurydice. Ovid tells us that the wedding torches of Hymen sputtered and smoked, but however much they were swung about they failed to blaze. In further witness of this ill-starred wedding, as Eurydice was crossing the lawn, she was bitten on the ankle by a poisonous serpent and perished on the spot. As is well known, Orpheus went to the underworld and sang so persuasively to Hades and Proserpina, the rulers there, that he was permitted to lead his bride back to the upper world. But at the last moment he failed to observe his instructions and looked back to make certain that she was following him. She was, indeed, but no sooner had he looked back than she turned and retraced her steps to the world of the dead.

> *Bracchiaque intendens prendique et prendere certans*
> *nil nisi cedentes infelix arripit auras.*
> *Iamque iterum moriens non est de coniuge quicquam*
> *questa suo (quid enim nisi se quereretur amatam?).*
> *Supremumque "vale," quod iam vix auribus ille*
> *acciperet, dixit revolutaque rursus eodem est.*

> Stretching out his arms to embrace her and to feel
> her embrace he, unhappy one, grasped nothing
> but the empty air. And now, again dying, she had
> no complaint against her husband (for what could
> she complain of except that she had been loved?).
> Uttering a last *vale*, which he could scarcely hear,
> she slipped back to that place she had just left.
> [Ovid, *Metamorphoses* 10.58–63]

---

[1]Latin of the third and fourth centuries A.D. is usually called Late Latin.

The ancient Greeks believed that women were especially susceptible to emotional disorders and that these disorders arose from the womb. Galen used the word *hysterikos*, hysterical, and seems to have used it to refer to suffering in the womb and the emotional upheaval caused by this distress. Hippocrates says, "When a woman suffers from hysterics or difficult labor, it is a good thing to sneeze" [*Aphorisms*, 5.35].

The two oviducts serve to convey the ovum from the ovary to the uterus. These tubes are called the fallopian tubes and are named for Gabriele Falloppio (1523–1562), the Italian anatomist who discovered the existence and the purpose of the ovaries and the tubes that bear his name. Like his teacher, Andreas Vesalius (1514–1564), the most important figure in European medicine after Galen and before Harvey, he was accused of vivisection of humans in his enthusiasm for research.

Another name for the fallopian tubes is the salpingian tubes, a term that is also used for the eustachian tubes of the ear (named for the sixteenth-century Italian anatomist Bartolommeo Eustachio). These two sets of tubes are named salpingian from the Greek word *salpinx, salpingos*, the war-trumpet, because of their shape.

Words in syring- and -syrinx have varied meanings in the terminology of medicine but usually refer to a cavity or hollow area, a fistula, or some other tubelike passage. The medical dictionary must be consulted to determine the meaning of these words. **Syringomyelia** is a disease of the spinal cord characterized by the development of cavities in the surrounding tissues; a **colpocystosyrinx** is a fistula between the bladder and the vagina; a **sialosyrinx** is a fistula into the salivary glands or a tube for draining these glands. **Syringosystrophy** (Greek *strophē*, turning, twisting) is a twisted condition of the oviduct. A **syringe** is an instrument for injecting fluids into body cavities and vessels, and a **microsyringe** is a syringe for injecting very small quantities of solutions.

In Greek, the *syrinx* was the shepherds' pipe, or pipes of Pan. Ovid, in the *Metamorphoses*, tells how the pipes of Pan came into existence. Once upon a time there lived on the mountain slopes of Arcadia in Greece a young, beautiful nymph of the woodland, and her name was Syrinx. One day, Pan, that rustic divinity, saw Syrinx and pursued her. The god had almost caught the unwilling nymph, when she prayed to her sisters for help. Pan did catch her; but when he held her, he found that in his arms there was only a bunch of reeds. While he sighed over his disappointment, his breath blowing through the reeds made a pleasing sound. He bound a number of the reeds of unequal length together and called them the syrinx, the pipes of Pan.

*"Hoc mihi concilium tecum" dixisse "manebit,"*
*atque ita disparibus calamis conpagine cerae*
*inter se iunctis nomen tenuisse puellae.*

"This union with you, at least, will remain,"
he said. And so pipes made of unequal
lengths of reeds joined together with wax
still keep the name of the nymph, *Syrinx.*
[Ovid, *Metamorphoses* 1.710–712]

Forms ending in -agogue entered English in the fourteenth century in words borrowed from Old French. Some of these words, like pedagogue and synagogue, had existed in Latin (*paedagogus* and *synagoga*), both of which had been borrowed from Greek (*paidagogos*, a slave who took children to school or who taught them at home, and *synagogē*, a place for gathering). The Greek words *agogos* and *agogē* are ultimately derived from the verb *agein*, lead *or* drive, which is cognate with the Latin verb *agere, actus*, with the same meanings. A **lithagogue** is an agent that expels calculi, usually from the urinary tract. A **uragogue** is an agent that expels urine—a diuretic.

The word **dyspareunia**, painful intercourse, has an interesting etymology. It is derived from an adjective, *dyspareunos* (*dys-*, unpleasant, painful, and *pareunos*, a lying with *or* beside, from *para-*, alongside, and *eunazesthai*, go to bed) that meant "ill- *or* badly mated." This adjective is found in Greek literature in a passage describing a bed.

In Sophocles' tragedy *Trachiniae* ("Women of Trachis," lines 794ff.), Hyllus, the son of the great Heracles, has come to the city of Trachis to report to Deianira, wife of Heracles, how her husband is dying just outside of the city, his flesh burned away by a magic cloak that Deianira has sent to him in ignorance of its dread powers. This cloak had been given to Deianira many years before by the centaur Nessus, whom Heracles had killed after he had attempted violence upon Deianira, then Heracles' bride. The centaur, dying, gave his cloak to the young bride and told her to give it to Heracles if she ever felt that his affections were fading. Now, many years later, Heracles has been away on a foreign conquest, and it is reported to Deianira that he is on the outskirts of the city and has requested a cloak to wear when offering sacrifices to the gods for a successful campaign. He has brought back with him as his prize the beautiful Iole, an oriental princess.

Deianira sent him the cloak that Nessus had given her, mindful of his advice. The cloak burned into the hero's flesh, and, as he lay dying in the greatest agony, he cursed his "ill-mated" wedding bed (*dyspareunon lektron*) and Deianira herself. Zeus, at length, rescued him from his suffering and brought him up to Mount Olympus as a god, with Hebe, the daughter of Zeus and Hera, as his companion for eternity.

*Epithelium* is the layer of cells that forms the epidermis of the skin and the surface of mucous and serous membranes. It was first discovered by the German histologist Jacob Henle (1809-1885). It is not clear why this type of tissue was named "membrane over the nipple" (Greek *thēlē*), except for the obvious fact that epithelial tissue does cover the nipple of the breast. *Endothelium*, the layer of cells that lines the vessels and organs of the cardiovascular system, was named by the Swiss physician Wilhelm His (1831-1904).

## EXERCISE 14

A. Analyze and define each of the following words.

1. galactagogue _____

2. hemagogue _____

3. sialagogue _____

4. archigaster _____

5. adrenarche _____

6. bromopnea _____

7. cervicovaginitis[1] _____

8. cervicobrachial _____

9. endocervix _____

10. colpocystocele _____

_____

[1]Latin *vagīna*, sheath, vagina

206

11. colpomyomectomy _____

12. colpostat _____

13. hydrocolpos _____

14. colpeurynter _____

15. colpatresia[1] _____

16. pachycolpismus _____

17. eccyesis _____

18. encyesis _____

19. galactocele _____

20. pneumogalactocele _____

21. galactostasis _____

22. galactotherapy _____

23. galactotoxism _____

24. neonate _____

25. antenatal _____

26. gonad _____

27. gonadal dysgenesis _____

28. gonadotrophic _____

29. gravida _____

30. nonigravida[2] _____

31. imperforate[3] hymen _____

[1]Greek *trēsis*, perforation
[2]Latin *nōnus*, ninth
[3]Latin *forāre, forātus*, pierce

32. hymenorrhaphy _____

33. hymenology _____

34. hysterogastrorrhaphy _____

35. hysterosalpingography _____

36. celiohysterectomy _____

37. delactation _____

38. superlactation _____

39. mammography _____

40. inframammary _____

41. mastadenitis _____

42. anisomastia _____

43. macromastia _____

44. micromazia _____

45. menostaxis _____

46. menostasis _____

47. cryptomenorrhea[1] _____

48. bromomenorrhea _____

49. metrocolpocele _____

50. metrorthosis _____

51. metreurynter _____

52. endometrium _____

_____
[1]Greek *kryptos*, hidden

53. pyophysometra _____

54. septimetritis _____

55. oophoron _____

56. oophorocystosis _____

57. perioophorosalpingitis _____

58. sclero-oophoritis _____

59. ovariohysterectomy _____

60. antepartum _____

61. parturition[1] _____

62. pachysalpingoovaritis _____

63. salpingosalpingostomy _____

64. hematosalpinx _____

65. physopyosalpinx _____

66. colpocystosyrinx _____

67. sialosyrinx _____

68. syringocystadenoma _____

69. syringosystrophy[2] _____

70. syringoma _____

71. syringomyelia _____

72. microsyringe _____

73. theloncus _____

[1]Latin *parturitiō*, *parturitiōnis*, childbirth
[2]Greek *strophē*, turning, twisting

74. polythelia _____

75. endothelium _____

76. epithelium _____

77. tocophobia _____

78. eutocia _____

79. oxytocia _____

80. intrauterine[1] _____

81. extrauterine _____

82. vaginismus _____

83. septipara[2] _____

B. Give the word derived from Greek and/or Latin elements that means each of the following. Verify your answer in the medical dictionary.

1. An agent that induces the secretion of milk (use the Latin form) _____

2. Inflammation within the cervix (uteri) _____

3. Inflammation (of the tissues) surrounding the vagina (use the Greek form) _____

4. Pregnancy in a fallopian tube _____

5. A toxic substance in milk (use Greek forms) _____

6. (Occurring) after birth (use Latin forms) _____

7. Surgical removal of an ovary (use Greek forms) _____

8. Plastic surgery of the nipple _____

9. Slow childbirth (use Greek forms) _____

10. Prolapse of the vagina (use Greek forms) _____

_____

[1]Latin *uterus*, uterus
[2]Latin *septem*, seven

11. (Agent) preventing offensive (body) odor _____

C. Give a clear, concise definition of each of the following italicized words.

1. Menorrhagia and *polymenorrhea* are not uncommon symptoms in chronic *salpingo-oovaritis* and are probably due to hormonal interference with ovulation, resulting in anovulatory cycles.

2. Except for prepubital girls, in whom urinary *gonadotropins* are normally undetectable, absence of gonadotropins in repeated specimens implies hypogonadotropism as a basis for *hypogonadism*.

3. From *menarche* to menopause, the functional units of the ovary release ova for fertilization and secrete various hormones responsible for the cyclic function of the reproductive tract and for a variety of nongenital metabolic effects.

4. Primary amenorrhea is the delay of menarche beyond age 18. In the absence of *thelarche* and *pubarche*,[1] diagnostic evaluation may begin by age 16.

5. Certain factors which predispose to *preeclampsia*[2] suggest uterine ischemia as a possible etiologic agent. Poor economic and social conditions also generally increase the frequency of complication, particularly in the young *primipara*.[3]

6. *Colposcopy* is not a substitute for cytologic examination, nor can it detect *occult*[4] neoplasia in the upper canal.

---

[1]Latin *pubēs*, *pubis*, pubic hair
[2]Greek *lampein*, shine
[3]Latin *prīmus*, first
[4]Latin *occulere*, *occultus*, cover, conceal

7. *Dyspareunia*[1] may be functional or organic or may be due to a combination of organic and emotional causes.

8. *Dysmenorrhea* rarely begins at menarche but has its onset one or more years later. It may be relieved by vaginal delivery of an infant; if not, it may continue through much of the woman's reproductive life and then fade, usually during the forties.

9. *Dystocia* may occur when the myometrial contractions are too weak or too strong, too frequent or too infrequent, too brief or too prolonged, or when they are irregular.

10. The cause of *endometrial* carcinoma is unknown, but abnormal *estrogen*[2] balance has been linked with its development.

11. *Salpingitis* may be acute or chronic and unilateral or bilateral. It accounts for 15 to 20 percent of gynecologic admission to large hospitals. It is more common in urban areas, especially where gonorrhea is prevalent, obstetric care is poor, and tuberculosis is not well controlled.

12. *Galactorrhea* is seen more often now than formerly, probably because of the wider use of tranquilizers and oral contraceptives.

13. *Hyperemesis gravidarum*[3] affects at least half of pregnant women in the USA.

---

[1]Greek *dyspareunos*, ill-mated; see the Etymological Notes to this lesson.
[2]Greek *oistros*, frenzy, madness
[3]*-arum* is the ending for the genitive plural of first-declension Latin nouns.

14. *Hymenotomy* and other plastic surgical procedures should be done only when obvious *gyna-tresia*[1] is present.

15. Primary or secondary amenorrhea may be caused by mechanical obstruction of the hymen or in the vaginal or cervical canal which prevents drainage of uterine secretions. Depending on the site and duration of obstruction, *hematocolpos*, *hematometra*, and/or hematoperitoneum may develop.

16. Observation, periodic uterine massage, and, when necessary, *oxytocin* administration, is required during the first hour.

17. *Bromidrosis* is caused by decomposition of the sweat and cellular debris by the action of bacteria and yeasts.

D. Answer each of the following questions.

1. *Hypercyesis* and *superfetation*[2] both mean the same thing. What do these words mean?

2. What is a *galactophore*? What is *galactase*?

3. What is a *tocodynamometer*?

---

[1] See page 207, footnote 1.

[2] Latin *fetus*, fetus

4. What is the meaning of *gonadotherapy*?

5. What is the meaning of *laparohysterosalpingo-oophorectomy*?

6. What is *gynecomastia*?

7. What is *xeromenia*? *xerotocia*?

8. What is the meaning of *hypovaria*?

9. What is *pseudocyesis*[1]?

10. What is the *mastoid process*?[2]

11. What is the meaning of *emmenia*?[3] What is the meaning of *emmeniopathy*? What is an *emmenagogue*?

---

[1]Greek *pseudēs*, false
[2]Latin *cēdere, cessus*, go
[3]Greek *emmēna*, menses, menstrual period

12. What is *icterus neonatorum?*[1]

## DRILL AND REVIEW

E. The meaning of each of the following words can be determined from its etymology. Determine the meaning of each and verify your answer in the medical dictionary.

1. cholagogue
2. ptyalagogue
3. lithagogue
4. helminthagogue
5. antisialagogue
6. antigalactagogue
7. hypnagogic
8. archenteron
9. archinephron[2]
10. bromidrosiphobia
11. cervical
12. endocervical
13. retrocervical
14. cervicectomy
15. cervicodynia
16. cervicovesical[3]
17. colpalgia
18. colpectasis
19. endocolpitis
20. paracolpitis
21. myocolpitis
22. colpocystitis
23. colpoxerosis
24. ankylocolpos
25. aerocolpos
26. pyocolpos
27. pyocolpocele
28. celiocolpotomy
29. colporrhexis
30. colpeurysis
31. acyesis
32. ovariocyesis
33. rhineurynter
34. osteoaneurysm
35. agalactia
36. dysgalactia
37. hypergalactia

38. oligogalactia
39. polygalactia
40. galactoid
41. galactopoietic
42. agalorrhea
43. neogala
44. antigalactic
45. galactischia
46. ischogalactic
47. galactophagous
48. galactophorous
49. natal
50. prenatal
51. neonatal
52. gonadectomy
53. gonadopathy
54. hypergonadism
55. gravid
56. pregravidic
57. multigravida[4]
58. sextigravida[5]
59. hymenitis
60. hymenectomy
61. hymenotome
62. hysteralgia
63. hysterocele
64. hysteroscopy
65. hystereurynter
66. hysteroptosis
67. hysteropexy
68. hysterotome
69. hysterectomy
70. laparohysterotomy
71. laparohysteropexy
72. ventrohysteropexy
73. panhysterocolpectomy
74. panhysterosalpingo-oophorectomy

---

[1] For words in -orum, see page 191, footnote 5.

[2] The nephron is the structural and functional unit of the kidney.

[3] Latin *vesīca*, (urinary) bladder

[4] Latin *multus*, many

[5] Latin *sextus*, six

75. lactocele
76. lactogenic
77. lactorrhea
78. lactation
79. hyperlactation
80. lactotoxin
81. lactiferous ducts
82. mammary
83. retromammary
84. mammectomy
85. mammoplasty
86. amastia
87. hypermastia
88. hypomastia
89. polymastia
90. mastitis
91. mastopathy
92. acromastitis
93. mastatrophy
94. mastadenoma
95. mastectomy
96. masthelcosis
97. mastochondroma
98. mastography
99. mastoncus
100. mastorrhagia
101. mastauxe
102. paramenia
103. amenorrhea
104. algomenorrhea
105. hypermenorrhea
106. hypomenorrhea
107. oligomenorrhea
108. menometrorrhagia
109. metralgia
110. endometritis
111. perimetritis
112. parametrium
113. parametritis
114. phlebometritis
115. pyometritis
116. exometritis
117. hydrometra
118. pyometra
119. hydrophysometra
120. pneumohydrometra
121. physohematometra

122. metromalacia
123. metrostenosis
124. metrotome
125. metrofibroma
126. metroptosis
127. metroplasty
128. metrectasia
129. metreurysis
130. metrostaxis
131. metratrophia
132. oophoralgia
133. oophororrhagia
134. oophoropathy
135. oophorauxe
136. oophoropexy
137. pyosalpingo-oophoritis
138. laparohystero-oophorectomy
139. hysterosalpingo-oophorectomy
140. ovoid
141. oviferous
142. ovarialgia
143. ovariocele
144. ovariocentesis
145. ovariectomy
146. ovariorrhexis
147. mesovarium
148. ovariosalpingectomy
149. salpingo-ovariectomy
150. perisalpingoovaritis
151. pachysalpingitis
152. myosalpingitis
153. hydrosalpinx
154. pyosalpinx
155. nulliparous
156. multipara
157. sextipara
158. oviparous
159. viviparous[1]
160. athelia
161. thelalgia
162. thelitis
163. thelorrhagia
164. endotheliolysin
165. endotheliotoxin
166. epithelioma
167. polytocous

---

[1]Latin *vivus*, living, alive

216

*If a carbuncle forms on the penis, it should first be bathed with water through a syringe. Then it should be burned with a salve made of copper ore mixed with boiled honey, or with fried sheep's dung mixed with honey. When the carbuncle falls off, use the same salve for ulcers in the mouth.* [Celsus, *De Medicina* 6.18.5]

## THE MALE REPRODUCTIVE SYSTEM

The principal organs of the male reproductive system are the testes (plural of testis) or testicles, the epididymides (plural of epididymis), the duct system, the penis, and accessory glands. In general, it is the function of the male reproductive system to manufacture sperm cells, or spermatozoa, and to convey these to the reproductive organs of the female through copulation. The two testes, the male gonads, are ovoid glands located in the scrotum which produce spermatozoa and the male hormone, testosterone. Each testis is divided into numerous lobules, each containing one to three seminiferous tubules within which spermatogenesis takes place.

The epididymis is a small structure located on the posterior surface of each testis consisting of a coiled mass of ducts enclosed within the tunica vaginalis. Spermatozoa are stored here until released in ejaculation. From the epididymis the sperm pass into the vas deferens, sometimes called the ductus deferens; the two seminal vesicles, located on either side of the prostate, secrete a mucoid substance which they empty into the vas deferens at ejaculation. The prostate gland secretes a thin, opalescent, alkaline fluid which is also added to the spermatozoa at this time. The thick, viscid fluid containing the spermatozoa and the mixed product of the accessory glands, the prostate and the seminal vesicles, is called semen. At ejaculation, semen passes into the ejaculatory duct, a short, narrow tube formed by the union of the vas deferens and the excretory duct of the seminal vesicles, and from here into the urethra, a canal that extends from the bladder to the tip of the penis, which serves as the passage for both urine and semen.

The epithelium of the seminiferous tubules of the testes can be destroyed through damage or disease. Inflammation of the testes, bilateral orchiditis (Greek *orchis, orchidos,* testis), from mumps may cause sufficient degeneration to result in sterility. Another cause of sterility can be increased temperature of the testes inhibiting spermatogenesis, and it is thought that the reason for the testes being located outside the body in the scrotum is to keep their temperature below that of the body. In addition to this, the scrotum is supplied with sweat glands which aid in keeping the testes cool in warm temperatures.

During the development of the male fetus, the testes are lodged within the body. Sometime before birth, in the late stages of gestation, the testes descend into the scrotum. Occasionally this descent does not take place, or it occurs incompletely so that one or both testes remain within the abdomen or somewhere along the line of descent. This is called **cryptorchidism.** Spermatogenesis

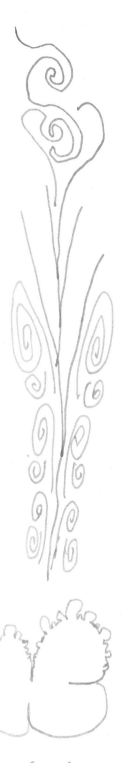

is not possible in a testicle that remains within the body, due, perhaps, to the destruction of epithelium from the heat of the body. Thus, operations are frequently performed to relocate in the scrotum the hidden testes. Such an operation (suturing the testicle to the tissue of the scrotum) is called **orchiorrhaphy** or **orchidopexy**.

In the usual quantity of semen ejaculated there is a total of some 400,000,000 sperm, any *one* of which is capable of fertilizing the ovum of the female. For reasons not understood, the ejaculate must contain this large number of sperm in order for a single one to find and fertilize the ovum. When the sperm count falls substantially below 50,000,000 infertility usually is the result.

## THE URINARY SYSTEM

The kidneys are a pair of organs lying on the left and right side of the upper abdominal cavity behind the peritoneum. Their function is to filter wastes from the blood and to maintain the proper acid-alkaline balance of the blood. End products of metabolism include the following: (1) those from proteins, mostly nitrogenous substances such as urea and uric acid; (2) detoxified material from the liver, such as drugs, antibiotics, alcohol, and other toxins; (3) all substances in the circulating blood that are present in amounts greater than needed, such as sugar, alkalines, and acids; (4) excess water.

On the medial side of each kidney is an indentation, the hilus, into which enter three structures: the renal artery, the renal vein, and the ureter. The renal artery, after entering the hilus, branches into smaller arteries which, in turn, branch into arterioles. These arterioles enter the nephrons of the kidney. The nephron is the functional unit of the kidney, and there are about one million nephrons in each kidney. Within each nephron there is a cluster of capillaries called the glomerulus. The walls of these glomeruli comprise collectively what is called the glomerular membrane. Blood plasma passes through this membrane, with blood cells and most of the protein excluded. The fluid that passes through the glomerular membrane is called the glomerular filtrate. This filtrate contains the metabolic wastes and other substances in excess of amounts needed by the body for its proper functioning. But the glomerular filtrate also contains substances that the body does need, such as the small amount of protein that is not filtered out by the glomerular membrane, as well as glucose and certain salts and acids, and these substances must be returned to the circulating blood. Still within the nephron, the glomerular filtrate passes through a series of passages called tubules, and, as it does, all but a small portion of it is reabsorbed into the blood, first through the capillaries of the nephron, and then into the venous system and into the renal vein. The portion of glomerular filtrate that does not re-enter the circulating blood is made up of waste material, and these wastes enter the large end of a funnel-shaped cavity in the hilus of the kidney called the renal pelvis. This fluid is now urine, and it passes out of the renal pelvis into the ureter to be carried to the bladder.

As the urine enters the ureters—there is one ureter leading from each kidney[1]—it is forced along its way by peristaltic contractions occurring at varying intervals from a few seconds to a few minutes. The urine enters the bladder through the ureteric orifices which open to allow passage of the urine and then close to prevent a reflux. Any impairment of the passage of urine from the kidneys to the bladder can result in stagnation of the urine with consequent precipitation of various calcium compounds which can accumulate into calculi, or kidney stones, in the ureters or, more commonly, in the pelvis of the kidney.

Urine is stored in the bladder until the volume reaches a certain amount, when the internal and the external urethral sphincters open to allow it to pass through the urethra. Emptying of the bladder by the passage of urine through the urethra is called micturition.[2]

---

[1]*Two veins, white in color, lead from the kidneys into the vesica; they are called by the Greeks ureters because they think that it is through them that the urine descends and flows into the vesica.* [Celsus, *De Medicina* 4.1.10]

[2]Latin *micturīre, micturītus*, urinate

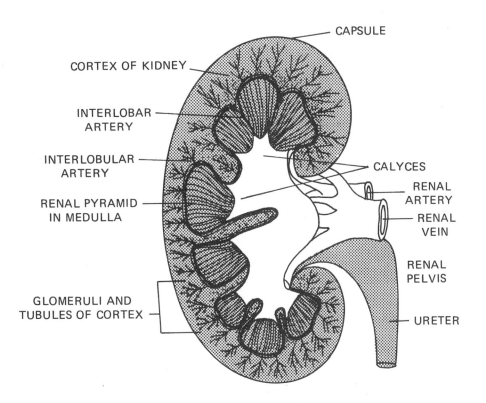

FIGURE 17. Longitudinal section through middle of kidney. (From *Taber's Cyclopedic Medical Dictionary*, ed. 14. F.A. Davis, Philadelphia, 1981.)

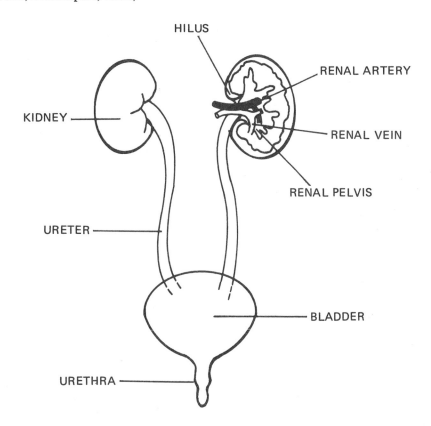

FIGURE 18. The kidneys and bladder. (Courtesy of Rosanne Martin, copyright 1977.)

# DISORDERS OF KIDNEY FUNCTION

Any kind of damage to the kidney that will impair its ability to cleanse the blood of metabolic wastes and toxins will result in abnormal kidney function, or renal insufficiency. Some disorders are congenital. **Bilateral renal agenesis** results in death within a few days after birth. Unilateral agenesis is not necessarily fatal, as one kidney is sufficient to sustain life.

Complete loss of function, acute renal failure, can result, often immediately, from kidney damage due to any number of causes. Among these are destruction of the cells of the tubules of the nephrons (tubular necrosis) from the toxic effect of various poisons, such as carbon tetrachloride and mercury, the latter often entering the body through the ingestion of fish from contaminated waters; crushing injury to the kidneys; shock, from burns or other injury, resulting in failure of the heart to pump blood in sufficient amounts to fill the needs of the various organs of the body, causing renal ischemia; interruption in the flow of blood through the nephrons due to stoppage of the tubules of the nephron caused by a mismatched blood transfusion. The reaction from transfusion of mismatched blood usually causes hemolysis, destruction of the erythrocytes, with the resultant release of abnormally large amounts of hemoglobin from the disintegrated red cells. The hemoglobin molecule is small enough to pass through the pores of the glomerular membrane, and the result is a heavy concentration of hemoglobin in the glomerular filtrate. It is thought that either this abnormally large amount of hemoglobin precipitates and blocks the normal passage of blood through the tubules of the nephron, or that the hemoglobin releases a vasoconstrictive agent that inhibits the flow of blood into the tubules. In either case, the result is the same: renal failure.

The immediate result of acute renal failure is a rapid concentration of urea, uric acid, potassium, and other undesirable substances in the blood. Failure to excrete nitrogenous wastes in the urea and uric acid causes the condition known as **uremia**, or **azotemia**. Failure to excrete potassium causes the condition called **hyperkalemia**.

Streptococcal infection, particularly in the respiratory tract, can result in acute glomerular nephritis, or **glomerulonephritis**. It is not the infection itself that causes any damage to the kidneys, but the glomeruli become inflamed in a reaction to the antibodies that are formed to combat the infection. The exact cause of this inflammation is not clearly understood, but the leukocytes that swarm in large numbers to combat this inflammation partially or totally block the normal passage of blood through the glomerular membrane, often rupturing the membrane, allowing erythrocytes to pass into the glomerular filtrate. All of this causes malfunction of the nephrons in varying degrees, sometimes resulting in acute renal failure. Usual symptoms of glomerulonephritis are **oliguria, hematuria, albuminuria**, and **edema**. Prompt treatment with an antibiotic, usually penicillin, to combat the glomerular inflammation will generally halt the disease within two or three weeks. But glomerulonephritis destroys large numbers of nephrons, and repeated attacks can lead to chronic glomerulonephritis, with continued destruction of the nephrons and eventual renal failure and death.

Inflammation of the renal pelvis is called **pyelitis**, but the disease invariably extends into the body of the kidney itself, the renal parenchyma. The proper term for the disease, when it affects both the pelvis and the body of the kidney, is **pyelonephritis**. Almost any pyogenic bacterium can cause this disease, which usually responds promptly to antibacterial therapy. Sometimes it is desirable to obtain an x-ray view of the movement of blood through the renal veins. This procedure, called an **intravenous pyelogram**, or IVP, involves injecting a radiopaque substance through the renal vein and taking a series of x-rays to observe its progress. An IVP may reveal calculi, lesions, or deformities in the pelvic area.

One of the most common causes of renal insufficiency is arteriosclerosis, often caused by atherosclerosis, fatty deposits in the walls of the arteries, followed by hardening of the fatty deposits and blockage of the vessels. As a result of sclerosis of the renal arteries, ischemia occurs, with consequent necrosis of the affected areas.

A disease concomitant with chronic renal insufficiency is anemia. It is thought that erythropoietin, a substance that stimulates the production of red blood cells in the bone marrow, is secreted in the kidneys. Insufficient kidney function results in insufficient erythropoietin production, with a consequent diminution in the number of erythrocytes. The exact mechanism of the production of erythropoietin is not fully understood, but renal insufficiency is usually accompanied by anemia.[1]

# THE ARTIFICIAL KIDNEY—RENAL DIALYSIS

In cases of kidney damage so severe that these organs cannot function efficiently enough to prevent fatal toxicity of the blood, resort can be made to renal dialysis. The artificial kidney operates on the same principle as the human kidney, but the filtering process is done outside the body. The functional unit of the artificial kidney is a porous membrane of cellophane that allows all of the blood to permeate it except erythrocytes and proteins. The circulating blood is withdrawn from the body from the radial artery of the arm and pumped through the "kidney," where it passes through the membrane, leaving behind red cells and proteins. Once through the membrane, the plasma passes into a liquid called the dialyzing fluid, which contains most of the constituents of normal plasma except the waste products of metabolism, principally urea. The toxic wastes in the plasma diffuse into the dialyzing fluid and remain there when the plasma, now rid of most of the waste matter, is returned through the membrane and into the body through the saphenous vein in the thigh, or some other suitable vein. To prevent coagulation of the blood in the artificial kidney, heparin is infused into the blood before it enters the dialysis machine; to insure proper coagulation after the blood re-enters the body, an agent to counteract the effects of the heparin is added to it.

# DIABETES MELLITUS

Diabetes mellitus, or sugar diabetes, is a chronic, incurable disease characterized by the inability, in varying degrees, to metabolize carbohydrates. This is due to inadequate production and secretion of insulin by the beta cells of the islets of Langerhans, clusters of cells in the pancreas (named after Paul Langerhans, a German pathologist, 1847–1888). Manifestations of the disease are elevated blood sugar (**hyperglycemia**) and sugar in the urine (**glycosuria**), and the symptoms of it include **polydipsia, polyuria**, loss of weight (despite polyphagia), fatigue, and pruritus (itching), especially in the genital region. When the course of diabetes is allowed to advance without proper treatment, nausea, vomiting, dyspnea, and delirium lead to deep coma resulting in death.

In many patients the only treatment required is a well-balanced diet, low in calories for those who are obese. Tests for blood sugar (glucose) should be made frequently, and if glucose concentration remains high in the blood and urine, it may be necessary to administer insulin. The isolation of insulin in 1921 by Doctors Frederick G. Banting, Charles H. Best, and James R. Macleod (for which Doctors Banting and Macleod were awarded the Nobel prize for medicine in 1923) has made it possible for diabetics to lead a normal life.

Insulin is thought to act as a stimulant for the intracellular transport of glucose into tissue cells, affecting the utilization of sugar in the cell by increasing its conversion to glycogen and fat and its oxidation to carbon dioxide and water; thus, diminished production of insulin leads to decreased carbohydrate utilization, with consequent hyperglycemia. The basic cause of the failure of the beta cells of the pancreas to secrete an adequate amount of insulin is unknown but may be due to inflammation of the pancreas, or invasion by malignant cells, or to a genetic disorder.

The Greek word *diabētēs* is found in the medical writings of Galen and of Aretaeus, both of the second century A.D., and is from the verb *bainein*, go, walk, pass, and means "a passing through," a reference to the immoderate passage of urine affecting those who have this disease.

---

[1]See page 236, footnote 3.

# VOCABULARY

| GREEK OR LATIN WORD | COMBINING FORM(S) | MEANING |
|---|---|---|
| *aktis, aktinos* | ACTIN- | [ray] radiation |
| *agra* | -AGRA | [hunting[1]] (sudden) pain, gout |
| *cortex, corticis* | *CORTIC-, CORTEX* | [bark, rind] outer layer (of an organ) |
| *kry(m)os*[2] | CRY(M)- | icy cold |
| *kryptos* | CRYPT- | hidden |
| *glykys* | GLYC- | sugar |
| *lagneia* | -LAGNIA | abnormal sexual excitation or gratification |
| *orchis, orchios* | ORCHI(D)-,[3] ORCH(E)- | testicle |
| *philein* | PHIL- | love; have an affinity for |
| *pyelos* | PYEL- | renal pelvis |
| *sēmen, sēminis* | *SEMIN-* | [seed] semen |
| *sperma, spermatos* | SPERM(AT)- | [seed] sperm, semen |
| *thyreos* | THYR-[4] | [shield] thyroid gland |
| *ouron* | UR- | urine,[5] urinary tract, uric acid[6] |
| *ourētēr* | URETER- | ureter |
| *ourēthra* | URETHR- | urethra |
| *vesīca*[7] | *VESIC-* | (urinary) bladder |
| *zōon* | ZO-[8] | animal, organism |

# ETYMOLOGICAL NOTES

The word kalium, the chemical name for the element potassium, was formed from the Arabic word *qali*, the name of the plant (now known in English as saltwort) from the ashes of which potash was made. Sir Humphry Davy (1778–1829) first separated potassium from potash, which

---

[1]The Greek word *agra* meant hunting or the catching of game; there was a word *podagra* which meant a trap for animals; this word later came to mean a disease of the feet of animals, and then gout, a painful, inflamed condition of a joint, in humans. Formations in English use this word as a suffix, as in odontagra, toothache (especially from gout), arthragra, acute pain in the joints, and so forth. The term podagra is used today to mean gout, especially of the foot or large toe.

[2]There were two forms of this word in Greek: *kryos* and *krymos*, with the same meaning.

[3]The combining form ORCHID- is used as if from a genitive case *orchidos*; the *-d-* dropped out of this word in the Greek language, leaving the genitive case *orchios*, with an alternate form *orcheōs*.

[4]The compound noun *thyroid* (shield-shaped) is also used as a combining form, meaning the thyroid gland, as in thyroidectomy and so forth.

[5]Latin *urīna*

[6]Words in uric- indicate the presence of uric acid, an acid that is formed as an end product of purine (protein) digestion. Uric acid is a common constituent of renal calculi and of the concretions of gout.

[7]The word vesicle, as well as words in vesicul-, is a modern formation (New Latin) as a diminutive of *vesīca*; these words mean either (1) a small sac containing fluid, especially a seminal vesicle, or (2) a small, blisterlike elevation on the skin containing serous fluid, as in the word vesicopustular.

[8]Words in azot- indicate the presence of nitrogen. This form is from a French word *azote*, nitrogen, coined by the scientist Lavoisier as though derived from the Greek negative prefix *a-* and *zōē*, life. See the Etymological Notes to this lesson.

previously had been considered an element, and gave it the name potassium. The Swedish chemist Berzelius (1779–1848) coined the name *kalium* and applied it to the newly isolated element. Such formations are called New Latin. The word alkali is from the Arabic *al-qaliy,* the calcined ashes of the plant *qali.*

The Greek word *nitron* and the Latin *nitrum* were probably borrowed from the Arabic *natrun,* sodium carbonate. The borrowing most likely took place in Egypt, where Nitriotes was the Greek name of a district where *nitron* was found in great quantities. The word is found in the Old Testament in Jeremiah 2.22 as Hebrew *nether.* In the King James version, the prophet says, "For though thou wash thee with nitre, and take thee much sope, yet thine iniquity is marked before me, saith the Lord God." The Hebrew word *nether* in the Old Testament is translated by *nitron* in the Septuagint and *nitrum* in the Vulgate.

The first use of the word nitrogen is found in 1790 as *nitrogène* in a work by the French chemist Jean Chaptal (1756–1832). It had been recognized by Lavoisier that this gas, which had been discovered as being one of the elements of the atmosphere by the British scientist Daniel Rutherford, would not support life, and for this reason Lavoisier named it *azote* (from the Greek negative prefix *a-* and *zōē,* life).

The Roman writer Pliny discourses at length about *nitrum,* soda. He says, "In the soda-beds of Egypt ophthalmia is unknown. Ulcers on those who visit there heal quickly, but if ulcers form on those who are already there, they are slow to heal. Soda mixed with oil causes those who are rubbed with that mixture to sweat; it also softens the flesh. . . . Soda is good for a toothache if it is mixed with pepper in wine. If it is boiled with a leek and then cooked down to make a dentifrice, it restores the white color to blackened teeth." [*Natural History* 31.115–117]

The word hilus, the indentation in the side of the kidney into which vessels enter, is a New Latin word formed from the Latin *hilum,* a rare word whose etymology is unknown. It forms the base of the noun *nihil,* nothing (as used in the English word nihilism, a doctrine of destruction). According to Festus, a Roman grammarian of the second century A.D., *hilum* meant "something that clings to the seed of a bean, from which we get the word *nihil.*" There was no Latin form *hilus,* and the earliest example of this word in English is found in 1840 in an anatomical treatise in which it is used to indicate a notch or fissure in an organ into which vessels enter. In botany, the word hilum is used to designate the point of attachment of a seed to its vessel—for example, the "eye" of a bean.

Glomeruli, clusters of capillaries within the nephrons of the kidneys, take their name from a New Latin word *glomerulus,* a diminutive of Latin *glomus,* ball of yarn. There was a verb *glomerāre* meaning wind into a ball *or* gather together. Vergil used this verb in the *Aeneid* to describe the souls of the dead gathered about the banks of the Styx, waiting to be ferried across to the realms of the dead by the boatman Charon.

> *quam multa in silvis autumni frigore primo*
> *lapsa cadunt folia, aut ad terram gurgite ab alto*
> *quam multae glomerantur aves, ubi frigidus annus*
> *trans pontum fugat et terris immittit apricis.*

> As many as the leaves that fall from trees
> in the first frost of the autumn, and as dense
> as the flocks of birds that gather together
> in flight when the season of cold drives them
> across the sea, sending them to sunny lands.
> [Vergil, *Aeneid* 6.309–312]

The term *goiter,* enlargement of the thyroid gland, comes from the French *goitre,* from Latin *guttur,* throat. Goiter is caused by a deficiency of iodine in the diet or by hyper- or hypo-function of the thyroid gland. Sometimes the condition is accompanied by abnormal protrusion of the eyeball; this is called ophthalmic goiter, or Graves' disease, named for Robert J. Graves, Irish physician (1797–1853). In areas where iodine is absent from the food supply, iodized salt is often used as prophylaxis.

## EXERCISE 15

A. Analyze and define each of the following words.

1. actinogen _____

2. actinotherapy _____

3. podagra _____

4. anconagra[1] _____

5. omagra[2] _____

6. cerebellar cortex _____

7. adrenal cortex _____

8. cryalgesia _____

9. cryotherapy _____

10. crymophilic _____

11. cryptotoxic _____

12. cryptopyic _____

13. glycopenia _____

14. glycopexic _____

15. glycophilia _____

16. glycosialorrhea _____

17. dysglycemia _____

18. hemophiliac[3] _____

19. hydrophilism _____

---

[1]Greek *ankōn*, elbow
[2]Greek *ōmos*, shoulder
[3]For hemophilia, see Supplementary Lesson I, Clotting.

20. necrophilism _____

21. coprophilic _____

22. orcheoplasty _____

23. orchidoncus _____

24. monorchidism[1] _____

25. synorchidism _____

26. pyelectasia _____

27. pyelocystostomosis _____

28. insemination _____

29. spermatopoietic _____

30. spermatoschesis _____

31. spermatozoon _____

32. oligospermia _____

33. thyroid _____

34. thyroidotoxin _____

35. thyroaplasia _____

36. thyrotropin _____

37. hyperthyroidism _____

38. glycuresis _____

39. anuresis _____

40. anazoturia[2] _____

_____

[1]Greek *monos*, one, single
[2]See the footnote to ZO- in the vocabulary of this lesson.

41. uroxanthin _____

42. urosepsis _____

43. uredema _____

44. dysuriac _____

45. uricolysis[1] _____

46. hyperuricemia _____

47. hyperuricuria _____

48. ureterocystostomy _____

49. ureteroureterostomy _____

50. urethratresia[2] _____

51. urethrostaxis _____

52. urethrotome _____

53. vesicocele _____

54. vesicoclysis _____

55. vesicula[3] _____

56. vesiculectomy _____

57. saprozoic _____

58. celozoic _____

59. protozoa[4] _____

60. zoophagous _____

---

[1]See the footnote on words in uric- in the vocabulary of this lesson.
[2]Greek *trēsis*, perforation
[3]See the footnote on *vesīca* in the vocabulary of this lesson.
[4]Greek *prōtos*, first

61. zoophyte _____

62. zooplasty _____

63. zootoxin _____

64. epizoon _____

65. hemocytozoon _____

66. zoolagnia _____

67. algolagnia _____

68. kleptolagnia[1] _____

69. kaliemia[2] _____

70. natremia[3] _____

B. Give the word derived from Greek and/or Latin elements that means each of the following. Verify your answer in the medical dictionary.

1. Poisoning of the blood due to radiation _____

2. Loss of sensation of cold _____

3. Hidden (subconscious) memory _____

4. Deficiency of sugar in the blood _____

5. Inflammation of the renal pelvis and bladder (use Greek forms) _____

6. Yellow (discoloration of the) urine _____

7. Relating to the bladder and the neck (of the uterus; use Latin forms) _____

8. Containing no animal (life) _____

9. Excessive amount of nitrogen in the urine (use Greek forms) _____

---

[1]Greek *kleptein*, steal
[2]See the Etymological Notes to this lesson.
[3]New Latin *natrium*, sodium, borrowed from Arabic *natrun*, sodium carbonate

10. Inflammation of a nerve (from exposure to) radiation (use Greek forms) _____

C. Give a clear, concise definition of each of the following italicized words.

1. The most common form of urethral stenosis is meatal stricture, congenital or acquired. In both sexes, *urethral meatotomy* is successful if upper tract damage has not occurred. In females, submeatal or distal urethral stenosis is a common cause of obstructive *uropathy* with *enuresis*, recurring infections, and *dysuria*; treatment is by internal urethrotomy, with a good prognosis.

2. *Diabetes mellitus*[1] is a metabolic disorder characterized by a relative or absolute insulin insufficiency. The clinical marker of the latter is the organism's inability to handle glucose normally. Glucosuria is one consequence of glucose intolerance and the attendant *hyperglycemia*.

3. Acute and chronic infections of the prostate are common in postpubescent males, frequently in association with urethritis. Fortunately, *seminal vesiculitis* is relatively uncommon, though an occasional seminal vesicle abscess may be seen in association with chronic prostatitis.

4. Decreased carbohydrate utilization and accelerated gluconeogenesis lead to hyperglycemia which results in an osmotic *diuresis*, consequent renal water, sodium, and potassium losses, and shifts in body water (e.g., intracellular dehydration).

5. *Azoospermia* may be associated with primary testicular disorders or complete obstructions of the seminal tract.

6. *Diuretics* should play only a small role in the treatment of nephrosis.

---

[1]Latin *mellītus*, of honey, from *mel, mellis*, honey; see the Etymological Notes to this lesson.

7. The importance of performing an intravenous *pyelogram* as part of the routine evaluation of hypertensive patients cannot be overemphasized.

8. *Seminiferous* tubular dysgenesis, or Klinefelter's syndrome, is a distinct form of male hypogonadism that occurs in approximately 1 in every 600 male births.

9. Reflex retching and sometimes vomitus may be induced from the pharynx. Furthermore, it occurs in appendicitis, gallbladder disease, and acute pancreatitis; in biliary, pancreatic, and renal colics; in various diseases of the female genital organs; in pregnancy; in acute *epididymitis*;[1] in peritonitis, or with intestinal parasites.

10. If there is no testicular descent, or if hernia persists, before age 5 or 6 years simultaneous *orchidopexy* and herniorrhaphy should be performed to insure subsequent normal testicular function. Delay in surgery may impair *spermatogenesis*, a critical factor when bilateral *cryptorchidism* occurs.

11. By *micturition*[2] cinecystourethrography, it has been demonstrated that vesicoureteral reflux is not rare in otherwise normal persons and that it is more common in persons with congenital anomalies, obstruction of urinary tract, or cystitis.

12. *Albuminuria*[3] is common in patients with diabetes. Sometimes in addition there may be other evidence of renal involvement such as a nephrotic syndrome or chronic renal failure.

---

[1]Greek *epididymis*, epididymis, from *didymos*, double, twin; a testicle

[2]As if from Latin *micturītus* as a perfect passive participle of Latin *micturīre*, urinate; this participle did not exist in Latin.

[3]Latin *albumen, albuminis*, white of an egg

13. Acute *glomerulonephritis*[1] occurs most commonly in children and adolescents. There is usually a history of a streptococcal throat infection one to three weeks previously. The onset is fairly sudden with malaise, shivering, and fever, and some patients complain of a pain in the loins or abdomen. Vomiting in children is common.

14. *Oligospermia* sometimes accompanies inflammatory conditions such as chronic prostatitis.

15. *Thyrotoxicosis* frequently affects the heart, particularly in the older age groups. The action of increased thyroid hormone is to raise the cardiac rate and output.

16. Childhood *pyelonephritis* is often associated with reflux of urine from the bladder on micturition and it interferes with the growth of the kidneys so that they never reach full size. Recurrent infection in children should therefore always be taken seriously.

17. No inflexible rules govern the use of diuretics. However, pretreatment evaluation of renal function and electrolyte balance is important not only because different compounds exert different effects on electrolyte metabolism, but also because alkalosis or acidosis, *hypokalemia*,[2] *hyponatremia*,[2] and *azotemia* can exist without producing symptoms.

D. Answer each of the following questions.

1. What is *actinic* dermatitis?

2. What is *renal decortication*?

---

[1]New Latin *glomerulus*, a diminutive of Latin *glomus, glomeris*, ball of yarn
[2]See the Etymological Notes to this lesson.

3. Why is *cortisone* so named?

4. What is *cryosurgery*?[1] What is meant by *cryothalamotomy*?[2]

5. What is *cryobiology*?

6. What is *colicystopyelitis*?

7. What is *zoanthropy*?[3]

8. What are *zoonoses*?[4] Give an example.

9. What are *coprozoa*? *ectozoa*? *entozoa*?

10. What is the difference in meaning between the words *vesical* and *vesicle*? Explain the form of each word.

---

[1]For the etymology of the word surgery, see the Etymological Notes to Lesson 2.

[2]Greek *thalamos*, inner chamber (of a house)

[3]Greek *anthropos*, man, human being. The best known form of zoanthropy is lycanthropy (Greek *lykos*, wolf).

[4]This plural word is formed as if from a singular *zoonosis*.

11. What is meant by the *vesical reflex*?

12. What is meant by *vesicoureteral reflux*?[1]

13. What is a *vesicovaginal*[2] *fistula*?

14. What is an *cinecystourethrogram*?[3]

15. What is *scopophilia*? *coprophilia*?

## DRILL AND REVIEW

E. The meaning of each of the following words can be determined from its etymology. Determine the meaning of each and verify your answer in the medical dictionary.

1. actinodermatitis
2. actinogenesis
3. actinogenic
4. arthragra
5. chiragra
6. ophthalmagra
7. odontagra
8. proctagra
9. cerebral cortex
10. corticoadrenal
11. pulmonary decortication
12. cryptogenic
13. cryometer
14. cryesthesia
15. crymodynia
16. crymotherapy
17. cryoaerotherapy
18. glycemia
19. aglycemia
20. glycolysis
21. glycogeusia
22. glycoptyalism
23. glycosialia
24. glycorrhachia
25. anorchism
26. polyorchidism
27. orchialgia
28. orchioneuralgia
29. orchectomy
30. orchidotomy
31. orchiorrhaphy
32. pyelitis

[1]Latin *fluere, fluxus*, flow

[2]Latin *vagīna*, vagina

[3]cine- is from Greek *kinein*, move; cf. the word cinema.

33. nephropyelitis
34. pyelography
35. pyeloscopy
36. pyelopathy
37. pyeloplasty
38. pyelotomy
39. pyelolithotomy
40. pyelostomy
41. aspermia
42. necrospermia
43. spermicide
44. spermatocidal
45. spermatolysis
46. spermatolysin
47. spermatolytic
48. spermatotoxin
49. pyospermia
50. thyrocardiac
51. thyroglossal
52. thyrolytic
53. thyroptosis
54. thyrotropic
55. thyrotome
56. thyrochondrotomy
57. thyroidotomy
58. thyroidectomy
59. hypothyroidism
60. paruria
61. polyuria
62. oliguria
63. ischuria
64. achromaturia
65. azoturia
66. hypoazoturia
67. erythruria
68. melanuria
69. hematuria
70. amyluria
71. adiposuria
72. oligohydruria
73. colibacilluria
74. seminuria
75. urocyanosis
76. urosepsis
77. urolithiasis
78. uropoiesis
79. uromelanin
80. uroerythrin
81. uropathogen
82. uropenia
83. uroschesis
84. uroncus
85. uropyonephrosis
86. urography
87. antidysuric
88. antidiuretic
89. uricemia
90. uricopoiesis
91. hypouricuria
92. uricolytic
93. uricocholia
94. hypouresis
95. natriuresis[1]
96. antinatriuresis
97. ureteralgia
98. interureteral
99. periureteritis
100. ureterocele
101. ureterolithiasis
102. ureterography
103. cystoureterogram
104. ureterectasis
105. ureteropyosis
106. ureteropathy
107. ureteroplasty
108. ureteropyeloplasty
109. ureterocolostomy
110. ureteroenterostomy
111. ureteroproctostomy
112. ureterovesicostomy
113. colpoureterotomy
114. urethralgia
115. urethrocystitis
116. urethrectomy
117. urethrorrhagia
118. urethrorrhaphy
119. urethropexy
120. urethremphraxis
121. urethreurynter
122. urethrismus
123. urethrophyma
124. aerourethroscope
125. paravesical
126. prevesical
127. vesicotomy
128. vesiculotomy
129. vesiculitis
130. vesiculogram
131. pyovesiculosis
132. prostatovesiculectomy
133. cystovesiculography
134. dermatozoon
135. hematozoon
136. enterozoic
137. coprozoic
138. zooid

---

[1]See page 227, footnote 3.

139. zoogenous
140. zoophobia
141. zoopathology
142. zoophilism
143. photophilic
144. thermophilic

145. cyanophilous
146. thrombophilia
147. pyrolagnia
148. osmolagnia
149. urolagnia

# THE HEMATOPOIETIC AND LYMPHATIC SYSTEMS

Blood is composed of a fluid called **plasma**, in which three types of cellular elements are suspended: **erythrocytes**, the red blood cells; **leukocytes**, the white blood cells; and **platelets**,[1] the elements that play an important role in the coagulation of blood. In addition to these, there are globules of fat and a number of chemical substances, among which are components called **coagulation factors**, elements that are essential to the clotting process. All of this adds up to about 22 percent solids and 78 percent water. The function of blood is to carry nutrients, principally oxygen, to the cells and tissues of the body, and to carry away wastes, principally carbon dioxide, from the cells and tissues for disposal. In addition to this primary function, blood plays an important part in the regulation of body temperature and in the defense mechanism against infection, especially through the phagocytic action of the leukocytes (see the section on Leukocytes).

## ERYTHROCYTES

In the adult, erythrocytes are formed in the bone marrow, principally that of the long bones of the legs, the bones of the ribs, and in the sternum (breastbone) and the vertebrae. In their immature form they have **nuclei** (singular, *nucleus*),[2] the essential agents in the development and growth of a cell, and are called **erythroblasts**.[3] It is only when they are mature and have expelled their nuclei that they are fully developed erythrocytes. They can then be called **akaryocytes**,[4] non-nucleated cells.

As was stated above, the primary function of erythrocytes is to carry oxygen to, and carbon dioxide away from, the cells and tissues of the body.[5] Oxygen is carried in the **hemoglobin** of the blood. This substance is composed of **hematin**, the iron-carrying portion, and **globin**,[6] a simple protein. Hemoglobin combines readily with oxygen to form an unstable compound called **oxyhemoglobin**, which is carried through the arterial system to all parts of the body, where the oxygen is released to the tissues. The average life of a red blood cell is about 4 months, after which it disintegrates. Hematin, the iron-bearing part of the cell, is carried to the liver and spleen for storage and later use of the iron.

An erythrocyte that has lost its hemoglobin is called an **achromatic erythrocyte**, a red blood cell without color. Any excess amounts of hemoglobin in the body as a result of overdestruction of the erythrocytes (**hemolysis**) is passed off in the urine and feces, thus, under normal circumstances, keeping the amount of hemoglobin in the system relatively stable. This principle of

---

[1] Greek *platē*, flat; -let is an English diminutive suffix derived from French.

[2] Latin *nucleus*, kernel (diminutive of *nux, nucis*, nut)

[3] Greek *blastos*, bud

[4] Greek *karyon*, nut, kernel

[5] For a thorough discussion of this function of blood, see Lesson 11, The Respiratory System.

[6] Latin *globus*, round body, globe

stability is called **homeostasis**;[1] when it is applied to the circulating blood, it means that production and destruction are mutually dependent upon each other and that the constituents and properties of the blood tend to remain stable. Any interference with this stability leads to one of the hemopathies.[2]

When there is insufficient hemoglobin in the bloodstream for an adequate supply of oxygen to the cells and tissues, a substance called **erythropoietin** is released into the bloodstream, and this stimulates the production of erythrocytes.[3] An insufficiency of oxygen in the body, a condition called **hypoxia** or **anoxia**, can be the result of no more than exposure to high altitudes, or it can be the result of disease, or of toxic substances, such as snake venoms, entering the bloodstream and causing hemolysis.

The normal number of erythrocytes averages about 5,500,000 per cubic millimeter[4] for males and about 4,500,000 for females. The total number in a person of average size is about 35 trillion. Determination of the number of erythrocytes in the blood is made by means of a **hematocrit**,[5] a centrifuge for separating the solid elements from the plasma in blood. The percentage of total blood volume that consists of erythrocytes is also called the hematocrit. Normal average for men is about 47 percent and for women, about 42 percent. A decrease below the normal number is called **erythropenia**, and an increase is called **erythrocytosis, polycythemia**,[6] **erythrocythemia**, or **erythremia**.

# LEUKOCYTES

Leukocytes can be classified into two groups, both possessing nuclei. One type contains **granules**,[7] minute, grainlike bodies located in the cytoplasm, the substance of a cell outside its nucleus; these cells are called **granulocytes**. Leukocytes without granules are called **agranulocytes**. Granular leukocytes, which readily accept certain kinds of dyes, are characterized and grouped according to the type of dye that will stain them. The granules of some leukocytes stain red, and these cells are called **eosinophils** (or eosinophilic leukocytes) from the acid dye that stains them, *eosin*, a red dye;[8] other cells stain blue and are called **basophils**[9] (or basophilic leukocytes) because the dye that stains them is a *basic*, or non-acidic—that is, alkaline—dye of a bluish color. Most leukocytes, however, take on a purplish color and are called **neutrophils**[10] (or neutrophilic leukocytes) because they can be stained only by neutral—that is, neither acidic nor alkaline—dyes, which are purple. An abnormal increase in the number of eosinophils in the blood is called

---

[1]Greek *homoios*, like

[2]Diseases of the blood are often referred to collectively as **blood dyscrasias** (Greek *krāsis*, a mixing).

[3]When, in 1906, the French scientists Carnot and Déflandre announced their theory that the circulating blood carried a substance *"hêmopoiêtin"* that stimulated the production of red blood cells, their work was largely ignored. But subsequent investigations, especially since 1950, have confirmed the presence of this substance. It is thought to be produced mainly in the kidneys, but there are other erythropoietin-producing tissues in the human body, the liver apparently being one. For a full discussion of this point see *Clinical Hematology*, Maxwell M. Wintrobe and others, 7th edition, Lea & Febiger, Philadelphia, 1974, p. 179ff.

[4]Usually abbreviated cu. mm.

[5]Greek *kritēs*, judge

[6]Polycythemia vera (Latin *verus*, true) is a chronic and deadly familial disease of unknown etiology characterized by an abnormal increase in the concentration of hemoglobin in the blood, as well as by an increase in total blood volume.

[7]Latin *grānulum*, diminutive of *grānum*, grain, seed

[8]The red dye eosin is named after Eos, the Greek goddess of the dawn, Homer's "rosy-fingered Dawn" (*rhododaktylos Eos*), a daughter of Hyperion and Theia, two of the Titans, children of the primeval couple Earth and Sky. Dawn's sister was Selene, goddess of the moon, and her brother was Helios, the sun-god.

[9]Greek *basis*, base

[10]Latin *neuter*, neither

eosinophilia, and a decrease is called **eosinopenia**. Abnormal increase or decrease in the number of basophils or neutrophils is called **basophilia** (or basocytosis), **basopenia** (or basocytopenia), **neutrophilia**, or **neutropenia**.

Most leukocytes, especially granulocytes, are **phagocytes**; that is, they have the ability to engulf and ingest particles of foreign substances or hostile bacteria, and this is their function in the body. When hostile bacteria invade the body, the production of leukocytes is greatly increased, and an increased number of leukocytes (leukocytosis) is usually an indication of bacterial infection. When the leukocytes themselves are destroyed by invading bacteria, the dead cells collect and form the whitish mass that we call pus. If a ready outlet to the surface of the body is not found for the pus, an abscess is formed. Normally, 1 cu. mm. of blood contains 5000 to 10,000 leukocytes. A decrease in number below 5000 is called **leukopenia**, and an increase above 10,000 is called **leukocytosis**.

## PLATELETS

Platelets are flat, round, or oval disks of microscopic size found in the blood. They number 200,000 to 300,000 per cu. mm. Sometimes called **thrombocytes**, they play an important part in the coagulation of blood, in the arrest of bleeding (**hemostasis**), and in the formation of blood clots. When there is damage to tissue, platelets adhere to each other and to the damaged parts, forming a protective mass around the injured part, thus stopping the loss of blood.

A decrease in the number of platelets, **thrombocytopenia**, can cause the condition known as **hemorrhagic diathesis**,[1] the tendency to bleed, which sometimes occurs in acute infections and in certain hemorrhagic diseases. The usual manifestation of this condition is **purpura**,[2] the spontaneous appearance of dark blue or purple patches on the skin and/or the mucosal surfaces of the mouth, due to hemorrhages into these areas. Such discolorations, if small, are called **macules**;[3] larger patches are called **ecchymoses**.[4] **Thrombocytosis**, increased platelet production, occurs after loss of blood following operations or violent injury to tissues.

## CLOTTING

When blood is exposed to air, it changes into a soft, jellylike mass, a blood clot, or *coagulum*.[5] This physical change from a liquid to a nonfluid mass is caused by a protein substance normally present in the plasma, **fibrinogen**. When blood escapes from the vessels that normally contain it, a substance called **thrombin** is formed from elements present in the blood. The thrombin acts upon the fibrinogen and converts it into **fibrin**, an insoluble, elastic, stringy substance, which forms a network in which platelets are caught. These platelets cling together, and a clot is formed. Clotting is slowed down by cold, by a deficiency of calcium, by the presence of certain mineral salts, and by the anticoagulant **heparin**, as well as by hemolytic agents such as snake venom.

**Hemophilia** is a hereditary blood disease that is carried by females who have this hereditary trait. Although only females are carriers of the disease, it occurs almost exclusively in males. It is characterized by a prolonged coagulation time—that is, the blood fails to clot in the normal

---

[1]Greek *diathesis*, disposition, from *dia-*, through, and *tithenai*, place

[2]Latin *purpura*, purple

[3]Latin *macula*, spot

[4]Greek *ekchymōsis* (Hippocrates), from *ek-*, out, and *chymos*, juice

[5]Latin *co(n)-*, together, *agere*, drive, and the diminutive suffix *-ulum*: "a little thing driven together"

time, and bleeding continues. The cause of this failure to coagulate is the deficiency of a factor in plasma necessary for coagulation of blood. This factor is usually called factor VIII, or the antihemophilic factor. Although there is no cure for hemophilia, factor VIII can be administered intravenously to stop bleeding.

# ANEMIA

Anemia is a condition in which there is a reduction in the normal number of red blood cells per cu. mm. or of the quantity of hemoglobin in the blood. This loss occurs when the equilibrium (homeostasis) between production and destruction of erythrocytes is disturbed. Anemia is not a disease but is a symptom of various diseases. It can be caused by a number of factors: excessive blood loss from disease or injury, excessive cell destruction (hemolysis), or decreased cell production. There are many types of anemia, some of which are listed below:

**achlorhydric anemia**: occurs principally in females in the thirties to fifties and results from *achlorhydria*, lack of hydrochloric acid in the gastric juice.

**aplastic anemia**: caused by failure of the bone marrow to develop properly (*aplasia*) or its destruction by myelotoxic agents such as benzene, arsenic, or x-rays. It also occurs in an idiopathic form.

**Cooley's anemia**:[1] resulting from inheritance of a trait that results in defective production of hemoglobin; also called **thalassemia**,[2] it occurs almost exclusively among peoples of the Mediterranean basin.

**iron-deficiency anemia**: results from the body's demand for more iron than can normally be supplied. Usually caused by chronic loss of blood, as in *hypermenorrhea*, abnormal increase in menstrual flow at regular periods.

**pernicious anemia**:[3] occurs usually in later adult life; characterized by *achlorhydria* (lack of hydrochloric acid in the gastric juice) caused by the reduced absorption of vitamin $B_{12}$.

**sickle cell anemia**: a hereditary hemolytic anemia characterized by large numbers of sickle-shaped erythrocytes (meniscocytes[4]) in the blood due to the presence of an abnormal type of hemoglobin (hemoglobin S) in these cells. Occurs almost exclusively in the African races.

# LEUKEMIA

Leukemia is a fatal disease of unknown origin affecting the hematopoietic organs of the body and characterized by an abnormal and unrestrained increase in the number of leukocytes in the blood. Most of the effects of the disease result from the failure of the bone marrow to function adequately; these effects include anemia, internal hemorrhage due to thrombocytopenia, a tendency to infections, and increasing exhaustion. Purpura and ostealgia, especially in children, and hepatosplenomegaly are common signs. The white cells increase in number to as many as 50,000 per cu. mm. There are many types of this disease, and they are generally classified on the basis of the duration of the disease—that is, acute or chronic—and/or the type of cell involved.

---

[1]named for Thomas Cooley, American physician (1871–1945)

[2]Greek *thalassa*, the sea

[3]Latin *perniciōsus*, destructive, from *perniciēs*, destruction

[4]Greek *mēniskos*, crescent

Some of the more common types include:
> **acute granulocytic leukemia**
> **acute lymphocytic leukemia**[1]
> **acute myelomonocytic leukemia**[2]
> **chronic granulocytic leukemia**
> **chronic lymphocytic leukemia**
> **monocytic leukemia**

# THE LYMPHATIC SYSTEM

The lymphatic system consists of a collection of tissues and vessels concerned with the production and circulation of **lymph**,[3] a colorless alkaline fluid containing proteins, salts, certain organic substances, and water. Lymph is carried in a network of very small and thin-walled vessels called **lymphatics**, or lymphatic capillaries. The cells present in lymph are called **lymphocytes**, which are white blood cells; there are no erythrocytes.

Lymph is formed all over the body in areas in tissues called **interstitial**[4] **spaces** and is gathered into the lymphatics, which carry it to two central points in the body where all of these vessels empty into either the right lymphatic duct, or the left, the thoracic duct. These two ducts empty into the venous system, thus returning the tissue fluid to the circulating blood. The function of the lymphatic system is twofold: (1) to return to the circulating blood proteins that have leaked out of the capillaries and into the tissues; (2) to filter foreign matter, especially bacteria, and to destroy it by the **phagocytic**[5] action of the lymphocytes.

All along the lymphatic vessels are accumulations of tissue called lymph **nodes**.[6] Within the nodes are spaces called lymph **sinuses**,[7] and, lining the walls of these sinuses are phagocytes called **reticuloendothelial cells**[8] which engulf and destroy foreign material and bacteria from the lymph as these substances pass through the nodes. It is this phagocytic activity in the nodes that causes the nodes to become swollen during severe bacterial infection. Lymph nodes are particularly abundant in the **axillae**[9] and neck, since the right and left lymphatic ducts empty into the right and left **jugular**[10] veins in the neck.

The phagocytes of the lymph nodes are able to destroy some cancer cells, but many of these malignant cells may be transferred to other parts of the body through the lymphatics, creating **metastases**,[11] secondary growths of malignancies spread from the site of a primary growth. This is the reason that in **radical**[12] mastectomy the axillary lymph nodes are also excised.

Inflammation of the lymph nodes is called **lymphadenitis**, and inflammation of the lymphatic vessels is called **lymphangitis**. Abnormal enlargement of the lymph nodes, called **lymphadenoma** or **lymphoma**, is one of the symptoms of **Hodgkin's**[13] **disease**, a form of carcinoma

---

[1]See the section on The Lymphatic System.

[2]Monocytes (Greek *monos*, single) are large mononuclear leukocytes.

[3]Latin *lympha*, clear water (probably borrowed from Greek *nympha*, water nymph).

[4]Latin *interstitium*, space between, from *inter-* and *-stituere*, stand

[5]Greek *phagein*, devour

[6]Latin *nodus*, knot

[7]Latin *sinus*, curve, hollow

[8]Latin *rēticulum*, diminutive of *rēte*, net, Greek *endon*, within, *thēlē*, nipple; lymph sinuses are lined with endothelial tissue.

[9]Latin *axilla*, armpit

[10]Latin *jugulum*, throat, neck

[11]singular, *metastasis*, from Greek *meta-*, change, *stasis*, position

[12]Latin *radix*, *radicis*, root

[13]named for Thomas Hodgkin, British physician (1798–1866)

characterized by inflammatory infiltration of lymphocytes into the bone marrow, resulting in disturbed hematopoiesis and anemia.

# VOCABULARY

| GREEK OR LATIN WORD | COMBINING FORM(S) | MEANING |
|---|---|---|
| *blastos* | BLAST- | [bud] primitive cell |
| *ēōs* | EOS-[1] | red (stain) |
| *globus* | *GLOB-* | round body, globe |
| *grānulum*[2] | *GRANUL-* | granule |
| *karyon* | KARY- | [nut] nucleus |
| *lympha* | *LYMPH-* | [clear water] lymph |
| *monos* | MON- | single |
| *neuter* | *NEUTR-* | neither[3] |
| *philos* | PHIL- | having an affinity for[4] |

# ETYMOLOGICAL NOTES

Greek and Latin are called cognate languages—literally, "coming into being together," since both of them are derived from a parent language called Indo-European. Thus, just as there are many words in the Romance languages (which are all derived from Latin) with similar form and meaning, so there are words in Greek and in Latin with these similarities. The -penia in erythropenia, for example, is from the Greek *penia*, poverty, need, and is related in this way to the Latin noun *penuria*, want, need, scarcity. Our words "penury," poverty, and "penurious," stingy, are from this Latin word. The same relation exists between Greek *leukos*, white, and Latin *lūx*, *lūcis*, light, as in the words "lucid," clear, and "translucent," transmitting light.

Another group of words with this same relationship is derived from the Greek verb *histanai*, stand, and the two Latin verbs *stāre*, *stātus*, stand, and *statuere*, *statūtus*, *-stituere*, *-stitūtus*, stand, set in place. These verbs have given us such words as hemostat, stasis, metastasis, homeostasis, station, statue, interstitial, constitution, and consistent.

Eosin, the red dye for which eosinophils have a special affinity, takes its name from the Greek word for the dawn, *ēōs*. In early Greek times Dawn was thought of as being a goddess, a daughter of Hyperion and Theia, two of the Titans, primeval children of Sky and Earth. Dawn's sister was Selene, the moon, and her brother was Helios, the sun. In the Homeric poems the new day was often heralded by the appearance of *rhododaktylos Eos*, rosy-fingered Dawn. On one occasion Eos fell in love with a mortal, Tithonus, a brother of Priam, king of Troy at the time of the Trojan War. She carried the young man away to her home in Ethiopia and secured immortality for him. But she neglected to obtain eternal youth for the unfortunate Tithonus, and deathless, he continued to age. Some say that he was eventually changed into a grasshopper, a creature that renews its youth by casting off its old skin.

Tennyson recalls the sad story of this youth in his poem *Tithonus* (1860) in which the unhappy lover asks Dawn to release him from immortality:

---

[1]Found in this terminology only in the form *eosin*; see page 236, footnote 8.

[2]*grānulum* is a diminutive of the Latin noun *grānum*, seed, grain.

[3]In this terminology words in neutr- refer to neutral dyes—those that are neither acid nor alkaline (basic).

[4]In this terminology words in phil- refer to the capacity of a cell to accept dye; a neutrophil is a cell that stains easily with neutral dyes.

*Yet hold me not forever in thine East;*
*How can my nature longer mix with thine?*
*Coldly thy rosy shadows bathe me, cold*
*Are all thy lights, and cold my wrinkled feet*
*Upon thy glimmering thresholds, when the steam*
*Floats up from those dim fields about the homes*
*Of happy men that have the power to die,*
*And grassy barrows of the happier dead.*
*Release me, and restore me to the ground.*
*Thou seest all things, thou wilt see my grave;*
*Thou wilt renew thy beauty morn by morn,*
*I in earth forget these empty courts,*
*And thee returning on thy silver wheels.*

Eos and Tithonus had two children, Emathion and Memnon. We know little about Emathion, but Memnon became king of the Ethiopians. In the closing phase of the Trojan War, Memnon came to the aid of the Trojans, leading his Ethiopian troops and wearing armor fashioned by the god Hephaestus himself. Shortly after his arrival he faced the great Greek hero Achilles in single combat and fell in the battle, mortally wounded. Ovid, in the *Metamorphoses*, tells us that Eos (Latin *Aurora*) appealed to Zeus to grant Memnon some special honor in death. The god agreed, and from the ashes that rose from Memnon's funeral pyre countless birds came into being, named Memnonides, Daughters of Memnon. The dew on the morning grass is said to be the tears shed daily by Eos for her unfortunate son.

Lymph, the clear, alkaline fluid found in the lymphatic vessels, is named from Latin *lympha*, clear water. This Latin word is a borrowing from Greek *nymphē* (or *nymphā*), young girl, maiden, nymph. Nymphs were female spirits of nature and were usually represented as living in either the mountains, where they were called oreads, in the woods, where they were called dryads, or in the waters, where they were called naiads. Some nymphs were singled out in mythology for the unusual events surrounding them and some do not appear to be oreads, dryads, or naiads. In Homer's *Odyssey*, the hero Odysseus spends seven years on the island of Ogygia, detained by the beautiful nymph Calypso, who wants to make him immortal so that he can dwell with her forever. But his thoughts are on his home and his wife Penelope and young son Telemachus. Eventually, he is released from this unusual bondage by orders of Zeus and does, at long last, after almost twenty years, return to his home, wife, and son.

Another well-known nymph was the oread Echo. She fell in love with a handsome young man named Narcissus, the son of a naiad, Liriope, and a river-god, Cephisus. Ovid tells us that when Narcissus was born, Liriope asked Tiresias, the blind prophet of Thebes, if her son would live to a ripe old age. Tiresias answered, "Only if he never knows himself."

Narcissus grew up to be a haughty young man and spurned all lovers. Finally, as the story goes, he, at last, fell in love with the image of a beautiful youth in a pool of clear water—himself. In his frustration at this hopeless love, he pined away until only a flower remained, a flower with a yellow center surrounded by white petals. His last words to himself were, *Heu, frustra dilecte puer*, Alas, dear boy, loved in vain. *Vale*, farewell. Echo repeated the same words to him. Ovid tells us that even in the Underworld his spirit gazes eternally at its image in the waters of the river Styx. Echo, desolate, mourning for her lost love, faded away until only her voice remained echoing through the hills and valleys, repeating whatever she heard spoken.

## EXERCISES

A. Analyze and define each of the following words and terms.

1. myeloblast _____

241

2. leukoblastosis _____

3. erythroblastosis fetalis[1] _____

4. eosin _____

5. hypereosinophilia _____

6. globin _____

7. hemoglobinocholia _____

8. hemoglobinuria _____

9. hemoglobinolysis _____

10. hematin _____

11. hematopoiesis _____

12. hematophage _____

13. hemolysin _____

14. hemopathology _____

15. erythropoietin _____

16. leukopoiesis _____

17. granulocyte _____

18. agranulocyte _____

19. lymphogranulomatosis _____

20. lymphoblast _____

21. lymphocytopenia _____

22. lymphocythemia _____

_____

[1]Latin *fētālis*, fetal, from *fētus*, offspring, fetus

242

23. lymphoma _____

24. lymphadenitis _____

25. lymphadenectasis _____

26. lymphagogue _____

27. lymphangioma _____

28. lymphangiectasis _____

29. lymphangitis _____

30. lymphaticostomy[1] _____

31. lymphocytotoxin _____

32. lymphopoiesis _____

33. akaryocyte _____

34. polykaryocyte _____

35. karyochromatophil _____

36. karyoclasis _____

37. karyophage _____

38. thrombin _____

39. thrombopenia _____

40. thromboclasis _____

41. ecchymoses[2] _____

42. hemorrhagic diathesis[3] _____

43. monocyte _____

_____

[1]From New Latin *lymphaticus*, lymphatic, a lymph vessel; for New Latin, see the Appendix.

[2]See page 237, footnote 4.

[3]See page 237, footnote 1.

44. monocytopenia _____

45. monocytosis _____

B. Give a clear, concise definition of each of the following italicized words.

1. Eosinophilic granuloma is a solitary lytic lesion occurring in young persons. It is cured by removal of the lesion, which contains many *eosinophils*.

2. In a number of patients who have a very large spleen as a result of congestion, *neutropenia* may develop. There is evidence to suggest that in this instance neutrophils are sequestered and probably destroyed by the large spleen.

3. Relative *polycythemia* is observed after severe loss of body fluids by vomiting, diarrhea, or perspiration or in diabetes insipidus if quenching of increasing thirst is prevented.

4. *Agranulocytosis* is a febrile disease with necrotizing lesions in the throat and sometimes other mucous membranes, marked prostration, and a septic course. It is encountered most frequently in women past middle age.

5. Pathological *leukocytosis* is most frequently a neutrophilic leukocytosis. It is one of the most important signs of acute infections, localized or generalized, especially those associated with accumulation of pus.

6. Symptomatic thrombocytopenia occurs in various diseases of the bone marrow that may impair the production of *megakaryocytes*, such as advanced stages of pernicious anemia, leukemia, aplastic anemia, multiple myeloma, or metastatic carcinomatosis of the bone marrow. It may or may not be associated with *purpura*.[1]

_____

[1]See page 237, footnote 2.

7. Infectious *mononucleosis* occurs sporadically or in small epidemics. It is, as a rule, benign in nature and characterized by irregular fever, sore throat, generalized *lymphadenopathy*, splenomegaly, and a well-defined morphologic and serologic alteration of the blood.

8. The normal number of *basophils*[1] of about 38 per mm. of blood is often and irregularly elevated in various diseases, particularly diseases of the hemopoietic system.

9. As the neutrophils encounter bacteria or other minute particles, they flow around them by their ameboid motion and engulf them. The engulfed bacteria are ordinarily digested by the enzymes present in the *granules* of the neutrophil.

10. Burning sensation of the tongue without grossly visible alteration is often a complaint in vitamin B deficiency or in *hyperchromic* or *hypochromic anemia*, or of heavy smokers and neurotics.

11. In man, severe exercise or administration of epinephrine will decrease the proportion of marginated cells and therefore induce *neutrophilia*.

12. After a relatively small injury to a blood vessel, vasoconstriction is an important early event in *hemostasis* before the formation of a clot.

13. Bleeding in association with *thrombocytosis* is limited to the myeloproliferative diseases, in which extremely high platelet levels are encountered and in which there is some evidence of qualitative platelet abnormalities.

---

[1]See page 236, footnote 9.

14. In symptomatic hypertension the *homeostasis*[1] of blood pressure is disrupted by a diseased organ. In constitutional hypertension a gradual decline of the homeostatic system develops.

15. Evaluation of the *hemoglobin* concentration in a particular individual requires careful consideration of any environmental or personal factors that may modify the hemoglobin concentration. For example, altitude has a predictable effect.

16. The *hematocrit*[2] is usually determined by spinning a blood-filled capillary tube in a centrifuge. The diluted blood specimen is passed through an electrical field and the disturbance in electrical conductivity acts as an indicator system.

17. Quite characteristic is the arthritis, usually of the knee or ankle, in *hemophilia*. Minute blows, which hardly can be avoided in daily life, produce hemorrhages with subsequent swelling and pain of the joint.

18. Various pigments from breakdown of red blood cells contribute to the xanthochromic appearance following intracranial bleeding. A high proportion of *oxyhemoglobin* is present with acute bleeding as contrasted with the greater amount of bilirubin found in specimens taken a longer time after hemorrhage.

19. Hemopericardium may also result from blood *dyscrasias*,[3] anticoagulant therapy, tumor, or pericarditis.

20. *Idiopathic aplastic anemia* is a disease characterized by varying degrees of bone marrow failure. Any or all marrow elements may be involved, and anemia, leukopenia, thrombocytopenia, or any combination may be produced. Leukopenia, especially *granulocytopenia*, carries a grave prognosis, since infection is a primary cause of death in these patients.

---

[1]See page 236, footnote 1.
[2]See page 236, footnote 5.
[3]See page 236, footnote 2.

# THE MUSCULOSKELETAL SYSTEM*

Muscle (Latin *musculus*, diminutive of *mus*, mouse; used in Latin to mean both a little mouse and a muscle) is a type of tissue composed of contractile cells or fibers whose outstanding characteristic is their elasticity—their ability to expand and contract. Three types of muscle tissue are differentiated in the body: smooth, striated (also called skeletal), and cardiac. Smooth muscle tissue forms the involuntary muscles, so named because they are not under control of the will. These muscles are found mainly in the internal organs—those of the digestive tract, the respiratory passages, the urinary ducts, and walls of blood vessels, for example. Cardiac tissue is the tissue of the muscle of the heart, and striated (or skeletal) muscle tissue composes the voluntary muscles—those that are under our control. It is these muscles that we are concerned with here. In anatomical terminology, muscles are called by their Latin name, *musculus* (plural, *musculi*) and are named for one of four of the following reasons:

1. After a physical characteristic of the muscle; **musculus bipennatus** (Latin *bi-*, two, *penna*, feather), so named because the muscle fibers flow down either side of a central tendon like the barbs on the two sides of a feather.

2. After the organ or part to which it is attached and which it controls: **musculi colli** (Latin *collum*, neck; genitive case, *collī*): muscles of the neck.

3. A combination of the preceding two: **musculus biceps brachii** (Latin *biceps*, two-headed, from *caput*, head, *brachium*, [upper] arm; genitive case, *brachiī*). The point of origin of a muscle is called the caput, or head. This muscle is bicipital—two-headed—attached to both the scapula and the coracoid (Greek *korax*, *korakos*, crow) process, a process (outgrowth) on the upper surface of the scapula resembling a crow's beak. The musculus biceps brachii flexes the forearm and supinates the hand—that is, turns the hand so that the palm faces upward.

4. After the function that the muscle performs: a muscle that lifts a part is a *levator*; one that flexes a part is a *flexor*; one that moves a part away from the central plane of the body is an *abductor*; one that moves a part toward the central plane of the body is an *adductor*, and one that extends a part is an *extensor*. These terms are generally (but not always) used in combination with the part that the muscle moves. Sometimes the muscle is described as being long (Latin

---

*This lesson differs slightly from previous ones, especially in the nature of the exercises. Words listed in the vocabularies of preceding lessons are not given here, and vocabulary words in this lesson are not listed in the Index of Combining Forms at the back of this text.

*longus*) or short (*brevis*): **musculus abductor**[1] **pollicis brevis** (*pollex, pollicis,* thumb) and **musculus abductor pollicis longus** abduct and assist in extending the thumb. **Musculus adductor longus** adducts the thigh. Note that it is not always possible to tell from the name of a muscle exactly which organ or part of the body it controls.

The names of muscles in their Latin form, as given in the preceding sections, are called *Nomina Anatomica*, anatomical names, usually abbreviated NA. This is anatomical terminology adopted as official by the International Congress of Anatomists at various meetings since 1950. The Tenth International Congress was held in Tokyo, in 1975, and the names adopted by this Congress were published in 1977.[2] Note that it is not only muscles that are given NA names, but also nerves, bones, and organs of the body.

## NOUN DECLENSION

In the naming of muscles, Latin nouns and adjectives are found in the forms of different grammatical cases and in both singular and plural number. The cases most commonly used are the nominative (the form found in the vocabularies) and the genitive, or possessive, case, in both singular and plural. Infrequently the accusative case is found; this is the case of the direct object of a verb or of a word with a verbal force, such as *attollens,* "lifting," in the muscle that lifts the ear: **musculus attollens auriculam**, where *auriculam* is the accusative case of *auricula,* ear.

To repeat what was stated in Lesson 8, there are five categories, called declensions, of Latin nouns, and two declensions of adjectives. Latin first-declension nouns end in *-a* and are feminine; second-declension nouns end in *-us* if masculine, and *-um* if neuter gender. Third-declension nouns may be either masculine, feminine, or neuter, and the nominative case (the vocabulary form) is not characterized by any particular ending. Nouns of the fourth and fifth declensions will not concern us here, with the exception of two fourth-declension nouns: *manus,* hand, is feminine, and the genitive singular is *manūs; genu,* knee, is neuter, and the genitive singular is *genūs.*

## A PARTIAL DECLENSION OF TYPICAL NOUNS

| Singular | | Plural | |
|---|---|---|---|
| Nominative | Genitive | Nominative | Genitive |
| *auricula,* f.,[3] ear | *auriculae* | *auriculae* | *auriculārum* |
| *digitus,* m., finger, toe | *digitī* | *digitī* | *digitōrum* |
| *labium,* n., lip | *labiī* | *labia* | *labiōrum* |
| *pēs,* m., foot | *pedis* | *pedēs* | *pedum* |
| *manus,* f., hand | *manūs* | *manūs* | *manuum* |
| *genū,* n., knee | *genus* | *genua* | *genuum* |

## LATIN ADJECTIVES

Latin adjectives are of two classes: they are either of the first and second declension, with endings like those of masculine, feminine, and neuter nouns of the first and second declensions—that

---

[1]The noun *abductor,* as well as other agent nouns in *-or* used in these exercises, is in apposition to the noun *musculus*—that is, it defines what kind of a muscle it is or what it does. It is easier to define these agent nouns as adjectives: the abductor muscle, that is, the muscle that abducts.

[2]See Supplementary Lesson III, Biological Nomenclature.

[3]The abbreviations m., f., and n., are for masculine, feminine, and neuter.

is, they assume these endings depending upon the gender of the nouns that they describe; or they are of the third declension and usually end in -*is*. The genitive singular of third-declension adjectives always ends in -*is*; thus, it is not always obvious whether a third-declension adjective, such as *brevis*, short (genitive, *brevis*), is in the nominative or genitive case. This must be determined from the way the adjective is used in the particular term in which it is found.

Adjectives that end in -*ior* are in the comparative degree: *superior*, higher; *inferior*, lower. This form is used for both masculine and feminine singular.[1] The genitive singular for both genders ends in -*is* (*superiōris*, *inferiōris*), and the nominative plural for both genders ends in -*ēs* (*superiōrēs*, *inferiōrēs*).

## THE ORDER OF WORDS

In Latin, nouns in the genitive case, the case of possession, usually follow the noun upon which they depend:

(nom. sing.)   (gen. sing.)
**musculus**     **laryngis**
"the muscle    *of* the larynx"   (that is, the laryngeal muscle)

(nom. pl.)    (gen. sing.)
**musculi**[2]    **thoracis**
"the muscles  *of* the thorax"   (that is, the thoracic muscles)

(nom. pl.)    (gen. sing.)
**musculi**      **dorsi**
"the muscles  *of* the back"   (that is, the dorsal muscles)

Adjectives follow the nouns that they describe:

**musculus bronchoesophageus**
"the bronchoesophageal muscle"

**musculus nasalis**
"the nasal muscle"

**musculi interspinales**
"the interspinal muscles"

**musculus adductor longus**
"the long adductor muscle"

**musculus adductor brevis**
"the short adductor muscle"

**musculi intercostales externi**
"the external intercostal (that is, between the ribs) muscles"

**musculi intercostales interni**
"the internal intercostal muscles"

**musculus verticalis linguae**
"the vertical muscle *of* the tongue"

---

[1]The comparative degree of neuter nouns ends in -*ius* (*superius*, *inferius*).
[2]Macrons are not placed over long vowels in this terminology.

**musculus longus colli**
"the long muscle *of* the neck"

**musculus transversus abdominis**
"the transverse muscle *of* the abdomen"

**musculi levatores costarum**
"the levator muscles *of* the ribs" (that is, muscles that raise the ribs)

**musculi incisivi labii inferioris**
"the incisive muscles *of* the lower lip"

**musculus obliquus internus abdominis**
"the internal oblique muscle *of* the abdomen"

**musculus abductor digiti quinti manus[1]**
"the abductor muscle *of* the fifth finger *of* the hand"

Sometimes the noun in the genitive case is enclosed between two adjectives:

**musculus extensor digitorum communis**
"muscle extensor *of* the fingers common" (that is, the common extensor muscle of the fingers)

**musculi levatores costarum longi**
"the long levator muscles *of* the ribs"

**musculi levatores costarum breves**
"the short levator muscles *of* the ribs"

**musculus obliquus capitis inferior**
"the lower oblique muscle *of* the head"

**musculus obliquus capitis superior**
"the higher oblique muscle *of* the head"


# SELECTED VOCABULARY FOR NAMES OF MUSCLES

| LATIN WORD | MEANING |
|---|---|
| *abductor*[2] | that which leads away, abductor |
| *accelerātor* | that which speeds up, accelerator |
| *adductor* | that which leads toward, adductor |
| *ala* | wing; *ala nasi*, wing of the nose, the lateral wall of each nostril |
| *angulus* | angle, corner |
| *anus* | anus, opening of the rectum |
| *arrector* | that which raises, erector |
| *articulāris* | joint (adj.), pertaining to joints |
| *attollens* | lifting |
| *attrahens* | moving toward |
| *auricula* | ear, the external portion of the ear |

---

[1] *manūs* is the genitive singular of the fourth declension noun *manus; quinti* (fifth) is in the genitive case in agreement with *digiti.*

[2] This word is not found in Latin of the classical period but has been formed on the model of other Latin words of similar construction. Such words (and terms), common in the terminology of anatomy and biology, are called New Latin. Several other words in this vocabulary are New Latin.

| | |
|---|---|
| *biceps* | two-headed |
| *brevis* | short |
| *buccinātor* | that which has to do with the cheek (*bucca*) |
| *constrictor* | that which narrows, constrictor |
| *corrugātor* | that which wrinkles, "wrinkler" |
| *cubitum* | elbow |
| *depressor* | that which lowers or depresses, depressor |
| *digitus* | finger, toe |
| *dīlātor* | that which widens, dilator |
| *extensor* | that which extends, extensor |
| *femur, femoris* | thigh |
| *flexor* | that which flexes or bends, flexor |
| *genu, genūs* | knee |
| *hallux, hallucis* | big toe |
| *index, indicis* | index (first) finger |
| *levātor* | that which raises, levator |
| *longus* | long |
| *manus, manūs* | hand |
| *medius* | middle |
| *mentālis* | of the chin (*mentum*) |
| *minimus* | smallest |
| *naris* | a nostril |
| *nasus* | nose |
| *opponens* | opposing |
| *palpebra* | eyelid |
| *pēs, pedis* | foot |
| *pilus* | a hair |
| *pollex, pollicis* | thumb |
| *pupilla* | pupil (of the eye) |
| *rotātor* | that which turns, rotator |
| *supercilium* | an eyebrow |
| *superior, superiōris* | upper, higher |
| *sura* | calf (of the leg) |
| *tensor* | that which tenses, tensor |
| *triceps* | three-headed |
| *tympanum*[1] | ear drum, tympanic membrane |

## ETYMOLOGICAL NOTES

The abductor and adductor muscles take their name from the Latin verb *ducere, ductus*, lead, draw. Related to this verb is the noun, *dux, ducis*, leader, commander, chief. The Italian honorific title *Il Duce*, the Chief, was accorded to Benito Mussolini upon his accession to the dictatorship of Italy in the years between the two World Wars. Adherents of his party belonged to the political organization called *Fascista*, Fascists, named for the symbol of the party, the *Fasci*, from Latin *fascēs*, a bundle of rods bound around an axe and carried in procession in front of the high magistrates of Rome. A related Latin word is *fascia*, band, bandage, which has given the name to the anatomical term fascia, the fibrous membrane covering, supporting, and separating muscles.

---

[1]borrowed from Greek *tympanon*, drum

251

The Latin word *cubitum*, elbow, is from the verb *cubāre, cubitus*, lie down. The sense was that, when reclining to dine, as the Romans did, the elbow was to lean upon. The verb meaning to recline at a dining table was *recumbere*, from *re-*, back, and *-cumbere*, lie down, an alternate form of *cubāre* which is used with prefixes. In Roman times the term *cubitum* also meant the distance from the elbow to the tip of the extended middle finger, a term of measurement: a cubit. The distance is variously calculated as being from 18 to 21 inches.

There is a number of words in current use all related to the verb *cubāre* and its alternate form *-cumbere*: cubicle, from *cubiculum*, a diminutive noun meaning "a (small) place for sleeping, bedroom." Procumbent means "leaning forward," and recumbent means "leaning backward." The incumbent is the one who is in office, and the expression "It is incumbent upon us" implies a burden "lying upon" us. The terms incubus and succubus refer to demons, or evil spirits, that visit one in the night for sexual intercourse. The incubus "lies upon" women, and the succubus "lies under" men. Today, the term incubus is used to refer to anything that is oppressive, something that weighs one down. Chickens incubate their eggs, and an incubator is an apparatus where eggs are artificially hatched, or it is a chamber used to provide a stable and healthful atmosphere for the development of premature or sick babes.

Latin *manus*, hand, has several interesting derivatives in English, among which are the words maneuver and manure, both with the same etymology, from *manus* and *opus, operis*, work, and both disguised as a result of their transition through French before entering the English language. Maneuver is from French *manoeuvre*, from Medieval Latin *manuopera*, something done by hand, from Latin *manuoperāre*, work by hand. Thus, a maneuver is literally "something done by hand." Today it means an evasive movement, a manipulation of affairs done for someone's advantage. (Note that the words manipulate and manipulation are from Latin *manipulus*, a handful.) Manure, barnyard refuse used as fertilizer, has the same ultimate etymology as maneuver but has suffered a secondary change in form during the Middle English period, the twelfth through fifteenth centuries. The Middle English form is *manouren*, a verb meaning to cultivate the land (by hand), with a secondary (and modern) meaning of using manure to enrich the soil. The second component of these words, *opus, operis*, has, of course, given us such words as operate, opera, operation, and inoperable.

The modern names for the bones of the body are those that were given by the ancient Roman anatomists and their successors in the Middle Ages and Renaissance. In some instances, the bones were named after some familiar object which they were thought to resemble, and, in others, there seems to be no etymology to the name or any reason for it—an arbitrary choice of words. Most of the names of bones are Latin words, but an appreciable number were borrowed from the early Greek scientists such as Hippocrates, Aristotle, or Galen.

The Latin words *digitus*, finger, toe, *ulna*, elbow, arm, *femur, femoris*, thigh, *humerus*, shoulder, *tibia*, shin bone, and *ilium*, flank, for example, were used only to designate these parts of the body. Later, they were given to the bones underlying these parts. Following is a partial list of bones that were named after familiar objects:

**clavicle**, collar bone: "little key." Latin *clavis*, key
**patella**, kneecap: "little dish." Latin *patena*, open dish, from *patēre*, lie open
**mandible**, jawbone: "capable of chewing." Latin *mandere*, chew
**fibula**, outer bone of leg: "safety pin." Latin *fibula*, brooch
**scaphoid**, a bone of the ankle and wrist: "boat-shaped." Greek *skaphē*, boat
**zygoma**, a bone of the cheek: "arch." Greek *zygon*, yoke
**trapezium**, a bone of the wrist: "little table." Greek *trapeza*, table.
**cuneiform**, a bone of the ankle: "wedge-shaped." Latin *cuneus*, wedge
**malleus**, ossicle ("little bone") of the middle ear: "hammer." Latin *malleus*, hammer
**incus**, ossicle ("little bone") of the middle ear: "anvil." Latin *incus*, anvil
**sacrum**, base of the vertebral column: "sacred thing." Latin *sacer*, sacred; this part of the body of animals was burned in offerings to the gods.
**lunate**, a bone of the wrist: "moon-shaped." Latin *lūna*, moon
**hamate**, a bone of the wrist: "hook-shaped." Latin *hama*, hook
**pisiform**, a bone of the wrist: "pea-shaped." Latin *pīsum*, pea

tarsus, ankle: "framework." Greek *tarsos*, wicker frame

**phalanges**, bones of the fingers *or* toes: "battle-line." Greek *phalanges*, plural of *phalanx*, a military unit. The Macedonian phalanx, a fighting group developed by Philip II, King of Macedonia and father of Alexander the Great, was made up of 256 men formed in a square 16 across and 16 deep and trained to maneuver with great dexterity on the field of battle.

## EXERCISES

Using the vocabulary for this lesson, determine the function of each of the following muscles.

1. musculus abductor[1] minimi digiti

2. musculus abductor digiti minimi pedis

3. musculus abductor hallucis

4. musculus abductor pollicis brevis

5. musculus abductor pollicis longus

6. musculus accelerator urinae[2]

7. musculus adductor hallucis

8. musculus adductor pollicis

9. musculi arrectores pilorum

10. musculus articularis cubiti

---

[1]When the second word of the names of muscles ends in *-or* (singular, or *-ores*, plural), this word is usually a noun that explains what the muscle does. All of the first five muscles above, for example, are abductor muscles. Whatever part of the body it is that they abduct is put in the genitive case. That is, each of these muscles is the abductor *of* something.

[2]Latin *urīna*, urine

11. musculus articularis genus

_____

12. musculus attrahens auriculam[1]

_____

13. musculus attollens auriculam

_____

14. musculus biceps brachii

_____

15. musculus femoris

_____

16. musculus buccinator

_____

17. musculus constrictor pharyngis inferior

_____

18. musculus constrictor pharyngis medius

_____

19. musculus constrictor pharyngis superior

_____

20. musculus corrugator supercilii

_____

21. musculus depressor anguli oris

_____

22. musculus depressor labii inferioris

_____

23. musculus dilator naris

_____

24. musculus extensor digiti minimi

_____

25. musculus extensor digitorum

_____

_____

[1]-am is the ending of the accusative singular for first-declension nouns.

26. musculus extensor hallucis brevis

_____

27. musculus extensor indicis

_____

28. musculus extensor pollicis brevis

_____

29. musculus flexor digiti minimi brevis pedis

_____

30. musculus flexor digiti minimi brevis manus

_____

31. musculus flexor digitorum brevis pedis

_____

32. musculus flexor hallucis brevis

_____

33. musculus flexor pollicis brevis

_____

34. musculus flexor pollicis longus

_____

35. musculus levator anguli oris

_____

36. musculus levator ani

_____

37. musculus levator labii superioris

_____

_____

38. musculus levator labii superioris alaeque nasi[1]

_____

39. musculus levator palpebrae superioris

_____

---

[1]*alaeque* means "and of the wing." *-que* affixed to a noun means that this noun is to be connected with the noun that precedes it with "and." This *-que* (called an enclitic) can be affixed to any form of a noun or adjective. The initials S.P.Q.R. frequently seen on Roman inscriptions stand for *Senatus Populusque Romanus*: The Senate *and* the Roman People.

40. musculus mentalis[1]

_____

41. musculus opponens digiti minimi

_____

42. musculus opponens pollicis

_____

43. musculi rotatores cervicis

_____

44. musculus sphincter ani externus

_____

45. musculus sphincter ani internus

_____

46. musculus sphincter pupillae

_____

47. musculus sphincter urethrae

_____

48. musculus tensor tympani

_____

49. musculus triceps brachii

_____

50. musculus triceps surae

_____

## THE SKELETON

The **skeleton** (Greek *skeleton*, dried up [sc. *sōma*, body]; that is, "a dried up body") is the bony framework of the body consisting of 206 bones. The distribution of these 206 bones is as follows:

skull: 8 bones
face: 14 bones
hyoid bone: a single U-shaped bone lying at the base of the tongue
ear: 6 ossicles—"little bones"
vertebrae: 26 bones

_____

[1]known also as musculus levator labii inferioris

ribs: 24 bones
sternum: the single breastbone
arms and shoulders: 10 bones
wrists: 16 bones
hands: 38 bones
legs and hips: 10 bones
ankles: 14 bones
feet: 38 bones
    See Figure 19 for a front and back view of the skeleton and the names of the major skeletal
bones.

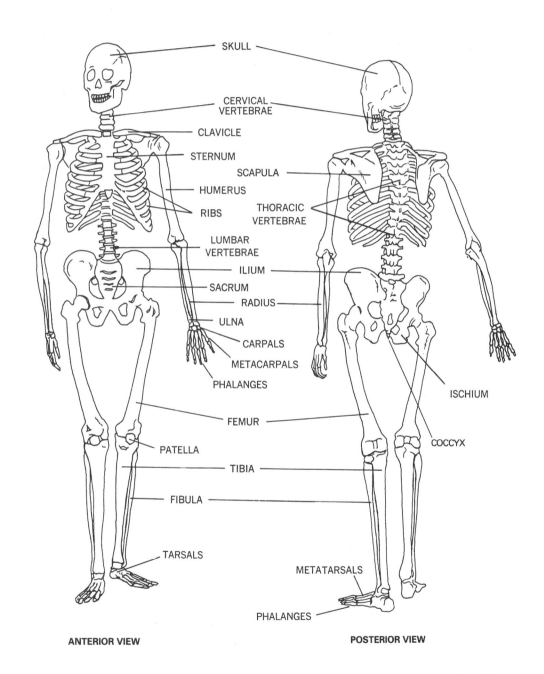

FIGURE 19. The skeleton: anterior and posterior views. (From *Taber's Cyclopedic Medical Dictionary*, ed. 15. F.A. Davis, Philadelphia, 1985.)

## EXERCISES

Indicate, in ordinary, everyday terms, the location of each of the following bones or groups of bones.

1. clavicle _____

2. sternum _____

3. humerus _____

4. lumbar vertebrae _____

5. metacarpals _____

6. patella _____

7. fibula _____

8. phalanges (two different sets) 1. _____ 2. _____

9. scapula _____

10. sacrum _____

11. radius _____

12. femur _____

13. tibia _____

14. ilium _____

15. metatarsals _____

# SUPPLEMENTARY LESSON **III**
# BIOLOGICAL NOMENCLATURE*

With the advance of human knowledge concerning the living organisms that inhabit the world around us—plants, birds, insects, fish, and all other living things, from the smallest, the virus, a minute organism not visible under ordinary light microscopy, to the largest, the whale—it became desirable to classify these living organisms into convenient groupings. Following this classification, the next, and immediate, desideratum was to give names to the members of each group. The term used for this classification is *taxonomy* (Greek *taxis*, arrangement, and *nomos*, law), and the term used for the naming of these groups is *nomenclature* (Latin *nomenclatura*, a calling by name, from *nomen*, name, *c[a]latus*, called, and *-ura*, a noun-forming suffix). The Latin noun *nomenclatura* was first used by Pliny, the Roman scientist, in his encyclopedic *Naturalis Historia* (Natural History), completed in A.D. 77. The groups that are distinguishable from each other, and thus classified, are called *taxa* (singular, *taxon*), and the allocation of names to these taxa is called nomenclature.

Nomenclature follows classification and is independent of it. But the objectives of each are the same: first, to provide a system whereby each and every living thing can be grouped according to shared characteristics, and, second, to give names to these groups so that they may be referred to and discussed intelligibly by all members of the scientific community *in all countries of the world*, regardless of the barriers to communication imposed by the different languages of these members. The language of biological, and, indeed, all scientific, nomenclature is Latin. Included in the term Latin are words borrowed from other languages, mainly ancient Greek, and given the *form* of Latin words, so that they look like Latin.

The reasons for the use of Latin as the language of scientific nomenclature are compelling. Latin ceased to be a spoken language centuries ago and, thus, is not subject to the changes that constantly influence living, spoken languages. It remains forever static. But perhaps the most cogent reason for the selection of Latin as a means of communication between the scientists of all nations is the fact that in the western world Latin had always been the language of the learned communities, whether the object of this learning was medicine, law, religion, philosophy, astronomy, or whatever. The monumental work of the British physician, William Harvey, on the circulation of the blood was written in Latin and published in 1628: *Exercitatio anatomica de*

---

*This lesson differs slightly from previous ones, especially in the nature of the exercises. Words listed in the vocabularies of preceding lessons are not given here, and vocabulary words in this lesson are not listed in the Index of Combining Forms at the back of this text.

259

*motu cordis et sanguinis* (An Anatomical Treatise concerning the Movement of the Heart and Blood). The Polish astronomer, Copernicus, wrote his great work, a treatise entitled *De Revolutionibus orbium coelestium* (Concerning the Revolutions of the Heavenly Bodies), in Latin in 1543, and the works of the Dutch theologian, Erasmus (1466–1536), were written in Latin.

It was the Swedish botanist Carl von Linné, better known as Linnaeus (1707–1778), who first formulated the principles that are still in use for botanical taxonomy and nomenclature. His *Genera Plantarum* and *Classes Plantarum* (Genera of Plants and Classes of Plants), published in 1737 and 1738, are considered to be the beginning of systematic classification and terminology for modern botany. Following other important publications, his *Philosophia Botanica* (1751) explained fully his system for botanical nomenclature, and the tenth edition of his *Systema Naturae* (1758) established the rules for zoological nomenclature. All of these works were written in Latin and, for the first time, laid down the rules for the formulation of all subsequent biological terminology.

The system, as elucidated by Linnaeus and in its simplest form, applied a binomial (Medieval Latin *binomius*, having two names; Latin *bi-*, two, and *nomen*, name) nomenclature to plants and animals. Each one is given two names in the form of Latin: the first naming the genus (Latin *genus, generis*, race, stock, kind) to which it belongs, and the second a name peculiar to a member of the genus to differentiate it from other members of the same genus. For example, there are many members of the cat family—the wild cat, the lion, the tiger, and so forth—obviously related to one another, and, just as obviously, not related to members of the dog family—the household dog, the wolf, the coyote, and so forth. The genus of cats is named *Felix*, and, in the binomial system, the wild cat is *Felix catus*; the lion, *Felix leo*; and the tiger, *Felix tigris*.

## SPECIES AND GENERA

The three binomial terms mentioned above for members of the cat family are names of **species** (Latin *species*, outward appearance). That is, all members of this group have a similar appearance. The first word of the name, *Felix*, is the **genus** (plural, *genera*) or **generic** name; the second, *catus, leo,* or *tigris*, is the **specific** name, which, following the generic name, indicates the species. To this group we can now add the name of its best-known member, *Felix domesticus*, the domesticated feline, our common household cat. Note that, in the names of species, the generic name is capitalized, while the specific name is not. Both names are customarily italicized, and it takes at least two words to name a species.

A species can be defined as a group of animals or plants that shares similar characteristics and is usually capable of interbreeding, although all members of each species are not identical in appearance. That is, all household cats look more or less alike, although they are not identical, and all tigers and lions look more or less alike, but household cats do not look much like either lions or tigers and cannot interbreed with these two species. All species of cats belong to the genus *Felix*. All species of bears belong to the genus *Ursus*. The polar bear (*Ursus maritimus*), the brown bear (*Ursus arctus*), and the grizzly bear (*Ursus horribilis*) are species that resemble each other, but none of them resembles any of the species of the genus *Felix*. The household dog, *Canis familiaris*, and the wolf, *Canis lupus*, are two species of the same genus. They resemble each other, but neither resembles any members of the genus *Felix* or *Ursus*.

It should be noted that the specific name in binomial nomenclature is not used by itself to refer to any plant or animal. The specific names *leo, tigris, maritimus, horribilis,* or *lupus* have no validity in this terminology standing alone.

## FAMILIES

The **family** is the name of the group that includes all the species of one genus. The name for the cat family is *Felidae* and includes all of the species. The name for the bear family is *Ursidae*, and that for the dog family is *Canidae*. Names for families consist of one name only, and, thus, are uninomial (Latin *unus*, one). Family names are capitalized and italicized. Under the Codes now in existence,[1] the names of families of animals are formed by adding *-idae* to the stem of the generic name, and names of families of plants are formed by adding *-aceae* to the stem of the generic name, with some exceptions: *Compositae*, *Palmae*, and *Cruciferae*.

## TAXONOMIC HIERARCHY

The grouping of taxa into species, genus, family, and so forth, follows what is called the Taxonomic Hierarchy (Greek *hieros*, sacred, *archein*, rule). The smallest group is the species. Species are grouped into genera, genera into families, families into orders, orders into classes, classes into phyla (or divisions), and phyla (or divisions) into kingdoms. The kingdom is the largest taxon. There are three kingdoms: animal, plant, and mineral.[2] The phylum (singular of phyla, from Greek *phylon*, clan, tribe) of invertebrate animals called *Arthropoda* is the largest animal phylum, containing over 700,000 species. It includes the crustaceans, insects, myriapods (centipedes and millipedes), arachnids (spiders and scorpions), and other, similar creatures. This phylum was well named: "jointed-feet," from Greek *arthros*, joint, and *pous*, *podos*, foot, as all of the members of this group have jointed exoskeletons, segmented bodies, and jointed appendages.

## THE FORM AND ETYMOLOGICAL SIGNIFICANCE OF NAMES

All of the Codes of Nomenclature require that scientific names be in the form of Latin words even, as noted above, if the terms employed are, in origin, of some language other than Latin—Greek, Arabic, or English, for example. Whatever their ultimate linguistic source, these names must follow the rules of Latin grammar—that is, the names must be in the proper Latin grammatical form. An adjective that modifies a noun, for example, must agree with the noun in gender and number—feminine singular, masculine plural, neuter singular, and so forth. In the binomial nomenclature for species, the specific name—the second of the two terms—may be an adjective; thus, it must agree in gender and number with the first, or generic name, which is always a noun.

    *Spirochaeta pallida* (the causative organism of syphilis) is a spiral, hairlike microorganism, and this is what its generic name means: Greek *speira*, spiral, *chaitē*, hair. It should be noted that the Greek form for this word would be *speirochaitē* (if it ever had existed in the ancient Greek language). But the rules of the Codes say that all of the names must be in the *form* of Latin. In the latinization of Greek words, the Greek diphthong *ei* usually becomes *i*, the diphthong *ai* usually becomes *ae* (often *e*), and a final *-ē* becomes *-a*. The reason for these changes is that Greek words, when borrowed into the Latin language in antiquity, were spelled in this way. The word *Spirochaeta* is a feminine noun (because the Greek noun *chaitē* was feminine) and is singular in number. The specific name, *pallida*, which identifies this particular spirochete from others of the same genus, is a Latin adjective in the form of the feminine singular, in agreement with the feminine singular noun *Spirochaeta*. The Latin adjective *pallida* means pale, pallid. Thus, *Spirochaeta pallida* means a pale, spiral, hairlike, microorganism. It belongs to the family *Spiro-*

---

[1]These Codes are drawn up in meetings of the appropriate international organizations and are called *Codes of Nomenclature*. The naming of animals is governed by the International Code of Zoological Nomenclature (ICZN), of plants, by the International Code of Botanical Nomenclature (ICBN), and of bacteria, by the International Code of Nomenclature of Bacteria (ICNB).

[2]Some taxonomists, however, recognize up to seven kingdoms, including bacteria, viruses, and fungi.

*chaetaceae*. It should be remembered that, while names of animal families end in *-idae* (*Felidae*, *Canidae*, *Ursidae*), the names of plant families (to which spirochetes belong) end in *-aceae*.

Another name for *Spirochaeta pallida* is *Treponema pallidum*. The generic name, *Treponema*, means the same etymologically as *Spirochaeta*. It is formed from the stem *trep-* of the Greek verb *trepein*, turn, twist, and the noun *nēma*, thread. The noun *nēma* was neuter gender and singular number; thus, the Latin adjective *pallidum*, the specific name, is in the form of the Latin neuter singular. *Treponema pallidum*, pale, twisted thread = *Spirochaeta pallida*, pale, spiral hair. The family name for the genus *Treponema* is *Treponemataceae* (the stem of the Greek noun *nēma* is *nēmat-*, and to this stem is added *-aceae* to form the family name).

The second term, the specific name, of the species does not have to be an adjective modifying the generic name. It may be a noun in the genitive (possessive) case, or it may be a noun in the nominative singular. Examples of specific names in the form of the Latin nominative singular include *Felix leo*, *Felix tigris*, and *Canis lupus*, where the Latin nouns *leo*, *tigris*, and *lupus* meant lion, tiger, and wolf. Examples of specific names in the form of the Latin genitive singular include *Bacillus anthracis* (*anthrax*, *anthracis*, carbuncle), the causative agent of anthrax, a disease of animals, and *Entamoeba coli* (*colon*, *colī*, colon), a species of nonpathogenic, parasitic amoeba normally found in the human intestinal tract.

It should be noted that uninomial names for genera, orders, classes, and phyla give no indication by themselves which taxon is referred to. Thus, for example, *Lepidoptera* is an order of the class *Insecta*, which includes the moths and butterflies. *Annelida* is the name of the phylum to which the earthworms belong. *Acanthocephala* is the name of a class of wormlike enterozoa, including the *Platyhelminthes*, a phylum of flatworms that includes the tapeworms. *Anoplura* is the name of the order that includes the common louse, and *Rhinosporium* is a genus of fungi.

A number of genera have been named after the individual who first realized their existence. These names have been put into the form of a Latin word—usually by the addition of either the suffix *-ia* or the diminutive *-ella*: *Salmonella* [Daniel E. Salmon, American pathologist, 1850–1914]; *Brucella* [Sir David Bruce, British bacteriologist, 1855–1931]; *Shigella* [Kiyoshi Shiga, Japanese physician, 1870–1957]; *Yersinia* [Alexandre Yersin, Swiss bacteriologist, 1863–1943]; *Giardia* [Alfred Giard, French biologist, 1846–1908]; *Wuchereria* [Otto Wucherer, German physician, 1820–1873].

# VOCABULARY

| GREEK OR LATIN WORD | COMBINING FORM | MEANING |
| --- | --- | --- |
| *akari* | ACAR- | mite |
| *albus* | ALB- | white |
| *amoibē* | AMOEBA | [change] amoeba |
| *anōphelēs*[1] | ANOPHELES | useless, harmful |
| *askos* | ASC- | sac, bag |
| *aspergere*[2] | ASPERG- | sprinkle |
| *aureus* | AURE- | golden-yellow |
| *blatta* | BLATTA | cockroach |
| *botulus* | BOTUL- | sausage |
| *bōs, bovis* | BOV- | ox, bull, cow |
| *canis* | CAN- | dog |
| *chaitē* | CHAET- | hair |
| *cīmex* | CIMEX | bug |
| *klōstēr* | CLOSTR- | spindle |

[1]Greek *an-* + *ōpheleia*, help

[2]Latin *ad-* + *spargere*, scatter

| | | |
|---|---|---|
| *culex* | *CULEX* | gnat |
| *daknein* | DECT- | bite |
| *dis* | DI- | twice, double |
| *duodenalis* | *DUODENAL-* | of the duodenum |
| *fēlineus*[1] | *FELINEUS* | of *or* belonging to a cat |
| *flāvus* | *FLAVUS* | golden-yellow |
| *fluere* | FLU- | flow |
| *Germanicus* | *GERMANIC-* | of Germany, German |
| *glaukos* | GLAUCUS | bluish-gray |
| *Helvetius* | *HELVET-* | Helvetian, Swiss |
| *hex* | HEX- | six |
| *latro* | LATR- | robber |
| *lectulus* | *LECTUL-* | couch, bed |
| *lepis, lepidos* | LEPID- | scale (of an animal) |
| *mactāre* | *MACT-* | kill, slaughter |
| *nēma, nēmatos* | NEMA, NEMAT- | thread |
| *niger* | *NIGER* | black |
| *opisthen* | OPISTH- | located in the back |
| *orchis* | ORCHIS | testicle |
| *orientalis* | *ORIENTAL-* | of the east, oriental |
| *pallidus* | *PALLID-* | pale, lacking color |
| *pestis* | *PEST-* | infectious disease; plague |
| *philos* | PHIL- | [loving] attracted to |
| *phtheir* | PHTHIR- | louse |
| *pīpīre* | *PIP-* | peep, chirp |
| *platys* | PLATY- | flat |
| *prōtos* | PROT- | first |
| *pteron* | PTER- | wing |
| *pūbes, pūbis* | *PUB-* | pubic region |
| *speira* | SPIR- | coil, spiral |
| *staphylē* | STAPHYL- | bunch of grapes |
| *stoma, stomatos* | STOMA, STOMAT- | mouth |
| *streptos* | STREPT- | twisted |
| *tabānus* | *TABAN-* | horsefly |
| *trepein* | TREP- | turn, twist |
| *typhos* | TYPH- | a kind of fever[2] |

# ETYMOLOGICAL NOTES

The language that was used by Linnaeus, as well as by other scientists and scholars of the Renaissance and the period following, that is, the period after c. 1500, is called New Latin. The Latin found in the writings of Cicero, Julius Caesar, and other literary figures of their time is called Classical Latin. While the language of this Classical Period (first century B.C. to second century A.D.) was kept alive by scholars, churchmen, and literary figures of these many centuries up to the Renaissance, the spoken tongue had changed so dramatically as to resemble Classical Latin in only the vaguest outlines. This is, of course, the phenomenon of the development of the Romance languages—Italian, Spanish, French—from the Latin spoken in the various parts of the great Roman empire. At any age and in any place, the spoken language differs from the literary language, just as today our everyday, informal speech tends to be more idiomatic than the language that we use in writing—certainly from the language of the literary figures of the day. The spoken language of the ancient Romans is called Vulgar Latin, from the adjective *vulgaris*, of the

---

[1]Latin *fēlēs*, cat

[2]mentioned by Hippocrates in one of his essays (*On Internal Diseases*) as being one of four types of fever

people, commonplace, from the noun *vulgus*, the people, the multitude. The first great document in Vulgar Latin was the Vulgate (from *vulgata editio*, the vulgar edition), the translation of the Scriptures from Greek by Jerome (later, Saint Jerome) in the early fifth century A.D.

Scientists and writers of the Renaissance and the period following, schooled in Classical Latin, tried to emulate the classical writers and to revive the style of Cicero and others. They were successful in varying degrees; while their Latin often lacks the polish of a Cicero, it is clear and straightforward and can be read with more or less ease by one who has a background in Classical Latin. Linnaeus' *Genera Plantarum*, *Classes Plantarum*, *Philosophia Botanica*, and *Systema Naturae* are good examples of this style. The language is called New Latin. Some of these new Latin writers went so far as to change their given names to the form of Latin. As noted above, Linnaeus' given name was Carl von Linné. Other well-known personages who Latinized their names include the composer Wolfgang Mozart, who changed his middle name, Gottlieb (God-loving), to Amadeus (Latin *amāre*, love, *deus*, god). The Polish astronomer of the fifteenth–sixteenth century, Nicolaus Koppernigk, changed his name to the familiar Copernicus, and the Swiss/German physician of the same period, Aureolus Theophrastus Bombastus von Hohenheim, already given a Latin name in part, preferred to be called Paracelsus, perhaps suggesting that he was the equal of, or even superior to, the early Roman physician, Celsus.

## EXERCISES

Using the vocabulary of this lesson, determine the etymological meaning of each of the following uninomial and binomial terms. Find the modern biological meaning of each of these terms in the medical dictionary.

1. Acarina _____

_____

2. Actinomyces bovis _____

_____

3. Ancylostoma duodenale _____

_____

4. Anopheles _____

_____

5. Arthropoda _____

_____

6. Ascomycetes _____

_____

7. Aspergillus flavus _____

_____

8. Aspergillus glaucus _____

_____

9. Aspergillus niger _____

_____

10. Blatta germanica _____

_____

11. Blatta orientalis _____

_____

12. Bordetella pertussis[1] _____

_____

13. Cimex lectularius _____

_____

14. Clostridium[2] botulinum _____

_____

15. Clostridium septicum _____

_____

16. Culex pipiens _____

_____

---

[1]Jules Bordet, Belgian physician (1870–1961)
[2]Here, the Greek-derived suffix -ium (*-ion*) is a diminutive ending: Clostr-id-ium, a little thing resembling a spindle.

17. Diplococcus pneumoniae _____

    _____

18. Diptera _____

    _____

19. Entamoeba coli _____

    _____

20. Entamoeba gingivalis _____

    _____

21. Hemiptera _____

    _____

22. Hemophilus influenzae[1] _____

    _____

23. Hexapoda _____

    _____

24. Lactobacillus helveticus _____

    _____

25. Lactrodectus mactans _____

    _____

26. Lepidoptera _____

    _____

27. Opisthorchis felineus _____

    _____

_____

[1]For the form of *influenza*, see The Form and Etymological Significance of Names, page 261.

266

28. Phthirus pubis _____

_____

29. Platyhelminthes _____

_____

30. Protozoa _____

_____

31. Salmonella[1] typhosa _____

_____

32. Sarcophagidae _____

_____

33. Shigella[2] dysenteriae[3] _____

_____

34. Spirochaeta pallida _____

_____

35. Staphylococcus albus _____

_____

36. Staphylococcus aureus _____

_____

37. Streptococcus pyogenes _____

_____

_____

[1]Daniel E. Salmon, American pathologist (1850–1914)
[2]Kiyoshi Shiga, Japanese physician (1870–1957)
[3]Greek *dysenteria*, dysentery

38. Tabanidae _____

_____

39. Treponema pallidum _____

_____

40. Trichinella spiralis _____

_____

41. Yersinia[1] pestis _____

_____

---

[1]Alexandre Yersin, Swiss bacteriologist (1863–1943)

# THE NERVOUS SYSTEM*

The human body, as we are all well aware, is the most complex of organisms in all nature, of infinitely more complexity than the entire universe around us. The factors that govern the operation of the universe are debatable, but the factors that govern the operation of the billions of cells that perform the several functions that keep our bodies in a normal, healthy condition—the condition called *homeostasis*—are well known. The effective functioning of our bodies is kept in control by two systems of communication, systems that, like telephone lines, receive and transmit messages to all parts of our bodies. These two communication systems are the *nervous system* and the *endocrine system*. In this lesson we shall discuss the nervous system, leaving the functions and operations of the endocrine system to later.

The nervous system may conveniently be divided into three parts: the *central nervous system* (abbreviated CNS), the *peripheral nervous system* (abbreviated PNS), and the *autonomic nervous system*. Each of these three systems is composed of cells called *neurons*. Some of these neurons are minute in length, measuring no more than a fraction of a millimeter, while others are up to a meter (39.37 inches) in length. The longer neurons are usually called *nerve fibers*. The terms neuron, or nerve cell, and nerve fiber are not to be confused with the term *nerve*, such as the trochlear nerve, which carries impulses (messages) between the brain and certain muscles of the eyes in both directions. Messages carried *from* the brain to any part of the body are called *efferent impulses*, while messages carried *to* the brain are called *afferent impulses*. A nerve consists of a bundle or a group of bundles of nerve fibers that connect the brain and the spinal cord with various parts of the body. A bundle of nerve fibers is called a *fasciculus* (diminutive of Latin *fascis*, bundle).[1]

---

*This lesson differs slightly from previous ones, especially in the nature of the exercises. Words listed in the vocabularies of preceding lessons are not given here, and vocabulary words in this lesson are not listed in the Index of Combining Forms at the back of this text.

[1]In Roman times, the *fasces*, plural of *fascis*, was an axe surrounded by a bundle of rods and carried before the highest magistrate as a symbol of his authority. The word Fascist (or *Fascista*, singular of *Fascisti*, in its Italian form) describes one of a group of Italian nationalists organized in 1919 to oppose Bolshevism in Italy. Under the title of the National Fascist Party (*partito nazionale fascista*) and led by Benito Mussolini, it assumed control of the Italian government in 1922.

# SUBDIVISIONS OF THE NERVOUS SYSTEM

The **central nervous system** (CNS) consists of the brain and the spinal cord with their nerves that control voluntary acts, such as walking and moving various parts of the body. Nerve tissue, which forms the brain, the spinal cord, and the nerves of both of these organs, is made up of two types of tissue called gray matter and white matter. Gray matter is composed of cells of nervous tissue (neurons), while white matter is composed of nerve fibers. White matter in the brain and spinal cord carries messages from various parts of the body or from the outside world—"afferent impulses"—to the cells of the gray matter of the brain to "ask" the brain to send out efferent impulses to cause the muscles of the body to react in any way whatever.

The brain is enclosed within the skull for protection, while the spinal cord is enclosed within the spinal column, or spine, composed of bony vertebrae. Care must be taken to distinguish the spinal *cord* from the spinal *column*. Mention has already been made of the *meninges* (see Lesson 3). These are three membranes that cover and protect the spinal cord and the brain and lie under the bony structures of the skull and the spinal column. The outermost of the three is a hard membrane called the *dura mater*. The innermost of the three is a soft membrane called the *pia mater*, and, lying between these two is a weblike membrane called the *arachnoid* or the *arachnoidea*. A blow to the head—even one that seems to be trivial—can result in bleeding in the area under the dura mater, an area called the subdural space. This bleeding, called *subdural hematoma*, may not be apparent for several days or even several weeks following the initial injury.

Inflammation of the meninges is called *meningitis*; if the inflammation is in the spine, it is called *spinal meningitis*, and if it is in the brain, it is called *cerebral meningitis*. The Greek word for the spinal cord was *myelos*, and the combining form is MYEL-. *Poliomyelitis* (Greek *polios*, gray), inflammation of the gray matter of the spinal cord, is the dread disease usually called simply "polio." Development of the Salk vaccine by Dr. Jonas E. Salk (1914– ), and later the Sabin vaccine, an oral vaccine developed by Dr. Albert B. Sabin (1906– ), has reduced the mortality from polio to an insignificant figure.

The **peripheral nervous system** (PNS) consists of nerves and masses of nervous tissue called ganglia (plural of ganglion). The peripheral system, so called because its nerves extend to peripheral—that is, out-lying—parts of the body, is an outgrowth of and is connected to the CNS, although its structures lie outside of both the brain and the spinal cord. Both the CNS and the PNS control the voluntary muscles of our bodies.

The **autonomic nervous system** is concerned with control of involuntary bodily functions. It regulates the action of the glands—the salivary, gastric, and sweat glands, as well as the adrenal medulla, which produces epinephrine. The autonomic nervous system is divided into two parts: the **sympathetic division** and the **parasympathetic division**, each with its own functions. Stimulation of the nerve fibers of the **sympathetic division** causes constriction of the vasomotor muscles, the muscles that surround the blood vessels of the body. This vasoconstriction causes a rise in blood pressure, erection of the hairs of the body, goose-flesh, dilation of the pupils of the eyes, depression of gastrointestinal activity, and acceleration of the action of the heart. These changes usually occur under the stimulation of fright.

Stimulation of the nerve fibers of the **parasympathetic division** produces vasodilation, a general fall in blood pressure, contraction of the pupils of the eyes, increased gastrointestinal activity, and slowing of the heart action.

Stimulation of the nerve fibers of the sympathetic and the parasympathetic systems is effected through the action of two substances: *norepinephrine*, a hormone, and *acetylcholine*, an ester. The endings of the nerve fibers of the sympathetic nervous system secrete norepinephrine; thus, these fibers are said to be *adrenergic* (named after adrenalin, the name given to synthetic epinephrine). Release of this hormone causes stimulation of the sympathetic system, and, thus, norepinephrine is said to be a *sympathetic mediator*, or, sometimes, an *adrenergic mediator*.

The endings of nerve fibers of the parasympathetic nervous system secrete acetylcholine, and, thus, are said to be *cholinergic*. It is the action of these two substances, norepinephrine and acetylcholine, that stimulates these two divisions of the autonomic system to produce the effects upon the body that they do—that is, vasoconstriction, for example, caused by the sympathetic division, and vasodilation, caused by the parasympathetic division.

## THE STRUCTURE OF THE NERVOUS SYSTEM

As was stated above, the nervous system is composed of nerve cells, called *neurons*, or, if of substantial length, *nerve fibers*. Neurons form the gray matter of the nervous system, while nerve fibers form the white matter. The neurons make contact with each other at points called *synapses* (from Greek *haptein*, touch). Through the synapses the neurons form a network of infinite complexity.

In addition to the synapses, the neurons have structures called *dendrites* (from Greek *dendritēs*, pertaining to a tree) and *axons* (from Greek *axōn*, axis). Dendrites, which under microscopy look like the branches of a tree, conduct impulses to the cell body. They form synaptic connections with dendrites of other neurons. The axons are structures—"processes" is the term used for both dendrites and axons—that conduct impulses away from the cell body. The axons are usually long and straight, and most end in synapses through which these impulses are conducted to other neurons. In other words, dendrites conduct *afferent* impulses, and axons conduct *efferent* impulses.

The brain contains approximately 50 *billion* neurons. Each neuron has contact with more than one synapse, perhaps as many as twenty synaptic contacts. This would bring the total number of synaptic contacts between neurons to the amazing figure of one trillion (1,000,000,000,000). In addition to the neurons, in the gray and white matter of the nervous system there are what are known as accessory cells, called *glia* cells (from Greek *glia*, glue), often called *neuroglia cells*. These glia cells bind the neurons in place and form supporting tissue for them. Tumors of the glia cells of the brain are not uncommon and are called *gliomas*, or *neurogliomas*. These tumors can often be removed by modern surgical techniques.

The **spinal cord** is a cylindrical structure about the thickness of a cigarette and about 18 inches in length. It runs through the spinal column from the base of the skull to just below the ribs. Thirty-one (or thirty-two) pairs of nerves issue from the spinal cord, and these spinal nerves conduct impulses between the brain and the trunk and limbs of the body. If the spinal cord is severed or damaged severely enough, sensation and control of all muscles below the point of the injury are lost. In the present state of medical knowledge, if the spinal cord is severed, the damage is irreparable, and permanent paralysis below the point of injury is the result.

The **brain stem** is the continuation of the spinal cord up into the skull. Although it is only about three inches in length, it contains several important structures, among which are the *medulla oblongata*, the *pons*, and the *midbrain*. The *medulla oblongata* (from Latin *medulla*, marrow, and *oblongata*, elongated), the lower part of the brain stem, is about one inch in length and contains structures that regulate heart action, breathing, circulation, and control of body temperature. The **midbrain**, also called the **mesencephalon**, is the upper part of the brain stem and contains structures that regulate senses of sight, touch, and hearing, as well as equilibrium and posture. The **pons** (from Latin *pons*, bridge) lies between the medulla and the cerebrum itself—that is, it bridges the area between these two structures. Functions of the pons include transmission of impulses from the fifth, sixth, seventh, and eighth cranial nerves, which control muscles of the face and of the eyes.[1]

At the upper end of the brain stem are two masses of nerve cells called the *thalami* (plural of *thalamus*, from Greek *thalamos*, inner chamber of a house). All sensory stimuli except olfactory—that is, the sense of smell—are received by the thalami: sensations of touch, pain, heat, cold, taste, sight, hearing, and others. These sensations are relayed by the thalami to the brain.

---

[1]The cranial nerves are discussed later in this lesson.

Just underneath the thalami is a structure called the *hypothalamus*. This structure controls certain metabolic activities, such as the maintenance of water balance, sugar and fat metabolism, and the regulation of body temperature.

The actual brain, the **cerebrum**, is divided into two halves, called the *cerebral hemispheres*. Within these two hemispheres are four masses of gray matter, called the *basal ganglia*. These ganglia control muscular movement, such as walking or lifting, and other voluntary movements. If these ganglia become damaged, the individual loses some control over these simple muscular movements, resulting in the disorders called cerebral palsy, Saint Vitus' dance, Bell's palsy, Parkinson's disease, and other abnormalities of voluntary muscular movement.

The **cerebellum** ("little brain") is an outgrowth of the brain stem and is located at the back of the skull. This portion of the brain exercises control over the locomotor system of the body, the system that governs voluntary muscular movements other than those under the control of the cerebral hemispheres.

The **cerebral cortex** is the name given to the covering of the outer surface of each cerebral hemisphere. The word *cortex* is from the Latin and, in that language, meant bark (of a tree). Other organs of the body have outer coverings called *cortices* (singular, *cortex*)—the adrenal gland, for example. But when the word cortex is used alone, the *cerebral cortex* is always meant. It is composed of gray matter, and, among the functions of the body over which it exercises control are sight, hearing, touch, smell, taste—the five senses—and motor control over certain muscles.

In addition to the functions just named, the cortex controls language, learning, and memory. The area of the cortex that controls language is called Broca's area (named after Pierre Paul Broca, a French surgeon of the nineteenth century). Damage to Broca's area causes loss of control over the muscles of speech, resulting in the abnormality called *expressive aphasia*. The individual so afflicted has difficulty in expressing himself or herself in speaking or writing, although there is no impairment of understanding or of intelligence. The patient simply cannot say or write what he or she wants to.

Another area of the cortex is called *Wernicke's* area (named after Karl Wernicke, a German neurologist of the nineteenth century). Damage to Wernicke's area results in the loss of comprehension of language, a condition called *receptive aphasia*.

It was noted above that the cortex exercises control over memory, but it is what is called short-term memory that is meant. Apparently what we call long-term memory is associated with another part of the brain, an area called the *hippocampus*[1]. Damage to the hippocampus results in the loss of the ability to remember anything for more than a short time—a day, or even a few hours.

# EPILEPSY

Epilepsy, from the Greek *epilēpsia*, seizure, was well known to the ancients and has been vividly described by Hippocrates, the Greek physician of the fifth century B.C., in a lengthy treatise on what he called "The Sacred Disease." This disease is caused by a disorder of cerebral function and is characterized by sudden, brief attacks of altered consciousness, motor activity, or sensory phenomena. The most common form of epileptic attacks are convulsive seizures. It is thought that epileptic seizures are mostly idiopathic—that is, they originate within the body and are usually due to a microscopic brain lesion occurring during birth or caused by trauma in later life, or they may be due to unexplained metabolic disturbances.

Epileptic seizures are classified into two types. *Grand mal* seizures are characterized by a loss of consciousness and falling; they generally last from 2 to 5 minutes. *Petit mal* seizures are of

---

[1]Greek *hippokampos*, a mythical sea horse, a creature with the head and neck of a horse and the body and tail of a fish

short duration, usually with a 10- to 30-second loss of consciousness. In light of present medical knowledge, there is no cure for epilepsy, but anticonvulsant drugs can help control the seizures.

## NERVE PLEXUSES

In certain areas of the body, nerves from the spine and the brain, of both the voluntary and the autonomic systems, join each other (anastomose is the term used) to form an interlacing network of nerves called a *plexus* (Latin *plexus*, a braid). The plural of plexus is either plexus or plexuses. Some characteristic plexuses and their location are listed here:

**brachial plexus**: lower part of the neck to the axilla (armpit)
**celiac plexus**: behind the stomach and in front of the aorta
**cervical plexus**: opposite the first four cervical vertebrae—that is, the top four of the seven vertebrae of the spinal column
**cystic plexus**: at the gallbladder
**esophageal plexus**: around the esophagus
**lumbar plexus**: psoas muscle (one of two muscles of the loins—the area known as the lumbar region)
**myenteric plexus**: the muscles that surround the walls of the intestine
**ophthalmic plexus**: around the ophthalmic artery and the optic nerve
**phrenic plexus**: accompanies phrenic artery to diaphragm
**pulmonary plexus**: root of the lungs
**renal plexus**: renal artery
**solar plexus**: celiac plexus
**vaginal plexus**: walls of the vagina

## THE CRANIAL NERVES

The **cranial nerves** are twelve pairs of nerves that have their origin on either side of the brain—that is, one of each pair arises in the left hemisphere, and one in the right. The name, the NA term,[1] the function, and distribution of these twelve pairs of nerves are listed here.

| Number | Name | NA term | Function | Distribution |
|--------|------|---------|----------|--------------|
| First | Olfactory | Nervi olfactorii | Smell | Nasal mucous membrane |
| Second | Optic | Nervus opticus | Sight | Retina |
| Third | Oculomotor | Nervus oculomotorius | Motor | Most muscles of the eyes |
| Fourth | Trochlear | Nervus trochlearis | Motor | Superior oblique muscles of the eye |
| Fifth | Trigeminal | Nervus trigeminus | Motor and chief sensory nerve of the face | Skin of face; tongue; teeth; muscles of mastication |
| Sixth | Abducent | Nervus abducens | Motor | Lateral rectus muscle of eye |
| Seventh | Facial | Nervus facialis | Motor | Muscles of facial expression |

[1]Nomina Anatomica. For an explanation of these NA terms, see Supplementary Lesson II, The Musculo-skeletal System.

| Eighth | Auditory | Nervus vestibulocochlearis | Hearing | Internal auditory meatus[1] |
| Ninth | Glosso-pharyngeal | Nervus glossopharyngeus | Motor and sensory | Sensation of pharynx and posterior third of tongue; parotid gland |
| Tenth | Vagus | Nervus vagus | Motor and sensory | Pharynx; larynx; heart; lungs; esophagus; stomach; abdominal viscera |
| Eleventh | Accessory | Nervus accessorius | Motor | Sternomastoid and trapezius muscles |
| Twelfth | Hypoglossal | Nervus hypoglossus | Motor | Muscles of tongue |

## SELECTED VOCABULARY FOR NAMES OF NERVES

| LATIN WORD[2] | MEANING |
|---|---|
| *antebrachium* | forearm |
| *anterior* (adj.[3]) | located in front, anterior |
| *auricularis* (adj.) | of the *auricula* (outer ear), auricular |
| *buccalis* (adj.) | of the *bucca* (cheek), buccal |
| *cutaneus* (adj.) | of the *cutis* (skin), cutaneous |
| *dorsalis* (adj.) | of *or* on the *dorsum* (back), dorsal |
| *femoralis* (adj.) | of the *femur* (thigh), femoral |
| *frontalis* (adj.) | of the *frons* (forehead), frontal |
| *intercostalis* (adj.) | between the *costae* (ribs), intercostal |
| *labialis* (adj.) | of the *labium* (lip), labial |
| *lacrimalis* (adj.) | of the *lacrima* (tear apparatus), lacrimal |
| *laryngeus* (adj.) | of the *larynx*, laryngeal |
| *lateralis* (adj.) | of *or* on the side (*latus, lateris*), lateral |
| *lingualis* (adj.) | of the *lingua* (tongue), lingual |
| *lumbalis* (adj.) | of the *lumbus* (loin), lumbar |
| *magnus* (adj.) | large |
| *mandibularis* (adj.) | of the *mandibula* (lower jaw), mandibular |
| *medialis* (adj.) | middle |
| *mentalis* (adj.) | of the *mentum* (chin), mental[4] |
| *nasus* | nose |
| *olfactorius* (adj.) | of the sense of smell (*olēre*, smell, *facere, factus*, make), olfactory |
| *\*ophthalmicus* (adj.) | of the eye (*ophthalmos*), ophthalmic |
| *palatinus* (adj.) | of the *palatum* (palate), palatine |
| *pes, pedis* | foot |
| *\*phrenicus* (adj.) | of the *phren* (diaphragm), phrenic |
| *spinalis* (adj.) | of the *spina* (spine), spinal |
| *\*splanchnicus* (adj.) | of the *splanchna* (viscera), splanchnic |

---

[1]Latin *meatus*, opening

[2]Words preceded by an asterisk [*] are derived from Greek nouns.

[3]Adjectives will be designated by this abbreviation. For a discussion of the forms of Latin adjectives, see the section on Latin Adjectives in Supplementary Lesson II, The Musculoskeletal System.

[4]Not to be confused with the homonym mental, of the mind (from Latin *mens, mentis*, mind)

| | |
|---|---|
| *subcostalis* (adj.) | beneath the *costae* (ribs), subcostal |
| *supraclavicularis* (adj.) | above the collarbone (*clavicula*, diminutive of *clavis*, key), supraclavicular |
| *suralis* (adj.) | of the *sura* (calf of the leg), sural |
| *\*thoracicus* (adj.) | of the *thorax*, thoracic |
| *\*tympanicus* (adj.) | of the *tympanum* (eardrum), tympanic |
| *ulnaris* (adj.) | of the *ulna* (inner bone of the forearm), ulnar |
| *\*zygomaticus* (adj.) | of the *zygoma* (cheekbone), zygomatic |

# ETYMOLOGICAL NOTES

The spinal cord and the brain are covered with three layers of protective membrane called the meninges (singular, meninx). Before the first century A.D., the Greek word *mēninx* was applied to any membrane of the body; Hippocrates used it to refer to the membrane of the eye, and Aristotle used it to refer to the eardrum. But, after the first century, the term came to be used exclusively to refer to the meninges in their modern anatomical sense. The three meninges are named the **pia mater**, the delicate inner covering, the **dura mater**, the tough outer coat, and the **arachnoid**, the membrane between these two. The arachnoid (resembling a web) takes its name from Greek *arachnē*, spider, web, because of its delicate structure. But the names pia mater, meaning devout mother in Latin, and dura mater, hard mother, make little sense until it is realized that they are translations from the Arabic.

By the fourth century A.D. the Roman empire was split into two halves, with Rome the capital in the west and Byzantium (later named Constantinople by the emperor Constantine, and today called Istanbul) in the east. The two halves were separated linguistically as well as geographically, with Latin the language of the west and Greek that of the east. Such writings as survived in the west in the period following this were preserved, for the most part, by the Roman church, and these were principally the Latin authors; Greek ceased to be taught in the schools, and the knowledge of this language gradually was lost, along with the works of Hippocrates, Aristotle, and others. Nevertheless, these works were very much alive in the east, not only in Byzantium/Constantinople, but in other lands of the eastern empire.

With the rise and spread of Islam during and following the seventh century, Arabic became the common language of almost the entire east. Works of the ancient Greek writers were now translated into Arabic and read in the great centers of learning all over the Islamic empire, including Spain. These Arabic translations, and Arabic literature in general, escaped the notice of most of western Europe for the simple reason that there were few who could read Arabic. Thus, by the early Middle Ages, practically all knowledge of ancient Greek literature, including the medical works, was unknown in the west.

In the eleventh and twelfth centuries, monks of the Roman church began translating some of the Arabic versions of the Greek writers into Latin. In Syria, a churchman known as Stephen of Antioch, produced a Latin translation of Galen from the Arabic version. At this time, only two of the three meninges—the ones that we call the dura and the pia—were known. Galen, writing in Greek, had named the outer (the dura) the *mēninx sklēra pacheia*, the hard, thick, membrane, and the inner (the pia), the *mēninx leptē*, the thin membrane. In the Arabic translation of Galen, the Greek terms were translated as hard mother and thin mother. The Arabic use of the word for mother to translate the Greek *mēninx* may have implied that the protection afforded the spinal cord by the meninges could be compared to the protection that a mother gives to her young. Stephen translated these two terms into the Latin *dura mater* and *pia mater*, "hard mother" and "devout mother." The *pia* (feminine of *pius*, devout, pious) should have been *tenuis*, thin, but Stephen, a monk, apparently decided that *pia* was a more appropriate term, and it has remained thus. The arachnoid membrane was not identified until the seventeenth century, when the Dutch anatomist Frederick Ruysch realized its existence and named it.

# EXERCISES

Using the selected vocabulary of this lesson as reference, determine the location of each of the following nerves.

1. Nervi auriculares anteriores[1] _____

2. Nervus auricularis magnus _____ _____

3. Nervus auricularis posterior _____

4. Nervus buccalis _____

5. Nervus cutaneus antebrachii lateralis _____

6. Nervus cutaneus antebrachii medialis _____

7. Nervus cutaneus antebrachii posterior _____

8. Nervus cutaneus brachii medialis _____

9. Nervus cutaneus brachii posterior _____

10. Nervus cutaneus brachii lateralis inferior _____

11. Nervus cutaneus brachii lateralis superior _____

12. Nervus cutaneus dorsalis lateralis pedis _____

13. Nervus cutaneus femoris lateralis _____

14. Nervus cutaneus femoris posterior _____

15. Nervus cutaneus surae lateralis _____

16. Nervus cutaneus surae medialis _____

17. Nervus femoralis _____

18. Nervus frontalis _____

19. Nervi intercostales _____

_____

[1]See the section on The Order of Words in Supplementary Lesson II, The Musculoskeletal System.

20. Nervi labiales anteriores _____

21. Nervi labiales posteriores _____

22. Nervus lacrimalis _____

23. Nervus laryngeus inferior _____

24. Nervus laryngeus superior _____

25. Nervus lingualis _____

26. Nervi lumbales _____

27. Nervus mandibularis _____

28. Nervus mentalis _____

29. Nervus nasopalatinus _____

30. Nervi olfactorii _____

31. Nervus ophthalmicus _____

32. Nervi palatini _____

33. Nervus phrenicus _____

34. Nervi spinales _____

35. Nervi splanchnici lumbales _____

36. Nervus subcostalis _____

37. Nervus sublingualis _____

38. Nervi supraclaviculares laterales _____

39. Nervi supraclaviculares mediales _____

40. Nervus suralis _____

41. Nervi thoracici _____

42. Nervus tympanicus _____

43. Nervus ulnaris _____

44. Nervus zygomaticus _____

# THE ENDOCRINE SYSTEM*

The state of equilibrium within our bodies when all organs are functioning perfectly is called *homeostasis* (from Greek *homoios*, like, and *stasis*, condition, state). The body is kept in homeostasis by two systems of communication which receive and transmit messages and instructions to all parts of the body. These two communication systems are the nervous system, described in the preceding lesson, and the **endocrine system** (from Greek *endo-*, within, and *krinein*, separate, secrete). The endocrine system of the body is made up of a group of glands that secrete **hormones** (from Greek *horman*, set in motion). When the need arises—that is, when any of these glands receive the appropriate message—the glands pour their secretions, the hormones, directly into the bloodstream that flows through the glands. Thus, these endocrine glands are known as *ductless glands*—that is, they do not transmit their secretions into ducts, as, for example, the sweat glands or the tear glands do. Glands that send their secretions through ducts are called **exocrine glands**.[1]

The hormones that are secreted in the endocrine glands are substances that, when carried to some other part or parts of the body by the bloodstream, stimulate these parts by chemical action to increased activity. Insulin, for example, is a hormone secreted by the islets of Langerhans in the pancreas. When the need arises—in this instance, when the level of blood sugar rises—insulin is secreted directly into the bloodstream and maintains proper metabolism of blood sugar.

The hormones secreted by the ductless glands may have a specific effect upon the body, as, for example, is the case with the gonads (the ovaries and testes), which are concerned with sexual development; or they may have a general effect upon the entire body, as is the case with the thyroid hormone, which regulates the rate of metabolism for the whole body. The principal endocrine glands and their functions follow.

---

*This lesson differs slightly from previous ones, especially in the nature of the exercises. Words listed in the vocabularies of preceding lessons are not given here, and vocabulary words in this lesson are not listed in the Index of Combining Forms at the back of this text.

[1]sometimes called **eccrine**, especially the eccrine sweat glands

# THE PITUITARY GLAND

Also called the *hypophysis cerebri*, this small gland (about the size of a bean) is situated at the base of the brain. It is divided into two distinct sections: the *anterior lobe* and the *posterior lobe*. A third division, called the *intermediate lobe*, seems to have no functions in man and other higher animals, although certain effects of it have been noted in cold-blooded creatures such as fish, amphibians, and reptiles. The anterior lobe is sometimes referred to as the master gland of the body, as its secretions stimulate other endocrine glands into increased (or decreased) activity. The **anterior lobe** of the pituitary secretes six principal hormones:

1. The **somatotrophic hormone** (STH), which regulates growth. Increased production of this hormone can cause *giantism*—abnormal growth—and/or *acromegaly*, abnormal enlargement of the hands, feet, jaw, and other extremities. Decreased production of STH can cause dwarfism and/or *acromicria*—abnormal smallness of the extremities.

2. The **adrenocorticotrophic hormone** (ACTH), which regulates the activity of the adrenal cortex, the outer layer of the adrenal gland. Secretions of the **adrenal cortex** include two groups of hormones that belong to the family of chemicals called *steroids*. The first of these two is a group called *mineralocorticoids*, which regulate the metabolism of sodium, an extremely important function, as an excess or a deficiency of sodium in the body can have serious results. The second of these hormones is a group of chemicals called *glucocorticoids*, which act mainly on the metabolism of glucose. This group of steroids is also effective in protecting the body against stress and in the promotion of the healing process.

In addition to these steroids the adrenal cortex secretes sex hormones—androgens in men and estrogens and progesterone in women.

3. The **thyrotrophic hormone** (TTH), which regulates the activity of the thyroid gland. The activities of this endocrine gland will be discussed in full below.

4. The (ovarian) **follicle-stimulating hormone** (FSH), which stimulates development of follicles in the ovaries and spermatogenesis in the testes. The ovarian follicles (from Latin *folliculus*, a little sac, diminutive of *follis*, sac) are spherical structures that produce an ovum every month in women of child-bearing age.

5. The **luteinizing hormone** (LH), which, in conjunction with FSH, induces secretion of estrogens and progesterone, female hormones, stimulates ovulation each month, and regulates the development of the *corpus luteum* (Latin, yellow body), a small yellow structure that develops within a ruptured ovarian follicle when the ovum is released each month.

6. The **luteotrophic hormone** (LTH), which maintains the mature corpus luteum. It also induces secretion of milk in the fully developed mammary gland and, because of this action, is often called the *lactogenic* hormone (from Latin *lac*, *lactis*, milk).

The **posterior lobe** of the pituitary gland secretes a hormone called *oxytocin* (from Greek *oxys*, rapid, and *tokos*, childbirth), which increases uterine contractions during labor. Another hormone secreted within the posterior lobe is *vasopressin*, which contracts the muscles of blood vessels and elevates blood pressure. Vasopressin also acts as an antidiuretic, preventing excessive loss of fluids through the kidneys.

# THE THYROID GLAND

The **thyroid gland** is situated at the base of the neck on both sides of the lower part of the larynx and upper part of the trachea. The name comes from Greek *thyreos*, shield: thyr-oid, "shield-shaped." As was noted above, the thyroid gland is stimulated by the thyrotrophic hormone (TTH, also called *thyrotropin*) secreted within the anterior lobe of the pituitary gland. The principle hormone secreted by the thyroid gland is **thyroxine**. Oversecretion of thyroxine produces the condition called *hyperthyroidism*. This increases the rate of basal metabolism, causing an increased demand for food to support this increased metabolic activity. Symptoms of hyperthyroidism include increased nervousness, tremor of the fingers, excessive sweating, increased heart rate, and weight loss. If the overproduction of this hormone is excessive, the condition called *thyrotoxicosis* results, the salient features of which are protruding eyes (*exophthalmos*) and, often, goiter (from Latin *guttur*, throat), enlargement of the thyroid, sometimes to the size of an orange or even larger.

Deficient production of thyroxin produces the condition called *hypothyroidism*, resulting in a lowered rate of basal metabolism. Symptoms of hypothyroidism are the opposite of those of *hyperthyroidism*: sluggishness, low blood pressure, slow pulse, and decreased muscular activity. However, goiter may accompany hypothyroidism as well as hyperthyroidism. The underlying cause of hyper- and hypothyroidism is associated with the maintenance of proper levels of iodine in the diet. In certain regions of the world the water is deficient in iodine salts, and hypothyroidism is endemic. In recent years, however, the use of iodized salt has reduced the incidence of hypothyroidism in areas where iodine salts are of low levels in the drinking water.

Severe lack of iodine in childhood produces the condition known as *cretinism*, characterized by lack of growth and mental development. The term *cretin* comes from Swiss French *creitin*, from Latin *Christianus*, Christian. Use of this term originated in Switzerland where, due to the fact that the land has long been geologically separated from the sea, the water lacks iodine salts. The Swiss are said to have used this term to indicate their realization that these creitins were, after all, children of God.

Hypofunction of the thyroid gland in older children and adults causes the condition called *myxedema* (from Greek *myxa*, mucus, and *edema*, swelling), characterized by anemia, edematous face and hands (caused by accumulations of mucus), coarse and thickened skin, drowsiness, and mental slowness.


# THE PARATHYROID GLANDS


The **parathyroid glands** are four in number and are located close to the thyroid gland. These glands secrete the *parathyroid hormone* (PTH), which regulates the metabolism of calcium and phosphorus. *Hypoparathyroidism* results in a fall in the level of blood calcium and a rise in the level of blood phosphorus. This condition is characterized mainly by loss of calcium in the teeth and bones, with resultant teeth defects and bone lesions. In general, the activity of the parathyroid glands is associated with proper maintenance of vitamin D in the body, as without normal levels of this vitamin, calcium cannot be properly utilized.

*Hyperparathyroidism* results in a rise in blood calcium and a fall in the level of blood phosphorus, characterized by muscular weakness and increased fragility of the bones caused by removal of calcium from the bones into the circulating blood. The presence of abnormal amounts of calcium in the blood (*hypercalcemia*) and the inability of the kidneys to excrete this excess can cause the deposition of calcium in the kidneys in the form of renal calculi—kidney stones—a condition known as *nephrolithiasis*.


# THE ADRENAL GLANDS


The **adrenal glands**, sometimes called the *suprarenal glands*, are two in number, one above each kidney. Each adrenal gland consists of two distinct parts: the outer covering, the *adrenal cortex*, and the inner structure, the *renal medulla*. As was stated above in the description of the functions of the pituitary gland, the **adrenal cortex** produces a hormone called the *adrenocorticotrophic hormone* (ACTH). This hormone stimulates the adrenal cortex to produce the chemical substances called *steroids*, principally those called *mineralocorticoids*, which help regulate the mineral content of the blood, and the *glucocorticoids*, which help maintain proper levels of glucose in the blood. Another important hormone secreted by the adrenal cortex is *cortisone*, important for its regulatory action in the metabolism of fats, carbohydrates, sodium, potassium, and proteins. Cortisone is manufactured synthetically and is used as an anti-inflammatory (*antiphlogistic*) agent.

Also secreted in small amounts in the renal cortex are *androgens*, the male hormones, and *estrogens* and *progesterone*, the female hormones. Irregularities in the production of these hormones can result in over- or under-sexual development in both males and females.

The **adrenal medulla** secretes three groups of chemical substances called *catecholamines: dopamine, norepinephrine,* and *epinephrine*. The principal effects of **dopamine** on the body are dilation of the arteries, increased cardiac output, with resultant increased flow of blood to the kidneys.

The principal effect of **norepinephrine** is constriction of the arterioles and venules—the ends of the arteries and veins, where they anastomose, or join, with the capillaries. This results in increased resistance to the flow of blood through the systemic circulation, which, in turn, causes elevated blood pressure and slowing of the heart action (*bradycardia*).

**Epinephrine** increases heart activity, dilates the bronchi (for which reason *adrenalin*, synthetic epinephrine, is useful in treating those suffering with asthma), increases the level of glucose in the blood, and diminishes the activity of the gastrointestinal system.

The adrenal medulla is under the control of the sympathetic nervous system, and, thus, is part of the autonomic system. The secretion of epinephrine and norepinephrine is closely related to emotional states. Fear, stress, and emergency situations can cause the sympathetic system to "send a message" to the adrenal medulla, which can result in immediate secretion of norepinephrine or epinephrine, whichever is needed in the particular situation, thereby giving a quick boost to the energy level of the body.

# THE ISLETS OF LANGERHANS

The **islets of Langerhans** are clusters of cells in the pancreas and are of three types: alpha, beta, and delta cells. The beta cells are found in the greatest number, and it is these that produce insulin.

**Insulin** (from Latin *insula*, island) is essential for the proper metabolism of blood sugar (glucose) and for the proper maintenance of glucose levels in the blood. Insufficient secretion of insulin results in deficient metabolism of carbohydrates and fats and brings on the conditions called *hyperglycemia*, excessive amounts of blood sugar, and *glycosuria*, the presence of glucose in the urine. These two conditions characterize the disease called diabetes.

Excessive secretion of insulin brings about the condition called *hypoglycemia*, characterized by acute fatigue, irritability, and general weakness. In extreme cases, *insulin shock*, as it is called, can bring about mental disturbances, coma, and even death.

The islets of Langerhans are named for Paul Langerhans, a German pathologist of the nineteenth century, who first realized their existence and function.

There are several forms of the disease **diabetes**, all characterized by excessive urination. The commonest type is *diabetes mellitus*, sugar diabetes. The cause of the disease is unknown. Heredity is thought by some to play a part in its development. But the disease is brought on, as was stated above, by failure of the beta cells of the pancreas to secrete insulin in adequate amounts. The principal symptoms of diabetes mellitus are elevated blood sugar (*hyperglycemia*), sugar in the urine (*glycosuria*), excessive urine production (*polyuria*), excessive thirst (*polydipsia*), and abnormally increased food intake (*polyphagia*).

Diabetes is a chronic, incurable disease, but its symptoms can be made tolerable and life prolonged by modern methods of treatment. The isolation of and eventual synthesization of insulin by the Canadian physicians Sir Frederick Banting and Charles H. Best (for which Banting became a Nobel laureate in 1923) has made it possible for diabetics to live with their disease by the administration of insulin by injection.

# THE GONADS

The **gonads** are the sex glands in both male and female. The male gonads, the testes, secrete spermatozoa, and the female gonads, the ovaries, produce an ovum each month during parturient, or child-bearing, years.

The **testes** (or **testicles**) produce the male hormone *testosterone*, an androgen that develops and maintains secondary male sex characteristics—muscular strength, development of hair on the body, and lowered voice.

The **ovaries** produce the female hormones *estrogen* and *progesterone*, which develop and maintain secondary female sex characteristics—development of the breasts, soft body, smooth skin, and high voice. For a discussion of ovulation, see Lesson 14 in this text, Gynecology.

# ETYMOLOGICAL NOTES

The Greek verb *krinein*, separate, which has supplied the -crine in the words endocrine and exocrine, has also given us other, nontechnical, words. The verb had the additional meanings in ancient times of pick out, choose, and then, judge. There was a noun, *krisis*, related to this verb, and the noun meant a separating, picking out, choosing. Extended meanings of this noun included trial, judgment, decision. From these varied, but related, meanings we get our word crisis, with its modern shades of meaning. Also related to the verb *krinein* was the noun *kritēs*, judge, arbiter; the adjectival form of this noun was *kritikos*, able to decide *or* judge; critical. This word was borrowed into Latin as the noun *criticus*, judge, critic. Another related word was *kritērion*, a means of judging, a standard; criterion.

Estrogen, the female hormone, takes its name from Greek *oistros*, an insect that infected cattle, plus the form *-gen*. This unusual etymology has at its root a secondary meaning of this noun: a sting, anything that excites, madness, frenzy, vehement passion. The term estrus (or oestrus) designates the cyclic period of sexual activity in females; thus, estrogen is the name of the hormone that causes or promotes the period of estrus. The ancients, of course, were unaware of the reasons for the cyclic periods of women between menarche and menopause, and the word *oistros* (Latin *oestrus*) was used by the writers in its original sense: that which excites (something *or* somebody) to action; a stinging insect. Vergil writes in the *Georgics* (3.146–148):

> *est lucos Silari circa ilicibusque virentem*
> *plurimus Alburnum volitans, cui nomen asilo*
> *Romanum est,* oestrum *Grai vertere vocantes, . . .*

"Around the groves of Silarus and around Alburnus green with oak trees there flies a creature which the Romans call *asilus*, but called *oestrus* by the Greeks."

Greek legend tells us of a young girl named Io, daughter of the river Inachus, who had the misfortune to be desired by Zeus. Just as he was about to consummate his desires, his wife, Hera, came upon the scene; in the instant before her appearance, Zeus changed Io into a heifer, a young cow. Hera, rightfully suspicious, asked that the creature be given to her. Zeus had no choice but to comply. Hera then stationed a hundred-eyed watchdog, Argus, to stand guard over the luckless Io. Zeus, unable to tolerate this state of affairs, sent his messenger, Hermes, with orders: "Kill Argus!" Hermes did as ordered, and Io was free, but still in bovine form. Hera took the hundred eyes of Argus and placed them in the tail of her favorite bird, the peacock. She then sent a stinging insect, the *oistros*, to drive poor Io in flight all over the face of the earth. Eventually Zeus restored her to human form, and she settled down in the land of Egypt, where she became the mother of a son, Epaphus, sired by Zeus.

## EXERCISES

Answer each of the following questions.

1. What are the functions of each of the following hormones, secreted in the anterior lobe of the pituitary gland?

   (a) the somatotrophic hormone (STH) _____

   (b) the adrenocorticotrophic hormone (ACTH) _____

   _____

   (c) the lactogenic hormone _____

2. What is the main function of the hormone *oxytocin*, secreted in the posterior lobe of the pituitary gland?

3. What effect does *vasopressin* have upon the body?

4. If there is excessive secretion of the hormone *thyroxine* by the thyroid gland, the result may be *thyrotoxicosis*. What is the meaning of each of the following two salient features of thyrotoxicosis?

   (a) exophthalmos _____

   (b) goiter _____

5. What is the cause of the condition known as *cretinism*?

6. *Myxedema* is a condition characterized by accumulations of mucus in the tissues of the face and hands. What is the cause of myxedema, as far as glandular function is concerned?

7. Hypoparathyroidism can result in the condition known as *hypercalcemia*. What is the meaning of this?

8. Hypercalcemia can result in *nephrolithiasis*. What is the meaning of this?

9. Cortisone, one of the hormones secreted in the adrenal glands, can be produced synthetically and is useful as an *antiphlogistic*. What is the meaning of this?

10. *Epinephrine*, secreted in the adrenal glands, can be produced synthetically. When it is produced in this way, what is it called?

11. What is the meaning of each of the following five principal symptoms of diabetes mellitus?

(a) hyperglycemia _____

(b) glycosuria _____

(c) polyuria _____

(d) polydipsia _____

(e) polyphagia _____

12. The hormone testosterone is an *androgen*. What is the meaning of this term?

13. What is the name given to glands that transmit their secretions through ducts, as is the case, for example, with the salivary glands?

14. What is the more usual term for the gland called the *hypophysis cerebri*?

15. What is the name given to the outside covering of the adrenal gland?

16. What is the name given to the inside portion of the adrenal gland?

17. Which endocrine gland is often called the master gland of the body? What is the reason for this?

18. What hormones provide sudden energy to the body in emergency situations?

19. Deficient secretion of the hormone STH can cause *acromicria*. What is the meaning of this term?

20. What hormone is secreted in the islets of Langerhans, and in what organ is this gland located?

21. What is the difference between the *endocrine* and the *exocrine* glands? What glands are commonly called *eccrine*?

# THE DEVELOPMENT
# OF THE ENGLISH LANGUAGE;
# NEW LATIN; THE ANCIENT
# MEDICAL WRITERS

The language that we call English began its development as an independent tongue with the migration of certain Germanic peoples from western Europe across the English Channel to Britain during the fifth and sixth centuries A.D. We know these invaders best as the Angles and the Saxons, two of many groups. Their language, or dialects, which we call Old English, or Anglo-Saxon, and which was a member of the Germanic family of Indo-European languages, gradually superseded the Celtic dialects in most of southern Britain. The earliest written records of Old English date to about the end of the seventh century, and even at this early date four distinct dialects are observable. These are called Northumbrian, Mercian, West Saxon, and Kentish. The first two of these are often grouped together and called Anglian. Many Old English words have survived, with the customary linguistic changes, into the English of today and have formed the basic vocabulary of our language. Such words are called native words, as opposed to words borrowed from other languages—mostly Latin, French, and Greek.

During the sixth century Britain had been converted to Christianity, and as the language of the Western Church was Latin, it was that language that was spoken, written, and read in the churches, schools, and monasteries, thus bringing large numbers of Latin words into the English language. The Norman conquest of England in 1066 brought a French-speaking ruling nobility to the royal court, and for about 150 years, Old French, as we call the language of this period, was the official spoken and written language of the governing class in England. But, despite this fact, few Old French words entered the English language during this period. However, in the 300 years following the expulsion of the Normans from England—from about 1200 to 1500—many words were borrowed from Old French. The vocabulary of this language was far richer than the limited vocabulary of English, and writers and educated people of England began to borrow heavily from French to provide words and concepts lacking in their own native language.

It was later, during the period of the Renaissance, that English words began to be formed directly from Latin (and Greek) and not borrowed through the intermediary of Old French. The English Renaissance began around A.D. 1500, and it was now for the first time that the literature of the ancient Greeks was read in England in the original language. Now the impoverished state of the English vocabulary was realized. How could one discuss or write about Aristotelian ethics, Stoic philosophy, or Epicureanism, for example, when English had no words for many of these philosophical concepts? The only recourse was to do what Cicero had done in his philosophical discourses: borrow the words in the language of the original writers, Greek in Cicero's case, both Latin and Greek in the case of the Renaissance philosophers. The ancient languages were now taught in the schools of England. Chapman translated Homer; Vergil and Plutarch were translated; King James authorized a translation of the Scriptures. And the beginnings of modern science were rapidly gaining ground.

As new theories and concepts in the sciences were realized, words had to be found to express these new ideas. The scientific men of the Renaissance and post-Renaissance—and indeed of this very day—borrowed their terminology from Greek and Latin writers.

In the field of medicine, by the time of the medieval period, much of the sophisticated knowledge epitomized in the writings of Hippocrates, Galen, Celsus, and others, had been lost or had degenerated into a mixture of magic and superstition. It was with the introduction of the writings of these early medical men into Europe that the scientists of the period paved the way for genuine scientific inquiry into the field of medical research. The works of Galen in particular led to a finer realization of scientific physiology and are to be considered the vivifying force that culminated in the turning point of modern medicine, the discovery of the circulatory system by William Harvey (1578–1657).

# NEW LATIN

The term New Latin is used to refer either to words that have been coined in modern times on the analogy of authentic Latin words, as, for example, *natrium*, the chemical name for sodium (borrowed from Arabic), or to authentic Latin words that have been given new meanings, as, for example, the word cancer, from *cancer*, crab, or the word bacillus, from *bacillus*, a small rod or staff. Biological terms are rich in New Latin, as in *Trichinella spiralis*, the species of Trichinella that causes trichinosis, or as in *Salmonella*, the genus of microorganisms named after the American pathologist Daniel E. Salmon.

# THE ANCIENT MEDICAL WRITERS

## HIPPOCRATES

Hippocrates, of the Greek island of Cos, a fifth-century B.C. contemporary of Socrates, is called The Father of Medicine. Although he is the most famous of the ancient physicians, very little is known about Hippocrates the man, and all that can be said about him is that he was a physician and that a large number of works have come down to us under his name. Modern scholars reject the authenticity of most of these works on various grounds. However, his importance and influence cannot be denied. He was the first that we know who freed medicine from the bonds of superstition and based its practice and theory upon scientific observation and reporting. The works that come to us under his name show that he understood quite well the workings of the human body and knew from his observations that there were certain morbid signs indicating what we would call disease, and that these morbid signs ran their course and led to either death or recovery. He also realized that the patient could aid in his own recovery by altering his way of living, but beyond this, and beyond the scientific reporting of what he observed, his theories are mostly conjecture, as when he says, "A woman does not get gout (*podagra*) unless menstruation is suppressed" [*Aphorisms* 6.29]. Hippocrates' greatest importance in the history of medicine is the influence that he exerted upon the later writer Galen.

# GALEN

Galen (A.D. 129–?199) was born in Pergamum in Asia Minor. After studying medicine at the Asclepium, the famed medical school in his native town, and in Smyrna and Alexandria, he came to Rome in 162 where, except for brief interruptions, he remained until his death, writing philosophical treatises and medical books. His fame and reputation were such that he became court physician to the emperor Marcus Aurelius. Galen wrote extensively on anatomy, physiology, and general medicine, relying upon his training—the best that was available in his time—and upon the dissection of human corpses and experiments upon living animals. It was the work of Galen above all other medical writers that profoundly influenced the physicians of the early Renaissance, and his theories on the flow of blood in the human body were not challenged until the discovery of the circulation of blood by William Harvey in the 17th century.

# CELSUS

Aulus Cornelius Celsus was a Roman encyclopedist who, under the reign of the emperor Tiberius (A.D. 14–37), wrote a lengthy work on the current state of knowledge of agriculture, military tactics, medicine, rhetoric, and probably philosophy and law. Apart from a few fragments of the other sections, only the portions on medicine have remained. In the introduction he deals with the history of medicine up to his own time and gives us valuable knowledge of Hellenistic theories. It is thought that Celsus was a layman writing for other laymen and not a professional physician, as it appears, especially in his discourses on surgery, that he had little first-hand experience in the field of medicine, relying upon material selected from different sources. Nonetheless, his anatomical observations are acute, even though marred by many inaccuracies and errors.

# INDEX OF PREFIXES AND SUFFIXES

## PREFIXES

Entries for Latin prefixes are in italic type.

a- (an- before a vowel or *h*): not, without, lacking, deficient

*ab-* (*a-* rarely before certain consonants; *abs-* before *c* and *t*): away from

*ad-* (*ac-* before *c*; *af-* before *f*; *ag-* before *g*; *al-* before *l*; *an-* before *n*; *ap-* before *p*; *as-* before *s*; *a-* before *sp-*; *at-* before *t*): to, toward

*ambi-*: both

amphi-, ampho-: on both sides, around; both

ana-: up, back, again

*ante-*: before, forward

anti- (ant- often before a vowel or *h*; hyphenated before *i*): against, opposed to, preventing, relieving

apo- (ap- before a vowel): away from

*bi-* (*bin-*, *bis-*): twice, double, both

cata- (cat- before a vowel or *h*): downward; disordered

*circum-*: around

*con-* (*co-* before *h*; *col-* before *l*; *com-* before *e*, *m*, and *p*; *cor-* before *r*): together, with; thoroughly, very

*contra-*: against, opposite

*de-*: down, away from, absent

di-: (rarely dis-): twice, double

dia- (di- before a vowel): through, across, apart

*dis-* (*di-* before *g*, *v*, and usually before *l*; *dif-* before *f*): apart, away

dys-: difficult, painful, defective, abnormal

ec- (ex- before a vowel): out of, away from

ecto- (ect- often before a vowel): outside of

en- (em- before *b*, *m*, and *p*): in, into, within

endo-, ento- (end-, ent- before a vowel): within

epi- (ep- before a vowel or *h*): upon, over, above

eso-: within, inner, inward

eu-: good, normal, healthy

*ex-* (*e-* before certain consonants; *ef-* before *f*): out of, away from

exo-: outside, from the outside, toward the outside

*extra-*, (rarely *extro-*): on the outside, beyond

hemi-: half, partial; (often) one side of the body

hyper-: over, above, excessive, beyond normal

hypo- (hyp- before a vowel or *h*): under, deficient, below normal

*in-* (*il-* before *l*; *im-* before *b*, *m*, and *p*; *ir-* before *r*): in, into

*in-* (*il-* before *l*; *im-* before *b*, *m*, and *p*; *ir-* before *r*): not

*in-* (*il-* before *l*; *im-* before *b*, *m*, and *p*; *ir-* before *r*): very, thoroughly

*infra-*: beneath, below

*inter-*: between

*intra-* (rarely *intro-*): within

meta- (met- before a vowel or *h*): change, after

*non-*: not

*ob-* (*oc-* before *c*; *op-* before *p*): against, toward; very, thoroughly

para- (often par- before a vowel): alongside, around, abnormal

*per-* (*pel-* before *l*): through; very, thoroughly

peri-: around, surrounding

*post-*: after, following, behind

*pre-*: before, in front of

pro-: before

*pro-*: forward, in front

pros-, prosth-: in place of

*re-*: back, again

*retro-*: backward, in back, behind

*se-*: apart, away from

*semi-*: half

*sub-* (*suf-* before *f*; *sup-* before *p*): under

*super-* (often *supra-*): over, above; excess

*trans-*: across, through

syn- (sym- before *b*, *p*, and *m*; *n* assimilates or is dropped before *l* and *s*): together, with, joined

# SUFFIXES

Suffixes form either nouns or adjectives (or, in rare instances, verbs). Most of the nouns in medical terminology are abstract, indicating a state, quality, condition, procedure, *or* process. Noun-forming suffixes that have specialized meanings, such as -itis, inflammation, will be so indicated. Adjectival suffixes usually have the generalized meaning of pertaining to, referring to, having to do with, in a condition *or* state of, caused by, causing, *or* located in. Only those meanings most commonly found are indicated here. Entries for Latin suffixes are in italic type.

-a: forms abstract nouns: *state, condition*

-*able*: forms adjectives: *capable of*

-ac (rare): forms adjectives: *pertaining to, located in*

-*ad*: indicates direction toward a part of the body: *toward*

-*al*: forms adjectives: *pertaining to, located in*

-*an*: forms adjectives: *pertaining to, located in*

-*ar*: forms adjectives: *pertaining to, located in*

-*arium*: denotes a place for something: *place for*

-*ary*: forms adjectives: *pertaining to*

-ary: denotes a place for something: *place for*

-ase: forms names of enzymes

-asia, -asis (rare): form abstract nouns: *state, condition*

-ate: forms names of chemical substances

-ate: forms adjectives: *having the form of, possessing*

-ce: forms abstract nouns: *state, condition*

-culus, -cula, -culum, -cle: form diminutives

-cy: forms abstract nouns: *state, condition*

-eal: forms adjectives: *pertaining to, located in*

-ean: forms adjectives: *pertaining to, located in*

-ellus, -ella,

-ella: forms names of biological genera

-ellus, -ella, -ellum: form diminutives

-ema: forms abstract nouns: *state, condition*

-esis, -esia: form abstract nouns: *state, condition, procedure*

-etic: forms adjectives, often from nouns in -esis: *pertaining to*

-ia: forms abstract nouns. In many instances -ia appears in English as -y: *state, condition*

-ia: forms abstract nouns: *state, condition*

-iac (rare): forms nouns: *person afflicted with*

-iasis: forms abstract nouns: *disease, abnormal condition*

-ible: forms adjectives: *capable of*

-ic: forms adjectives: *pertaining to, located in*; many words in -ic have come to be used as nouns

-ic: forms adjectives: *pertaining to*

-ics, -tics: form nouns indicating a particular science or study: *science* or *study of*

-id: see -oid

-id: forms adjectives: *pertaining to*: often has the meaning *in a state* or *condition of*

-ide: forms names of chemical substances

-ile: forms adjectives: *pertaining to*

-ile: forms adjectives: *capable of*

-illus, -illa, -illum: form diminutives

-in, -ine: form names of substances

-ine: forms adjectives: *pertaining to, located in*

-ion: forms abstract nouns: *the act of*

-ism: forms abstract nouns: *state, condition, quality*

-ismus: forms abstract nouns: *state, condition; muscular spasm*

-ist: forms nouns: *a person interested in*

-ite: forms names of chemical substances

-itic: forms adjectives: *pertaining to; pertaining to inflammation*; often these adjectives are used as nouns

-itis: forms nouns indicating an inflamed condition: *inflammation*

-ium (rarely -eum): forms nouns: *membrane, connective tissue*

-ive: forms adjectives: *pertaining to*

-lent: forms adjectives: *full of*

-ma: forms nouns: (often) *abnormal* or *diseased condition*; sometimes forms names of substances

-ment: forms nouns: *agent* or *instrument*

-oid, (rarely) -ode, -id: forms words (both nouns and adjectives) indicating a particular shape, form, or resemblance: *resembling*

-olus, -ola, -olum, -ole: form dimunitives

-oma: forms abstract nouns: usually *tumor*; occasionally *disease*

-one: forms names of chemical substances

-or: forms nouns: *agent* or *instrument*

-orium: forms nouns: *place for* (something)

-ory: forms adjectives: *pertaining to*

-ory: forms nouns: *place for* (something)

-ose: forms adjectives; also used to form names of chemical substances: *full of, resembling*

-osis: forms abstract nouns: *abnormal* or *diseased condition*
-otic: forms adjectives from nouns in -osis: *pertaining to*
*-ous*: forms adjectives: *pertaining to, characterized by, full of*
-sia: forms abstract nouns: *state, condition*
-sis: forms abstract nouns: *state, condition*
-ter: forms nouns: *instrument, device*
-tic: forms adjectives from nouns in -sis: *pertaining to*; many words in -tic have come to be used
    as nouns
-tics: see -ics
*-ty*: forms abstract nouns: *state, condition*
*-ulus, -ula, -ulum, -ule*: form diminutives
*-ure, -ura*: form nouns: *result of* (an action)
*-us*: forms nouns: *condition, person* (sometimes a malformed fetus)
-y: forms abstract nouns: *state, condition*
*-y*: forms abstract nouns: *state, condition*

# SELECTIVE GLOSSARY OF ENGLISH—GREEK/LATIN

The following glossary presents the Greek and Latin words necessary for the formation of medical terms asked for in part B of most of the exercises in this text. It is not comprehensive and contains only those forms needed for completion of the exercises. Verbs are given in the form of the present infinitive, along with the appropriate combining form. Nouns and adjectives are given in their dictionary form. Appropriate prefixes are listed. Only those suffixes with specialized meanings (*-itis*, inflammation, *-ium*, membrane, and so forth) are given, along with compound suffix-forms that are necessary (*-genic*, producing, *-logy*, the study of, and so forth); otherwise, suffixes are not listed, and the student is expected to supply the appropriate noun-forming or adjectival suffix where necessary. Combining forms are printed in capital letters; prefixes, suffixes, and combining suffix-forms are in lower case. Entry words for Latin forms, as well as all Latin elements, are in italic type.

abdomen: (*lapara, koilia*) LAPAR-, CELI-
abdominal wall: (*lapara*) LAPAR-
*above: (superior) -SUPERIOR*
absence: a(n)-
*across: trans-*
*after: post-*
*agent: -e*
agent that induces secretion: (*agōgos*) -AGOGUE
air: (*aēr*) AER-
all: (*pas*) PAN-
animal: (*zōon*) ZO-
*apart: dis-*
(have an) appetite: (*oregein*) OREC-
*arm: (bracchium) BRACHI-*
around: peri-
*around: circum-*
artery: (*arteria*) ARTERI-
*back: re-*
backward: retro-

bacterium: (*baktērion*) BACTERI-
*behind: (posterior) POSTER-, POSTERIOR, retro-*
bend: (*flectere*) FLEX-
between: inter-
bile: (*cholē*) CHOLE-
(give) birth: (*gignere, parere*) GENIT-, *-PARTUM*
bladder: (*kystis*) CYST-
*bladder: (vesīca) VESIC-*
blood: (*haima*) -EM-
blood clot: (*thrombos*) THROMB-
blood vessel: (*angeion*) ANGI-
blue: (*kyanos*) CYAN-
body: (*sōma*) SOMAT-
bone: (*osteon*) OSTE-
bronchus: (*bronchos*) BRONCH-
calculus: (*lithos*) LITH-
carbon dioxide: (*kapnos*) CAPN-
*carry: (ferre) FER-*

cartilage: (*chondros*) CHONDR-
causing: -genic, -genous
*cecum: (carcus) CEC-*
*cervix: (cervix) CERVIC-*
*chest: (pectus) PECTOR-*
childbirth: (*tokos*) TOC-
cold: (*kryos*) CRY-
colon: (*kolon*) COL-
color: (*chrōma*) CHROM(AT)-
cornea: (*keras*) KERAT-
corpse: (*nekros*) NECR-
*cut: (caedere, secāre) -CIS-, SECT-*
dark: (*melas*) MELAN-
death: (*thanatos*) THANAT-
defective: dys-
deficiency: a-, hypo-
deficient: (*oligos*) OLIG-
development: (*telos*) TEL-
difficult: dys-
dilation: -ectasis, -ectasia
diminished: a(n)-, hypo-
discharge: -rrhea
disease: (*pathos*) PATH-
disintegration: -lysis
dislocation: -ectopia
duct: (*angeion, dochos*) ANGI-, -DOCH-
*duodenum: (duodēnī) DUODEN-*
ear: (*ous*) OT-
enzyme: -ase
equal: (*īsos*) IS-
esophagus: (*oisophagos*) ESOPHAG-
every (thing): (*pas*) PAN-, PANT-
excessive (amount): hyper-
extremity: (*akron*) ACR-
eye: (*ophthalmos*) OPHTHALM-
eyelid: (*blepharon*) BLEPHAR-
falling: -ptosis
fallopian tube: (*salpinx*) SALPING-
fat: (*lipos*) LIP-
fear: (*phobos*) PHOB-
feeling: (*aisthēsis*) ESTHE-
fever: (*pyr, pyretos*) PYR-, PYRET-
*fever: (febris) FEBR-*
finger: (*daktylos*) DACTYL-
fissure: -schisis
flow: (*rhein*) RHE-
fluid: (*hydōr*) HYDR-
foot: (*pous*) POD-
force: (*dynamis*) DYNAM-
form: (*morphē, plassein*) MORPH-, PLAS-
formation of: -iasis
formation of a passage: -stomy
*front: (anterior) ANTER-*
fungus: (*mykēs*) MYC-
*fungus: (fungus) FUNG-*

gall: (*cholē*) CHOLE-
gland: (*adēn*) ADEN-
hair: (*thrix*) TRICH-
half: hemi-
hard: (*skleros*) SCLER-
hear: (*akouein*) ACU-
heart: (*kardia*) CARDI-
hemorrhage: -rrhagia
hernia: (*kēlē*) -CELE
hidden: (*kryptos*) CRYPT-
*ileum: (ileum) ILE-*
incision: -tomy
incomplete: a(n)-
increased: hyper-
inflammation: -itis
inhibiting: anti-
instrument for cutting: -tome
instrument for examining: -scope
instrument to record: -graph
intestine: (*enteron*) ENTER-
iris: (*īris*) IRID-
iron: (*sidēros*) SIDER-
jaw: (*gnathos*) GNATH-
*jejunum: (jejunus) JEJUN-*
kidney: (*nephros*) NEPHR-
*kidney: (rēn) REN-*
*kill: (caedere) -CID-*
lack: a(n)-
large: (*megas, makros*) MEGAL-, MACR-
larynx: (*larynx*) LARYNG-
lens: (*phakos*) PHAC-
life: (*bios*) BI-
ligament: (*desmos*) DESM-
light: (*phōs*) PHOT-
limb: (*melos*) MEL-
lip: (*cheilos*) CHEIL-
*little: (use diminutive suffix)*
liver: (*hēpar*) HEPAT-
loss: a(n)-
lung: (*pneumōn*) PNEUMON-
male: (*anēr*) ANDR-
many: (*polys*) POLY-
measure: (*metron*) METR-
membrane: -ium
meninges: (*mēninx*) MENING-
milk: (*gala*) GALACT-
*milk: (lac) LACT-*
mind: (*psychē*) PSYCH-
*mouth: (ōs) OR-*
movement: (*kinēsis*) KINES-
mucus: (*myxa, blennos*) MYX-, BLENN-
muscle: (*mys*) MY-
narrow: (*stenos*) STEN-
*neck (of the uterus): (cervix) CERVIC-*
nerve: (*neuron*) NEUR-

296

new: (*neos*) NE-
nipple: (*thēlē*) THEL-
nitrogen: (*azote*) AZOT-
no: a(n)-
nose: (*rhis*) RHIN-
nourishment: (*trophē*) TROPH-
offensive odor: (*brōmos*) BROM-
opening: (*stoma*) STOM-
originating: -genous
*out: ex-*
outside: exo-
ovary: (*oophoron*) OOPHOR-
pain: (*algos, odynē*) ALG-, ODYN-
paralysis: -plegia
people: (*dēmos*) DEM-
perspiration: (*hidrōs*) HIDROT-
pharynx: (*pharynx*) PHARYNG-
plastic surgery: -plasty
pleural cavity: (*pleura, thōrax*) PLEUR-,
　THORAC-
poison: (*toxon*) TOX-
*pour: (fundere) FUS-*
(be) pregnant: (*kyein*) CYE-
preventing: anti-
producing: -genic, -genous
prolapse: -ptosis
prostate gland: (*prostatēs*) PROSTAT-
pulse: (*sphygmos*) SPHYGM-
puncture: (*kentein*) CENTE-
pupil: (*korē*) CORE-
pus: (*pyon*) PY-
radiation: (*aktis*) ACTIN-
rapid: (*tachys*) TACHY-
red: (*erythros*) ERYTHR-
remember: (*mimnēskein*) MNE-
renal pelvis: (*pyelos*) PYEL-
resembling: -oid
*right: (dexter) DEXTR-*
rupture: -rrhexis
sensation: (*aisthēsis*) ESTHE-
*shape: (forma) -FORM*
*skin: (derma) DERM-, -DERMA, DERMAT-*
sleep: (*hypnos*) HYPN-
slow: (*bradys*) BRADY-
small: (*mikros*) MICR-
*small: (use diminutive suffix)*
soft: (*malakos*) MALAC-
specialist in the study of: -logist
spider: (*arachnē*) ARACHN-
spinal cord: (*myelos*) MYEL-
spine: (*rhachis*) RHACH-
spleen: (*splēn*) SPLEN-
*spleen: (liēn) LIEN-*

starch: (*amylon*) AMYL-
stomach: (*gastēr*) GASTR-
strength: (*sthenos*) STHEN-
study: -logy
substance: -in
substance producing: -gen
sugar: (*glykys*) GLYC-
supernumerary: (*polys*) POLY-
surgical removal: -ectomy
surrounding: peri-
suture: (*rhaptein*) -RRHAPH-
swallow: (*phagein*) PHAG-
sweat: (*hidrōs*) HIDR-
taste: (*geuein*) GEUS-
tear: (*dakryon*) DACRY-
thick: (*pachys*) PACHY-
thorax: (*thōrax*) THORAC-
through: dia-
*through: per-*
tissue: (*histos, histion*) HIST-, HISTI-
together: syn-
*tongue: (lingua) LINGU-*
tonsil: (*amygdalē*) AMYGDAL-
tooth: (*odous*) ODONT-
*toward: -ad*
treat: (*therapeuein*) THERAP-
tumor: -oma
turning: (*tropē*) TROP-
ulcer: (*helkos*) HELC-, -ELC-
umbilicus: (*omphalos*) OMPHAL-
unable: a-
*under: sub-*
urine: (*ouron*) UR-
uvula: (*staphylē*) STAPHYL-
vagina: (*kolpos*) COLP-
*varix: (varix) VARIC-*
vein: (*phleps*) PHLEB-
*vein: (vēna) VEN-*
vertebra: (*spondylos*) SPONDYL-
*vessel: (vas) VAS-*
*virus: (vīrus) VIRU-*
viscus: (*splanchnon*) SPLANCHN-
vision: (*ōps*) OP-
voice: (*phonē*) PHON-
vomit: (*emein*) EME-
water: (*hydōr*) HYDR-
*with: con-*
within: endo-
*within: intra-*
woman: (*gynē*) GYNEC-
worm: (*helmins*) HELMINTH-
x-ray examination: -graphy
yellow: (*xanthos*) XANTH-

# INDEX OF COMBINING FORMS

In this index will be found an alphabetical listing of the combining forms found in the vocabulary of Lessons 1–15 and Supplementary Lesson I, along with their basic meaning, the number of the lesson in which the word is found, and the vocabulary form of the Greek or Latin word. It should be noted that only current medical meanings are given. Certain words (anthrax, herpes, larynx, and so forth) that are not properly combining forms are listed here; others (cervix, edema, thorax, and so forth) are given in their vocabulary form even though they are used both as separate terms and as combining forms (for example, endocervix, acroedema, hemothorax). Combining forms for Latin words are in italic type.

## A

ACOU- hear 5 *akouein*
ACOUS- hear 5 *akouein*
ACR- extremities 2 *akron*
ACTIN- radiation 15 *aktis*
ACU- hear 5 *akouein*
ACUS- hear 5 *akouein*
ADEN- gland 7 *adēn*
ADIP- fat 8 *adeps*
AER- air, gas 7 *aēr*
AGOG- leading, drawing forth 14 *agōgos*
-AGRA (sudden) pain, gout 15 *agra*
ALEX- ward off (disease) 6 *alexein*
ALEXI- ward off (disease) 6 *alexein*
ALG- pain 1 *algos*
ALGES- sensitivity to pain 1 *algēsis*
ALVE- hollow, cavity 11 *alveus*
AMNI- fetal membrane, amniotic sac 5 *amnion*
AMYGDAL- tonsil 11 *amygdalē*
AMYL- starch 10 *amylon*
ANCYL- fused, stiffened; hooked 6 *ankylos*
ANDR- man, male 6 *anēr*

ANGI- (blood) vessel, duct 1 *angeion*
ANGIN- choking pain; angina pectoris 10 *angina*
ANKYL- fused, stiffened; hooked 6 *ankylos*
ANTER- front, in front 9 *anterior*
ANTHRAC- coal; anthrax 11 *anthrax*
ANTHRAX anthrax 11 *anthrax*
AORT- aorta 10 *aortē*
APHRODIS- sexual desire 6 *Aphrodisios*
APHRODISI- sexual desire 6 *Aphrodisios*
ARACHN- spider, web; arachnoid membrane 3 *arachnē*
ARCH- beginning, origin 14 *archē*
-ARCHE beginning, origin 14 *archē*
ARCHI- beginning, origin 14 *archē*
ARCT- compress 10 *arctāre*
ARCTAT- compress 10 *arctāre*
ARTERI- artery 1 *arteria*
ARTHR- joint 1 *arthron*
ATHER- fatty deposit 10 *athērē*
ATRI- atrium 10 *atrium*
AUR- ear 8 *auris*
AUT- self 4 *autos*

AUX- increase, grow 11 *auxein*
-AUXE abnormal growth 11 *auxein*
-AUXIS abnormal growth 11 *auxein*

## B

*BACILL*- bacillus 8 *bacillus*
BACTER- bacterium 11 *baktērion*
BACTERI- bacterium 11 *baktērion*
BI- life 1 *bios*
*BILI*- bile 12 *bilis*
BLAST- primitive cell I *blastos*
BLENN- mucus 7 *blennos*
BLEPHAR- eyelid 13 *blepharon*
BOL- a throwing 10 *bolē*
*BRACHI*- (upper) arm 9 *bracchium*
BRADY- slow 1 *bradys*
BROM- stench, offensive odor 14 *brōmos*
BRONCH- bronchus 11 *bronchos*
BRONCHI- bronchus 11 *bronchos*
*BURS*- bursa 8 *bursa*

## C

*CALC*- stone, calcium, lime (salts) 8 *calx*
*CAPILL*- capillary 10 *capillus*
*CAPIT*- head 8 *caput*
CAPN- carbon dioxide 11 *kapnos*
CARCIN- carcinoma, cancer 2 *karkinos*
CARDI- heart 1 *kardia*
[CARDI- cardia 12 *kardia*]
*CEC*- cecum 12 *caecus*
-CEL- hernia, tumor 2 *kēlē*
CEL- abdomen 7 *koilia*
CELI- abdomen 7 *koilia*
CENTE- pierce 5 *kentein*
CEPHAL- head 1 *kephalē*
-CEPT- take 9 *capere*
*CEREBR*- brain 8 *cerebrum*
*CERVIC*- neck (of the uterus), cervix uteri 14
   *cervix*
*CERVIX* neck (of the uterus), cervix uteri 14
   *cervix*
CHEIL- lip 7 *cheilos*
CHEIR- hand 2 *cheir*
CHIL- lip 7 *cheilos*
CHIR- hand 2 *cheir*
CHLOR- green 3 *chlōros*
CHOL- bile, gall 2 *cholē*
CHOLE- bile, gall 2 *cholē*
CHONDR- cartilage 3 *chondros*
CHOROID- choroid 13 *chorioeidēs*
CHROM- color, pigment 5 *chrōma*
CHROMA- color, pigment 5 *chrōma*
CHROMAT- color, pigment 5 *chrōma*
-CID- cut, kill 9 *caedere*
-CIP- take 9 *capere*

CIRS- dilated and twisted vein, varix 10 *kirsos*
-CIS- cut, kill 9 *caedere*
CLA- break (up), destroy 7 *klan*
CLAS- break (up), destroy 7 *klan*
-CLAST something that breaks *or* destroys 7
   *klan*
-CLUD- close 10 *claudere*
-CLUS- close 10 *claudere*
CLY- rinse out, inject fluid 12 *klyzein*
CLYS- rinse out, inject fluid 12 *klyzein*
COCC- coccus 11 *kokkos*
-COCCUS coccus 11 *kokkos*
COL- colon 2 *kolon*
COLI- the colon bacillus (*Escherichia coli*) 2
   *kolon*
COLON- colon 2 *kolon*
COLP- vagina 14 *kolpos*
CONI- dust 11 *konis*
COPR- excrement 12 *kopros*
*COR* heart 10 *cor*
*CORD*- heart 10 *cor*
*CORE*- pupil 13 *korē*
*CORTEX* outer layer 15 *cortex*
*CORTIC*- outer layer 15 *cortex*
*COST*- rib 8 *costa*
CRANI- skull 1 *kranion*
CREAT- flesh 12 *kreas*
*CRESC*- grow 9 *crēscere*
-CRET- grow 9 *crēscere*
CRY- icy cold 15 *kryos*
CRYM- icy cold 15 *krymos*
CRYPT- hidden 15 *kryptos*
*CUSP*- point 10 *cuspis*
-CUSPID point 10 *cuspis*
CYAN- blue 2 *kyanos*
CYCL- circle; ciliary body 13 *kyklos*
CYE- be pregnant 14 *kyein*
CYST- bladder, cyst 2 *kystis*
CYSTI- bladder, cyst 2 *kystis*
-CYSTIS bladder, cyst 2 *kystis*
CYT- cell 1 *kytos*

## D

DACRY- tear; lacrimal sac *or* duct 13 *dakryon*
DACTYL- finger, toe 3 *daktylos*
DEM- people, population 6 *dēmos*
DERM- skin 3 *derma*
-DERMA skin 3 *derma*
DERMAT- skin 3 *derma*
-DESIS binding 7 *desis*
DESM- ligament 7 *desmos*
*DEXTR*- right (side) 10 *dexter*
DIPLO- double 11 *diploos*

300

DIPS- thirst 5 *dipsa*
-DOCH- duct 12 *dochos*
*DORS-* back (of the body) 8 *dorsum*
DROM- a running 6 *dromos*
*DUC-* lead, conduct 9 *ducere*
*DUCT-* lead, conduct 9 *ducere*
*DUODEN-* duodenum 12 *duodēnī*
DYNAM- force, power 7 *dynamis*

### E

EDEMA swelling 5 *oidēma*
EDEMAT- swelling 5 *oidēma*
-ELC- ulcer 3 *helkos*
-EM- blood 2 *haima*
EME- vomit 5 *emein*
ENCEPHAL- brain 1 *enkephalon*
ENTER- (small) intestine 2 *enteron*
EOS- red (stain) I *eōs*
ER- sexual desire 6 *Erōs*
ERG- action, work 2 *ergon*
EROT- sexual desire 6 *Erōs*
ERYTHR- red, red blood cell 1 *erythros*
ESOPHAG- esophagus 12 *oisophagos*
ESTHE- sensation, sensitivity, sense 4 *aisthē-sis*
ESTHES- sensation, sensitivity, sense 4 *ais-thēsis*
EURY- widen, dilate 14 *eurynein*
EURYN- widen, dilate 14 *eurynein*
*EXTERN-* outer 8 *externus*

### F

*FAC-* make 9 *facere*
*FACI-* face, appearance, surface 9 *faciēs*
*FACIES* face, appearance 9 *faciēs*
*FEBR-* fever 9 *febris*
*FEBRIS* fever 9 *febris*
*FEC-* excrement 12 *faex*
-*FECT-* make 9 *facere*
*FER-* carry, bear 9 *ferre*
*FIBR-* fiber, filament 8 *fibra*
-*FIC-* make 9 *facere*
-*FICI-* face, appearance, surface 9 *faciēs*
*FISTUL-* fistula 8 *fistula*
*FLECT-* bend 9 *flectere*
*FLEX-* bend 9 *flectere*
-*FORM* shape 10 *forma*
*FUNG-* fungus 9 *fungus*
*FUS-* pour 9 *fundere*

### G

GAL- milk 14 *gala*
GALACT- milk 14 *gala*
GASTR- stomach 2 *gastēr*
GEN- come into being; produce 4 *gignesthai*

GENE- come into being; produce 4 *gignes-thai*
*GENIT-* bring forth, give birth 9 *gignere*
*GER-* carry, bear 9 *gerere*
*GEST-* carry, bear 9 *gerere*
GEUS- taste 12 *geuein*
GEUST- taste 12 *geuein*
*GINGIV-* gum (of the mouth) 12 *gingiva*
*GLOB-* round body, globe I *globus*
GLOSS- tongue 12 *glōssa*
GLYC- sugar 15 *glykys*
-GN- be born 14 *(g)nascī*
GNATH- (lower) jaw 7 *gnathos*
GNO- know 5 *gignōskein*
GNOS- know 5 *gignōskein*
GONAD- sex glands 14 *gonad*
GRAM- a record 4 *gramma*
*GRANUL-* granule I *grānulum*
GRAPH- write, record 4 *graphein*
*GRAVID-* pregnant 14 *gravidus*
*GURGITAT-* flood, flow 10 *gurgitāre*
GYN- woman, female 6 *gynē*
GYNEC- woman, female 6 *gynē*

### H

HELC- ulcer 3 *helkos*
HELMINT- (intestinal) worm 6 *helmins*
HELMINTH- (intestinal) worm 6 *helmins*
HEM- blood 2 *haima*
HEMAT- blood 2 *haima*
HEPAT- liver 2 *hēpar*
HERPES herpes 13 *herpēs*
HERPET- herpes 13 *herpēs*
HIDR- sweat 3 *hidrōs*
HIDROT- sweat 3 *hidrōs*
HIST- tissue 3 *histos*
HISTI- tissue 3 *histion*
HYDR- water, fluid 3 *hydōr*
HYMEN- membrane; hymen 14 *hymēn*
HYPN- sleep 3 *hypnos*
HYSTER- uterus 14 *hystera*

### I

IATR- healer, physician; treatment 4 *iatros*
ICTER- jaundice 3 *ikteros*
IDI- of one's self 4 *idios*
-IDR- sweat 3 *hidrōs*
*ILE-* ileum 12 *ileum*
*INFERIOR-* below 9 *inferior*
*INSUL-* island 8 *insula*
*INTERN-* inner 8 *internus*
IR- iris 13 *īris*
IRID- iris 13 *īris*
IS- equal 3 *īsos*
ISCH- suppress, check 7 *ischein*

## J

JEJUN- jejunum 12 *jejunus*

## K

KARY— nucleus I *karyon*
KERAT- cornea 13 *keras*
KINE- move 4 *kinein*
KINES- movement, motion 4 *kinēsis*
KINESI- movement, motion 4 *kinēsis*
KONI- dust 11 *konis*

## L

LAB- slide, slip 9 *labī*
LABI- lip 11 *labium*
LACT- milk 14 *lac*
-LAGNIA abnormal sexual excitation *or* gratification 15 *lagneia*
LAL- talk 5 *lalein*
LAPAR- abdomen, abdominal wall 5 *lapara*
LAPS- slide, slip 9 *labī*
LARYNG- larynx 11 *larynx*
LARYNX larynx 11 *larynx*
LAT- carry, bear 9 *ferre*
LATER- side 9 *latus*
LEI- smooth 7 *leios*
LEP- attack, seizure 7 *lēpsis*
LEUK- white, white blood cell 1 *leukos*
LEX- read 5 *legein*
LIEN- spleen 12 *liēn*
LINGU- tongue 12 *lingua*
LIP- fat 2 *lipos*
LITH- stone, calculus 1 *lithos*
LOG- word, study 1 *logos*
LY- destroy, break down 4 *lyein*
LYMPH- lymph I *lympha*
LYS- destroy, break down 4 *lyein*

## M

MACR- (abnormally) large *or* long 2 *makros*
MALAC- soft 1 *malakos*
MAMM- breast 14 *mamma*
MAN- be mad 7 *mainesthai*
MAST- breast 14 *mastos*
MAZ- breast 14 *mazos*
MEAT- passage, opening, meatus 8 *meātus*
MEGA- (abnormally) large *or* long 2 *megas*
MEGAL- (abnormally) large *or* long 2 *megas*
MEL- limb 7 *melos*
MELAN- dark, black 2 *melas*
MEN- menstruation 14 *mēn*
MENING- meningeal membrane, meninges 3 *mēninx*
-MENINX meningeal membrane, meninges 3 *mēninx*
MES- mesentery 12 *mesos*

## (continued)

-METER instrument for measuring 7 *metron*
METR- measure 7 *metron*
METR- uterus 14 *mētra*
-METRA uterus 14 *mētra*
MICR- (abnormally) small 2 *mikros*
MNE- remember 5 *mimnēskein*
MON- single I *monos*
MORPH- form, shape 7 *morphē*
MY- muscle 3 *mys*
MYC- fungus 3 *mykēs*
MYCET- fungus 3 *mykēs*
MYEL- bone marrow, spinal cord 3 *myelos*
MYS- muscle 3 *mys*
MYX- mucus 4 *myxa*

## N

NARC- stupor, numbness 3 *narkē*
NAT- be born 14 *(g)nascī*
NE- new 5 *neos*
NECR- corpse; dead 3 *nekros*
NEMAT- thread (worm) 6 *nēma*
NEPHR- kidney 1 *nephros*
NEUR- nerve, nervous system 1 *neuron*
NEUTR- neither I *neuter*
NO- mind, mental activity, comprehension 5 *nous*
NOM- law 7 *nomos*
NOS- disease, illness 6 *nosos*

## O

OCUL- eye 13 *oculus*
ODONT- tooth 6 *odous*
ODYN- pain 2 *odynē*
OLIG- few, deficient 3 *oligos*
OMPHAL- navel, umbilicus 7 *omphalos*
ONC- tumor 2 *onkos*
ONYCH- fingernail, toenail 3 *onyx*
OOPHOR- ovary 14 *oophoron*
OP- vision 13 *ōps*
OPHTHALM- eye 13 *ophthalmos*
OPS- vision 13 *ōps*
OPT- vision; eye 13 *optos*
OR- mouth, opening 9 *ōs*
ORCH- testicle 15 *orchis*
ORCHE- testicle 15 *orchis*
ORCHI- testicle 15 *orchis*
ORCHID- testicle 15 *orchis*
OREC- have an appetite 5 *oregein*
OREX- have an appetite 5 *oregein*
ORTH- straight, erect; normal 4 *orthos*
OS mouth, opening 9 *ōs*
OSM- sense of smell; odor 12 *osmē*
OSPHR- sense of smell 12 *osphrēsis*
OSS- bone 9 *ossa*
OSTE- bone 1 *osteon*

-SCHE- suppress, check 7 *ischein*
-SCHISIS split 6 *schizein*
SCHIST- split 6 *schizein*
SCHIZ- split 6 *schizein*
SCLER- hard 1 *skleros*
SCOP- look at, examine 4 *skopein*
*SECT-* cut 9 *secāre*
*SEMIN-* semen 15 *sēmen*
SEP- be infected 4 *sēpein*
*SEPT-* wall, partition 10 *saeptum*
SIAL- saliva, salivary duct 12 *sialon*
SIDER- iron 11 *sidēros*
SIGM- sigmoid colon 12 *sigma*
*SIN-* sinus 10 *sinus*
*SINISTR-* left (side) 10 *sinister*
*SINUS-* sinus 10 *sinus*
SIT- food 7 *sītos*
SOM- body 3 *sōma*
-SOMA body 3 *sōma*
SOMAT- body 3 *sōma*
*SOMN-* sleep 9 *somnus*
SPASM- spasm 2 *spasmos*
SPERM- sperm, semen 15 *sperma*
SPERMAT- sperm, semen 15 *sperma*
SPHINCTER- sphincter muscle 12 *sphinctēr*
SPHYGM- pulse 10 *sphygmos*
*SPIR-* breathe 11 *spīrāre*
*SPIRAT-* breathe 11 *spīrāre*
SPLANCHN- internal organ, viscus 12 *splanchnon*
SPLEN- spleen 2 *splēn*
SPONDYL- vertebra 6 *spondylos*
STA- stand, stop 7 *histanai*
STAL- send 10 *stellein*
STAPHYL- uvula, palate; staphylococci 11 *staphylē*
STAT- stand, stop 7 *histanai*
-STAXIA dripping, oozing (of blood) 6 *staxis*
-STAXIS dripping, oozing (of blood) 6 *staxis*
STEAR- fat, sebum, sebacious glands 5 *stear*
STEAT- fat, sebum, sebacious glands 5 *stear*
STEN- narrow 1 *stenos*
STHEN- strength 3 *sthenos*
STOL- send 10 *stellein*
STOM- mouth, opening 2 *stoma*
STOMAT- mouth, opening 2 *stoma*
STREPT- streptococci 11 *streptos*
*SUD-* sweat 11 *sudor*
*SUDOR-* sweat 11 *sudor*
*SUPERIOR-* above 9 *superior*
*SYNOV-* synovial fluid, synovial membrane or sac 8 *synovia*
*SYNOVI-* synovial fluid, synovial membrane or sac 8 *synovia*

SYRING- fistula, cavity, oviduct, sweat glands, syringe 14 *syrinx*
-SYRINX fistula, cavity, oviduct, sweat glands, syringe 14 *syrinx*

## T

TA- stretching 4 *tasis*
TACHY- rapid 1 *tachys*
TAX- (muscular) coordination 7 *taxis*
TEL- end, completion 4 *telos*
TEN- tendon 4 *tenōn*
TENON- tendon 4 *tenōn*
TENONT- tendon 4 *tenōn*
THAN- death 6 *thanatos*
THANAT- death 6 *thanatos*
THE- place, put 6 *tithenai*
THEL- nipple 14 *thēlē*
THELE- nipple 14 *thēlē*
THERAP- treat medically, heal 4 *therapeuein*
THERAPEU- treat medically, heal 4 *therapeuein*
THERM- heat, (body) temperature 7 *thermē*
THORAC- chest cavity, pleural cavity, thorax 11 *thōrax*
THORAX chest cavity, pleural cavity, thorax 11 *thōrax*
THROMB- blood clot 10 *thrombos*
THYR- thyroid gland 15 *thyreos*
TOC- childbirth, labor 14 *tokos*
TOM- a cutting, slice 4 *tomē*
TON- tone, tension 4 *tonos*
TOP- place 10 *topos*
TOX- poison 1 *toxon*
TOXI- poison 1 *toxon*
TRACH- trachea 11 *trachys*
TRACHE- trachea 11 *trachys*
TRACHY- trachea 11 *trachys*
TRICH- hair 6 *thrix*
TROP- turning 7 *tropē*
TROPH- nourishment 6 *trophē*
*TUM-* be swollen 9 *tumēre*
*TUME-* be swollen 9 *tumēre*
*TUSS-* cough 8 *tussis*
TYPHL- cecum 12 *typhlos*

## U

UR- urine, urinary tract, uric acid 15 *ouron*
URETER- ureter 15 *ourētēr*
URETHR- urethra 15 *ourēthra*

## V

*VACC-* cow 8 *vacca*
*VAG-* the vagus nerve 10 *vagus*